THERAPEUTIC MUSHROOMS FOR DIABETES MELLITUS

Current Evidences and Future Scope

THERAPEUTIC MUSHROOMS FOR DIABETES MELLITUS

Current Evidences and Future Scope

Edited by

Uzma Azeem, PhD

Khalid Rehman Hakeem, PhD

APPLE ACADEMIC PRESS

First edition published 2023

Apple Academic Press Inc.
1265 Goldenrod Circle, NE,
Palm Bay, FL 32905 USA

760 Laurentian Drive, Unit 19,
Burlington, ON L7N 0A4, CANADA

CRC Press
6000 Broken Sound Parkway NW,
Suite 300, Boca Raton, FL 33487-2742 USA

4 Park Square, Milton Park,
Abingdon, Oxon, OX14 4RN UK

Library and Archives Canada Cataloguing in Publication

Title: Therapeutic mushrooms for diabetes mellitus : current evidences and future scope / edited by Uzma Azeem, PhD, Khalid Rehman Hakeem, PhD.
Names: Azeem, Uzma, editor. | Hakeem, Khalid Rehman, editor.
Description: First edition. | Includes bibliographical references and index.
Identifiers: Canadiana (print) 20230171346 | Canadiana (ebook) 20230171435 | ISBN 9781774912225 (hardcover) | ISBN 9781774912232 (softcover) | ISBN 9781003332046 (ebook)
Subjects: LCSH: Diabetes—Alternative treatment. | LCSH: Edible mushrooms—Therapeutic use. | LCSH: Diabetes. | LCSH: Diabetes—Etiology.
Classification: LCC RC661.A47 T44 2023 | DDC 616.4/6206—dc23

Library of Congress Cataloging-in-Publication Data

CIP data on file with US Library of Congress

ISBN: 978-1-77491-222-5 (hbk)
ISBN: 978-1-77491-223-2 (pbk)
ISBN: 978-1-00333-204-6 (ebk)

Dedication

This book is dedicated to my beloved Mother **"Hajrah Begum"**, who left this world so early. To me, she was the whole world. She was the most loving, humble, compassionate, understanding, family-orientated woman and one of the most beautiful souls one could ever meet. I am going to miss you so much, Mom. I pray to Allah (SWT) to bless your soul and grant you, **Jannatul-Firdous** (the highest level of heaven).

—Prof. (Dr.) Khalid Rehman Hakeem

About the Editors

Uzma Azeem, PhD

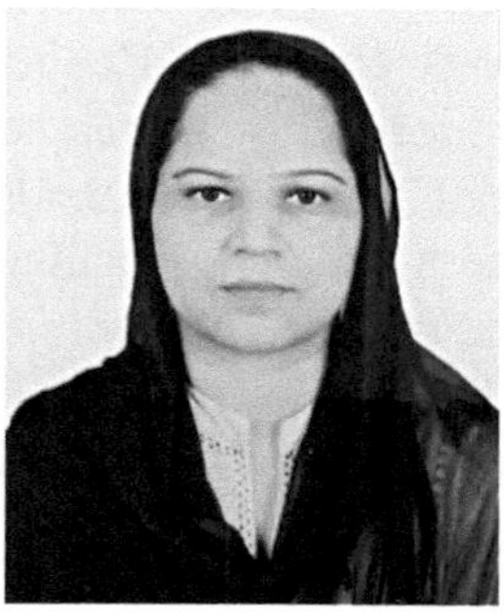

Uzma Azeem, PhD, is affiliated with the Sanmati Government College of Science Education and Research, Ludhiana, Punjab, India. She was formerly Assistant Professor in the Department of Botany and Environmental Sciences at Sri Guru Granth Sahib World University, Punjab, India. To date, she has authored 11 papers published in peer-reviewed national and international journals and one book, *Fungi for Human Health: Current Knowledge and Future Perspectives* (Springer Nature). Dr. Azeem earned her MPhil and doctorate in Botany with specialization in Mycology and Plant Pathology at Punjabi University, India. She was awarded a Maulana Azad National Fellowship for Minority Students during 2011–2016 by the University Grants Commission, New Delhi, India.

Khalid Rehman Hakeem, PhD

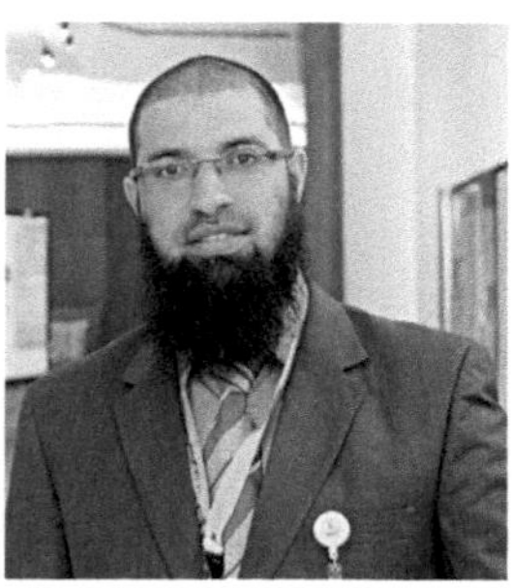

Khalid Rehman Hakeem, PhD, is Professor at King Abdulaziz University, Jeddah, Saudi Arabia. After completing his doctorate (botany, specialization in plant eco-physiology and molecular biology) from Jamia Hamdard, New Delhi, India, he worked as a lecturer at the University of Kashmir, Srinagar, India, at Universiti Putra Malaysia, Selangor, Malaysia, where he was a Postdoctorate Fellow and Fellow Researcher (Associate Professor) for several years. Dr. Hakeem has more than 10 years of teaching and research experience in plant eco-physiology, biotechnology and molecular biology, medicinal plant research, plant-microbe-soil interactions, as well as in environmental studies. He is the recipient of several fellowships at both national and international levels. He has served as a visiting scientist at Jinan University, Guangzhou, China. Currently, he is involved with several international research projects with various government organizations. To date, Dr. Hakeem has authored and edited more than 80 books with international publishers. He also has to his credit more than 180 research publications in peer-reviewed international journals and 75 book chapters in edited volumes. At present, Dr. Hakeem serves as an editorial board member and reviewer for several high-impact international scientific journals. He is included in the advisory board of Cambridge Scholars Publishing, UK. He is also a fellow of the Plantae Group of the American Society of Plant Biologists, member of the World Academy of Sciences, member of the International Society for Development and Sustainability, Japan, and member of the Asian Federation of Biotechnology, Korea.

Contents

Contributors

Ahmad Ali
Department of Life Sciences, University of Mumbai, Vidyanagari, Santacruz [East], Mumbai 400098, India

Hina Alim
Department of Life Sciences, University of Mumbai, Vidyanagari, Santacruz [East], Mumbai 400098, India

Hale Alvandi
Department of Life Science Engineering, Faculty of New Sciences and Technologies, University of Tehran, Tehran, Iran

Amita
Department of Botany, Punjabi University, Patiala 147002, Punjab, India

Elham Ansari
Department of Life Science Engineering, Faculty of New Sciences and Technologies, University of Tehran, Tehran, Iran

Mohd Yaqub Bhat
Plant Pathology, Mycology and Microbiology Laboratory, Department of Botany, University of Kashmir, Srinagar 190006, Jammu and Kashmir, India; E-mail: myaqub35@gmail.com

Shiveena Bhatia
Chitkara College of Pharmacy, Chitkara University, Punjab, India

Kundan Singh Bora
University Institute of Pharmaceutical Sciences, Chandigarh University, Gharuan, Mohali 140413, Punjab, India

Asif Hamid Dar
Plant Pathology, Mycology and Microbiology Laboratory, Department of Botany, University of Kashmir, Srinagar 190006, Jammu and Kashmir, India

Lena Ahmed Saleh Al-Faqeeh
Maulana Azad Collage of Arts, Science and Commerce, Dr. Rafiq Zakaria Campus, Rauza Bagh, Aurangabad, M.S., 431001, India; E-mail: lenaalfaqeeh8@gmail.com

Mariano Torres-Gómez
Interdisciplinary Group for the Development of Ethnomycology in Mesoamerica A.C. (GIDEM), Coyoacan, Mexico
Research Institute in Ecosystems and Sustainability (IIES), National Autonomous University of Mexico (UNAM), Antigua Carretera a Patzcuaro No. 8701, Ex Hacienda de San Jose de la Huerta, 58190. Morelia, Michoacan, Mexico; E-mail: mtorres@cieco.unam.mx

Bahman Ebrahimi-Hoseinzadeh
Department of Life Science Engineering, Faculty of New Sciences and Technologies, University of Tehran, Tehran, Iran

Zahra Beagom Mokhtari Hosseini
Department of Chemical Engineering, Faculty of Petroleum and Petrochemical Engineering, Hakim Sabzevari University, Sabzevar, Iran

Nayeema Jan
Plant Pathology, Mycology and Microbiology Laboratory, Department of Botany, University of Kashmir, Srinagar 190006, Jammu and Kashmir, India

Harwinder K
Department of Botany, Akal University, Talwandi Sabo 151302, Bathinda, Punjab, India

Soheil Kianirad
Department of Life Science Engineering, Faculty of New Sciences and Technologies, University of Tehran, Tehran, Iran

Wasim Sajad Malik
Plant Pathology, Mycology and Microbiology Laboratory, Department of Botany, University of Kashmir, Srinagar 190006, Jammu and Kashmir, India

Varsha Mahesh Mayekar
Department of Life Sciences, University of Mumbai, Vidyanagari, Santacruz [East], Mumbai 400098, India

Mridu
Department of Biotechnology, Dyal Singh College, Karnal 132001, Haryana, India; E-mail: mriduphd@gmail.com

Anees Un Nisa
Plant Pathology, Mycology and Microbiology Laboratory, Department of Botany, University of Kashmir, Srinagar 190006, Jammu and Kashmir, India

Nimisha Patel
Department of Life Sciences, University of Mumbai, Vidyanagari, Santacruz [East], Mumbai 400098, India; E-mail: patelnimisha916@gmail.com

Latif A. Peer
Plant Pathology, Mycology and Microbiology Laboratory, Department of Botany, University of Kashmir, Srinagar 190006, Jammu and Kashmir, India

Aadil Rashid Sheikh
Plant Pathology, Mycology and Microbiology Laboratory, Department of Botany, University of Kashmir, Srinagar 190006, Jammu and Kashmir, India

Richa Shri
Department of Pharmaceutical Sciences and Drug Research, Punjabi University, Patiala 147002, Punjab, India; E-mail: richashri@pbi.ac.in; rshri587@hotmail.com

Pallaki Shrikhandia
Plant Pathology, Mycology and Microbiology Laboratory, Department of Botany, University of Kashmir, Srinagar 190006, Jammu and Kashmir, India

Varinder Singh
Chitkara College of Pharmacy, Chitkara University, Punjab, India

Mehrajud din Talie
Plant Pathology, Mycology and Microbiology Laboratory, Department of Botany, University of Kashmir, Srinagar 190006, Jammu and Kashmir, India

Abdul Hamid Wani
Plant Pathology, Mycology and Microbiology Laboratory, Department of Botany, University of Kashmir, Srinagar 190006, Jammu and Kashmir, India

Ashrafalsadat Hatamian-Zarmi
Department of Life Science Engineering, Faculty of New Sciences and Technologies, University of Tehran, Tehran, Iran; E-mail: hatamian_a@ut.ac.ir

Abbreviations

AACP	alkali soluble *Agrocybe cylindracea* polysaccharide
AAMP	associated migratory cell protein
AAMP	alkali soluble polysaccharides of *Amillariella mellea*
AAPs	*Auricularia auricular* polysaccharides
ABM	Agaricus blazei Murrill
ABMP	Agaricus blazei polysaccharide
ABP	*Agaricus* bisporus polysaccharides
ABTS	2, 2′-azino-Bis-3-ethylbenzothiazoline-6-sulfonjic acid
AGE/AGEs	advanced glycated end product(S)
AGRP	alkali soluble *Gomphidius rutilus* polysaccharide
AHMP	alkali soluble polysaccharides *Hypsizygus marmoreus*
AICAR	5-aminoimidazole-4-carboxamide ribonucleoside
Akt	protein kinase B
ALP	alkaline phosphatase
ALT	alanine aminotransferase
AMPK	adenosine monophosphate-activated protein kinase
AP-1	activator protein 1
APEP	alkali soluble *Pleurotus eryngii* polysaccharides
APOP	alkali soluble *P. ostreatus* polysaccharides
AR	aldose reductase
AST	aspartate aminotransferase
ATGL	adipose triglyceride lipase
BafA1	bafilomycin A1
BGL	blood glucose level
BHA	butylated hydroxyanisole
BHT	butylated hydroxytoluene
BUN	blood urea nitrogen
CAT	catalase
CCRV	*Coprinus comatus* rich in vanadium
CNS	central nervous system
DM	diabetes mellitus
DMEM	Dulbecco's Modified Eagle's Medium
DMSO	dimethyl sulfoxide

DPP	pileus of *Dictyophora rubrovolvata*
DPPH•	1,1-diphenyl-2picrylhydrazyl
ECL	enhanced chemiluminescence
ECPs	extracellular polysaccharides
EDTA	ethylenediamine tetra acetic acid
EPO	ergosterol peroxide
EPS	extracellular polysaccharides
FBG	fasting blood glucose
FBGL	fasting blood glucose level
FBS	fetal bovine serum
FG	high glucose and fatty acids
FITC	fluorescein isothiocyanate
FOXO	Forkhead Box O
FPG	fasting plasma glucose
FRAP	ferric-reducing antioxidant power
FTIR	Fourier Transform Infrared Spectroscopy
G6PD	glucose-6-phosphate dehydrogenase
GAA	glacial acetic acid
GA-C1	ganoderic acid-C1
GA-C2	ganoderic acid-C2
GA-Df	ganoderic acid-Df
GC-MS	gas chromatography-mass spectroscopy
GDM	gestational diabetes mellitus
GDM-STZ	gestational diabetes mellitus induced by streptozotocin
GFP	*Grifola frondosa* polysaccharide
GFP-LC3	green fluorescent protein-light chain 3
GLP	glucagon-like peptide
GLP-1	glucagon-like peptide 1
Gl-PS	*Ganoderma lucidum* polysaccharide
GLUT 4	glucose transporter Type 4
GLUT2	glucose transporter 2
GPCR	G-protein coupled receptor
GPx/GSH-Px	glutathione peroxidase reduced
GSIS	glucose-stimulated insulin secretion
GSK 3	glycogen synthase kinase 3
GSK-3β	glycogen synthase kinase-3β
GTT	glucose tolerance test
H2DCFDA	2′,7′-dichlorodihydrofluorescein diacetate

H_2O_2	hydrogen peroxide
HbA1c	glycosylated hemoglobin
HDL	high-density lipoprotein
HEPES	4-(2-hydroxyethyl)-1-piperazineethanesulfonic acid
HMW	high molecular weight fraction
HNF-1α	hepatocyte nuclear factor-1 alpha
HOMA-IR	homeostatic model assessment for insulin resistance
HPLC	high performance liquid chromatography
HSL	hormone-sensitive lipase
HSP	*Hirsutella sinensis* polysaccharide
IC50	half-maximal inhibitory concentration
ICPs	intracellular polysaccharides
IDDM	independent diabetes mellitus
IDF	International Diabetes Federation
IFN-α	interferon alfa
IgG	immunoglobulin G
IL-1β	Interleukin 1 Beta
IL-6	Interleukin 6
IR	insulin resistance
IRS-1	insulin receptor substrate-1
IRS2	insulin receptor substrate-2
ITT	insulin tolerance test
JNK1c-Jun	N-terminal kinase-1
KCl	potassium chloride
LC3	light chain 3
LCMS	liquid chromatography mass spectrometry
LDL	low-density lipoprotein
LDL-C	LDL cholesterol
LMW	low molecular weight fraction
MALDI	matrix-assisted laser desorption/ionization
MAPK	mitogen-activated protein kinase
MDA	malondialdehyde
MEM	minimal essential medium
MET	one metabolic equivalent
MgCl2	magnesium chloride
MMV	medium molecular weight fraction
NAC	N acetyl cysteine
NADPH	nicotinamide adenine dinucleotide phosphate-H

NAG	urinary N-acetyl-beta-D-glucosaminidase
2-NBDG	2-deoxy-2-[(7-nitro-2, 1, 3-benzoxadiazol-4-Yl) amino]-D-glucose
NF-κB	nuclear factor-Kb
NIDDM	nonindependent diabetes mellitus
NMR	nuclear magnetic resonance
NOD	nonobese diabetic
OGTT	oral glucose tolerance test
ORAS	Oxygen Radical Absorption Capacity
OS	oxidative stress
PA	palmitic acid/palmitate
PAGE	polyacrylamide gel electrophoresis
P-Akt	Phospho-Akt
PBST	phosphate-buffered saline with Tween 20
PDX-1	Pancreatic Duodenal Homeobox-1
PEP	*Pleurotus eryngii* polysaccharide
P-GSK-3β	Phospho-GSK-3beta
PI3K/PI-3-P	phosphotidyl inositol-3 Kinase
PIO	polysaccharides Inonotus obliquus
PKC	protein kinase-C
PLP	*Phellinus linteus* polysaccharide
PMSF	phenylmethylsulfonyl fluoride
PPAR-gamma/ PPAR-γ	peroxisome proliferator-activated receptor gamma
PTP1B	protein tyrosine phosphatase 1-B
RBC	red blood cell
ROS	reactive oxygen species
SCFAs	short-chain fatty acids
Scr	serum creatinine
SDS	sodium dodecyl sulfate
sGOT	serum glutamic oxaloacetic transaminase
sGPT	serum glutamic pyruvic transaminase
SOD	superoxide dismutase
STZ	streptozotocin
T1DM	Type 1 diabetes mellitus
T2DM	Type 2 diabetes mellitus
TBARS	thiobarbituric acid reactive substance
TC	total cholesterol

TF	transcription factor
TG	triglyceride
TNF-α	tumor necrosis factor alpha
UV	ultra violet
WBC	white blood cell

Preface

Diabetes mellitus is a chronic syndrome diagnosed by a persistent rise in blood glucose concentration. The world today is facing a major problem of diabetes mellitus because of sedentary lifestyles and eating habits. Less physical activity leads to hyperglycemia, resulting in a persistent rise in blood glucose level. This condition leads to many other secondary disorders. Moreover, people suffering from different health disorders, including diabetes mellitus, are more prone to COVID-19 infection.

Diabetes mellitus is of two types: (1) type I (insulin dependent) and (2) type II (insulin independent). In order to combat diabetes mellitus type II, various drugs such as miglitol, voglibose, metformin, acarbose, etc. are available in the market. These drugs act by different pathways to decrease and maintain the blood glucose levels. However, these drugs are costly and have various side effects such as abdominal distention, flatulence, meteorism, diarrhea, etc. Insulin injections are also in common use against hyperglycemia. The use of insulin injections is painful and sometimes causes injury and infection at the site of injection.

Therefore, current research aims at exploring the natural antidiabetic resources (1) to avoid side effects of antidiabetic drugs, (2) to replace insulin injections, and (3) to find novel, oral, and cheap antidiabetic products.

Several mushrooms have been used in folk medicine against diabetes mellitus for ages. Mushrooms are enriched with various bioactive constituents with antidiabetic efficacy such as polysaccharides, terpenes, sterols, etc. The extracts as well as bioactive constituents through different mechanisms exhibit antidiabetic action.

This volume, *Therapeutic Mushrooms for Diabetes Mellitus: Current Evidences and Future Scope*, focuses on the prevalence, causes, and management of diabetes mellitus type II. It sheds light on the traditional uses of mushrooms against diabetes in human history; antidiabetic bioactive components of mushrooms; their mechanisms of action; in vitro, in vivo, and clinical studies on antidiabetic mushrooms; the role of mushrooms in gestational diabetes mellitus; and clinical and various antidiabetic market product of mushrooms. It gives an insight into the role of mushrooms such as *Ganoderma lucidum, Innotus obliquus, Grifola frondosa, Phellinus species*, etc. against diabetes mellitus. It highlights the use of mushroom powder, extracts, and their bioactive components for the management of diabetic syndromes and discusses various in vitro, in vivo, and clinical studies performed to lower hyperglycemia and other diabetes-associated secondary abnormalities. The book also provides information regarding the mushrooms-based antidiabetic market products.

The volume first provides information about diabetes mellitus, its causes, treatments available, natural resources for the management of diabetes mellitus, history of use of mushrooms especially against diabetes. The middle part of the book is composed of chapters highlighting (1) the presence of bioactive constituents of antidiabetic mushrooms, (2) the mechanisms of action of these antidiabetic mushroom components, and (3) *in vitro* and gestational diabetes mellitus studies performed using antidiabetic mushrooms. The last portion of the book lays emphasis on (1) *in vivo* studies and clinical trials done using antidiabetic mushrooms and the available antidiabetic market products of mushrooms.

Academicians, research scholars, medicos, pharmaceutical industry professionals as well as students will find it a rich resource on therapeutic mushrooms for diabetes mellitus for the development of novel and cheap antidiabetic products with few or no side effects.

—Editors

Acknowledgments

The editors would like to extend their special thanks to all the authors for giving their valuable ideas and time to accomplish this volume of the book.

CHAPTER 1

Diabetes Mellitus: A Health Syndrome

LENA AHMED SALEH AL-FAQEEH

Maulana Azad Collage of Arts, Science and Commerce,
Dr. Rafiq Zakaria Campus, Rauza Bagh, Aurangabad, MS 431001, India
E-mail: lenaalfaqeeh8@gmail.com

ABSTRACT

Diabetes mellitus (DM) is a lifelong metabolic disorder, which affects people around the world. Ancient Egyptians were the first people who described diabetes as a mysterious disease. It has been estimated that by 2045, 629 million people will be diabetic patients. The three common types of diabetes are type 1, type 2, and gestational DM. Diabetes results from insufficient insulin secretion or poor insulin-directed form beta cells in pancreas. Symptoms of diabetes can include weight loss, polydipsia (increased thirst), and polyuria (frequent urination). Complications like blindness, cardiovascular disease, and even death can occur if diabetes is not treated. It can be diagnosed by fasting plasma glucose, random plasma glucose, and oral glucose tolerance tests. Treatment of DM includes insulin injections, oral antidiabetic pills, controlling lifestyle, and using of some remedies like herps to help in controlling high blood sugar. Prevention and management of DM depend on several factors including avoiding of carbohydrates and meat intake, avoiding of tobacco and alcohol along with using appropriate medications.

Therapeutic Mushrooms for Diabetes Mellitus: Current Evidences and Future Scope. Uzma Azeem, Khalid Rehman Hakeem, (Eds.)

1.1 DIABETES MELLITUS (DM)

DM is a metabolic disorder characterized by increasing blood glucose level (hyperglycemia). Diabetes is due to either pancreas do not produce enough insulin (lack of insulin) or body cells do not respond properly to the insulin produced (insulin dysfunction). It is a global health problem and it has been estimated that 629 million people will be diabetic patients by 2045.[1,2]

1.1.1 HISTORY OF DM

Term of DM come from Greek word "diabainein" that means "to siphon or pass through" and Latin word "mellitus" that means "sweetened with honey."

- In 1500 BC, ancient Egyptian are the first people who describe diabetes as a disease with recurring urination. It was first documented in the Eberes papyrus by George Eberes.
- In the 6th century BC, Sushruta, an Indian physician, noticed the sweet nature of urine in such patients and because of its sweetness it attracted ants. He termed the condition Madhumeha (honey urine).
- In the first century AD, a Greek physician, Aretaeus of Cappadocia, stated the word diabetes (Greek, 'siphon'). He described the disease as increasing of thirsty and drinking of water and increasing of urination.
- In 1675, Thomas Willis (British doctor) added the word mellitus (honey sweet). He observed what had been known for many centuries elsewhere, that the urine of diabetic patients is sweet.[3–7]

1.1.2 DM CAUSES

The causes of diabetes are complex and majority of diabetes cases begin with one of two processes:

1.1.2.1 AUTOIMMUNE

This form includes type 1 diabetes in which immune system in human body mistakenly destroy the pancreas beta-cells that produce insulin. In general, this form develops in children and young adults. Autoimmune diabetes causes can include family history, genetics, viruses, or other environmental factors.

1.1.2.2 METABOLIC

Uncontrollable risk factors and unhealthy lifestyle factors such as genetics, age, family history, obesity, overeating, and physical inactivity can impair the body's ability to use insulin (insulin resistance). Metabolic forms of diabetes include type 2 diabetes that accounts for 90–95% of diabetic cases and gestational diabetes, which can be develop in any previously nondiabetic woman during pregnancy due to hormonal changes. Type 2 diabetes is widely diagnosed in adults.[8]

1.1.3 ECONOMIC BURDEN AND GLOBAL PREVALENCE OF DIABETIC MELLITUS

DM is a very costly illness and has profound consequences in terms of long-term microvascular and macrovascular complications, which shorten life expectancy and quality of life at the same time. DM poses a significant economic burden in terms of the costs to the health care system, the indirect costs resulting from the loss of the patient's disability and premature mortality.[9–12] The incidence and prevalence of DM around the world are still increasing each day. One in 11 adults in the world currently have diabetes (most of cases are type 2) and it is estimated that by 2040, it will be to rise to 1 in 10 adults.[13] Common cases of DM (especially type 2) are in developed countries, where the majority of patients are aged between 45 and 64 years. The greatest increase in prevalence is, however, expected to occur in Asia and Africa, where most patients will probably be found by 2030. For example, in India, China, Egypt, Brazil, and Japan, the estimated diabetic people by 2030 will reach to 79.7, 42.3, 6.7, 11.3, and 8.9 million diabetic cases.[14]

1.1.4 TYPES OF DM

1.1.4.1 TYPE 1 DM

Type 1 DM accounts 5–10% of diabetes cases. It results from pancreatic beta-cell destruction, leading to body failure to produce enough insulin.

The rate of beta-cell destruction is quite variable, being rapid in some individuals (mainly infants and children) and slow in others (mainly adults). It was previously referred to as "insulin-dependent DM" or "juvenile-onset diabetes."

1.1.4.2 TYPE 2 DM

This is the most common form of diabetes and its accounts for 90–95% of all diabetes cases. It results from defect of insulin secretion due to peripheral resistance. It's previously referred to as "noninsulin-dependent diabetes" or "adult-onset diabetes."[15,16]

1.1.4.3 GESTATIONAL DM

Gestational DM arises in pregnant women during second or third trimester of pregnancy. Insufficient insulin production during pregnancy to meet the extra needs leads to gestational diabetes. The women affected with this type are about 20–50%.[17]

1.1.4.4 OTHER SPECIFIC TYPES OF DM

These types include a wide variety of relatively uncommon conditions, primarily specific genetically defined forms of diabetes or diabetes associated with other diseases or drug use. It comprises less than 10% of DM cases.[18]

1.1.4.4.1 Prediabetes

Prediabetes is a condition when levels of blood sugar are higher than normal but not high enough to be diagnosed as diabetes. If it is not controlled, it can become type 2 diabetes.[19,20]

1.1.5 RISK FACTORS FOR DM

As in any disease, there are many risk factors that contributing to getting diabetes. Risk factors for DM include gender, family history of diabetes, ethnicity, injury to the pancreas (such as infection, tumor, surgery, or accident), genetic factors and autoimmune disease, age (risk increases with elder people), physical stress (such as surgery or illness), high blood pressure, abnormal blood triglyceride or cholesterol levels, smoking, physical inactivity, obesity, use of certain medications including steroids, diet, salt intake, low vegetables and fruits intake and low dietary fiber intake stress.[21–24]

1.1.6 SYMPTOMS OF DIABETES

The classic signs and symptoms include polydipsia (increased thirst), polyuria (frequent urination), weight loss, polyphagia, increased hunger, fatigue, blurry vision, sexual dysfunction among men over 50 years, headache, slow healing of cuts, gum's infection and swollen, itchy skin, and numbness or tingling, especially in the hands and feet.[25,26]

1.1.7 COMPLICATION OF DIABETES

If patient do not control its diabetes, a complication may occur.[27,28] DM causes two types of complications acute and chronic. Acute complications include hypoglycemia, diabetic ketoacidosis, and hyperosmolar hyperglycemic nonketotic coma while chronic complications include retinopathy, nephropathy, neuropathy, and cardiovascular and peripheral vascular disease (Fig. 1.1A and B).[29]

1.1.8 DIAGNOSIS OF DM

Diabetes can be detected in urine analysis. If excess amount of glucose present, blood test should be carried out to confirm that the patient is diabetic or not. DM in blood can be diagnosed by testing any one of the following:

1.1.8.1 FASTING PLASMA GLUCOSE (FPG)

For this test, 8 hours fasting is required. If blood glucose test results exceed 126 mg/dl on two or more tests on different days, this confirms a diagnosis of diabetes (Table 1.1).[30]

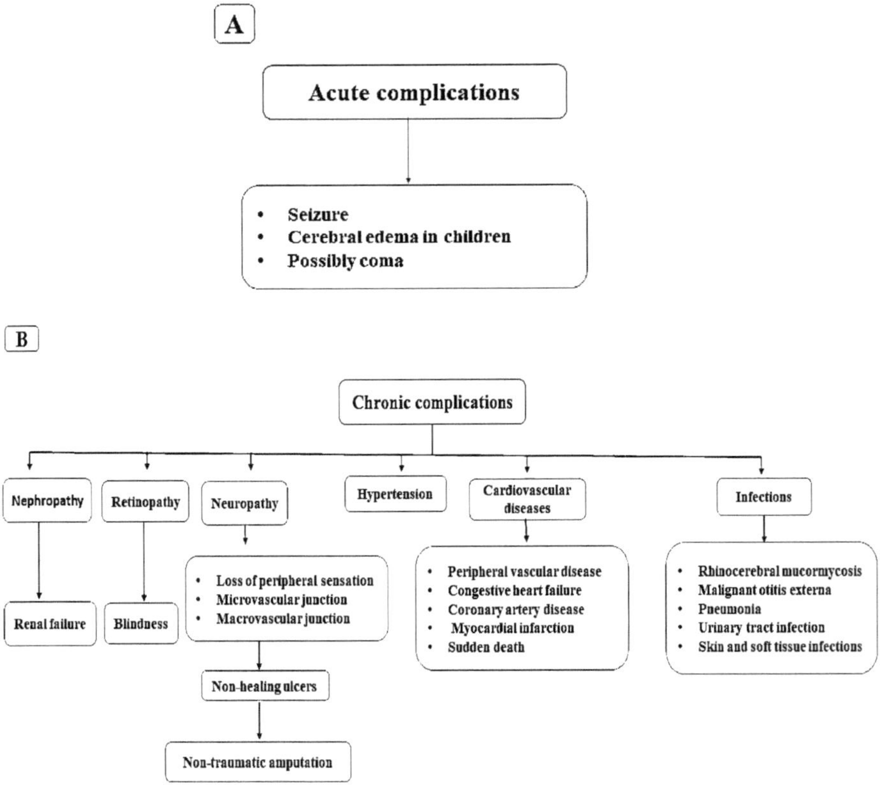

FIGURE 1.1 (A) Acute complications of DM and (B) chronic complications of DM.

1.1.8.2 RANDOM PLASMA GLUCOSE TEST

The simplest test requires no fasting before taking the test. If 200 or more than 200 mg/dl of blood glucose, this is an indication of diabetes. More tests are required to confirm diabetes.

1.1.8.3 ORAL GLUCOSE TOLERANCE TEST (OGTT)

This test is performed when fasting plasma test is 110–125 mg/dl and plasma glucose test is 160–200 mg/dl.[31] After determination of fasting plasma glucose level, 75 g of glucose is given to patients orally (100 g for pregnant women). The blood glucose is tested every 30 min, 1 h and 2 or 3 h. Also, medical history of patients should be reviewed.[32,33]

TABLE 1.1 Test Ranges of Diabetes Mellitus.

	Fasting plasma glucose (FPG) (mg/dl)	Oral glucose tolerance test (OGTT) (mg/dl)
Normal	≤99	≤139
Prediabetic	100–125	140–199
Diabetic	≥126	≥200

1.1.9 TREATMENT

- DM type 1 is treated with regular exogenous insulin injections (multiple doses per day), exercise, following a special diet, and yoga.[34]
- DM type 2 is usually treated with oral tablets such as thiazolidinediones, repaglinide, biguanides (it is known by metformin that remains the initial oral antidiabetic of choice, especially with type 2 diabetes), glinides, sulfonylureas, tolbutamide, rosiglitazone, phenformin, and troglitazone.[35,36] Although, these drugs have a side effect on patients and may probably increase the incidence of acute hepatitis, hepatic injury, and renal tumors.[37,38] Besides oral tablets sometimes insulin injections are also required. Also, diabetes treatments include changing of lifestyle, diet modification, weight regulation, regular exercising, and using of alternatives therapies such as herbal therapy can be included in treatment of DM type 2.[39–41]

1.1.10 PREVENTION AND MANAGEMENT OF DIABETES

There are some factors that help in prevent or delay diabetes type 2. Exercise, losing weight, following a proper diet which include reducing carbohydrate intake (carbohydrate have the most effect on blood glucose and insulin), reducing or avoiding consuming refined cereals, sugars and red meat, and intake of food supplements such as probiotics, fish oil is recommended to prevent the appearance of diabetes. For type 1 diabetes, there are no preventive measurements.[41,42]

To manage diabetes, following an active lifestyle which includes regular physical, avoiding cigarette smoking and stopping alcohol intake with the using of proper medication will help in management of diabetes.[42]

1.1.11 CONCLUSION

DM is a global health syndrome. During years more people become diabetic patients. DM is an important predictor of cardiovascular disease and mortality due to its complications. All forms of diabetes increase the risk of long-term complications. DM can be diagnosed by FPG and OGTT. Treatment of DM includes insulin injection, antidiabetic pills with following a proper lifestyle and sometimes using of herbal extracts which can help in decrease level of glucose in blood.

KEYWORDS

- **diabetes mellitus**
- **causes**
- **types signs and symptoms**
- **treatment**
- **prevention and management**

REFERENCES

1. Zheng, Y.; Bai, L.; Zhou, Y.; Tong, R.; Zeng, M.; Li, X.; Shi, J. Polysaccharides from Chinese Herbal Medicine for Anti-diabetes Recent Advances. *Int. J. Biol. Macromol.* **2019,** *121*, 1240–1253.
2. Ganesan, K.; Chung, S. K.; Vanamala, J.; Xu, B. Causal Relationship between Diet-Induced Gut Microbiota Changes and Diabetes: A Novel Strategy to Transplant *Faecalibacterium prausnitzii* in Preventing Diabetes. *Int. J. Mol. Sci.* **2018,** *19* (3720), 1–28.

3. Ian, F. G. Diabetes Mellitus: A Brief History, Epidemiology, Definition and Classification. *Clin. Exp. Optom.* **1999,** *82* (2–3), 102–105.
4. MacCracken, J.; Hoel, D. From Ants to Analogues: Puzzles and Promises in Diabetes Management. *Postgrad. Med.* **1997,** *101*, 138–140, 143–145, 149–150.
5. Tipton, M. C. Susruta of India, an Unrecognized Contributor to the History of Exercise Physiology. *J. Appl. Physiol.* **2008,** *108*, 1553–1556.
6. Frank, L. L. Diabetes Mellitus in the Texts of Old Hindu Medicine (Charaka, Susruta, Vagbhata). *Am. J. Gastroenterol.* **1957,** *27*, 76–95.
7. Ahmed, A. M. History of Diabetes Mellitus. *Saudi Med. J.* **2002,** *23*, 373–378.
8. Riaz, S. Diabetes Mellitus. *Sci. Res. Essays* **2009,** *4* (5), 367–373.
9. Ashcroft, F. M.; Ashcroft, S. J. H. Insulin. *Molecular Biology to Pathology*; Oxford University Press: Oxford, 1992; pp 266–284.
10. Collins, F, M. Current Treatment Approaches to Type 2 Diabetes Mellitus Successes and Shortcomings. *Am. J. Manage. Care* **2002,** *8* (16), S460–S471.
11. Olokoba, A. B.; Obateru, O. A.; Olokoba, L. B. Type 2 Diabetes Mellitus: A Review of Current Trends. *Oman Med. J.* **2012,** *27* (4), 269–273.
12. Kirigia, J. M.; Sambo, H. B.; Sambo, L. G.; Barry, S. P. Economic Burden of Diabetes Mellitus in the WHO African Region. *BMC Int. Health Hum Rights* **2009,** *9*, 6.
13. Sone, H. Diabetes Mellitus. *Encyclopedia of Cardiovascular Research and Medicine*; Elsevier: Amsterdam, 2017; pp 9–16.
14. Wild, S.; Roglic, G.; Green, A.; Sicree, R.; King, H. Global Prevalence of Diabetes: Estimates for the Year 2000 and Projections for 2030. *Diabetes Care* **2004,** *27*, 1047–1053.
15. American Diabetes Association. Classification and Diagnosis of Diabetes: Standards of Medical Care in Diabetes. *Diabetes Care* **2020,** *43* (1), S14–S31.
16. American Diabetes Association (ADA). Classification and Diagnosis of Diabetes: Standards of Medical Care in Diabetes. *Diabetes Care* **2018,** *41* (1), S13–S27.
17. Spitaler, M. M.; Graier, W. F. Vascular Targets of Redox Signaling in Diabetes Mellitus. *Diabetologia* **2012,** *45*, 476–494.
18. Baynes, H. W. Classification, Pathophysiology, Diagnosis and Management of Diabetes Mellitus. *J. Diabetes Metab.* **2015,** *6*, 541.
19. Selvin, E.; Rawlings, A. M.; Bergenstal, R. M.; Coresh, J.; Brancati, F. L. No Racial Differences in the Association of Glycated Hemoglobin with Kidney Disease and Cardiovascular Outcomes. *Diabetes Care* **2013,** *36*, 2995–3001.
20. Selvin, E. Are There Clinical Implications of Racial Differences in HbA1c? A Difference, to Be a Difference, Must Make a Difference. *Diabetes Care* **2016,** *39*, 1462–1467.
21. Fagninou, N. A.; Tougan, P. U.; Nekoua, M.; Fachina, R.; Koutinhouin G. B.; Yessoufou, A. Diabetes Mellitus: Classification, Epidemiology, Physiopathology, Immunology, Risk Factors, Prevention and Nutrition. *Int. J. Adv. Res.* **2019,** *7* (7), 855–863.
22. Fletcher, B.; Gulanick, M.; Lamendola, C. Risk Factors for Type 2 Diabetes Mellitus. *J. Cardiovasc. Nurs.* 2002, *16* (2), 17–23.
23. Patil, R.; Gothankar, J. Risk Factors for Type 2 Diabetes Mellitus: An Urban Perspective. *Indian J. Med. Sci.* **2019,** *71* (1), 16–21.

24. Chan, J. C.; Malik, V.; Jia, W.; Kadowaki, T.; Yajnik, C. S.; Yoon, K. H.; Hu, F. B. Diabetes in Asia: Epidemiology, Risk Factors, and Pathophysiology. *JAMA* **2009,** *301* (20), 2129–2140.
25. Suresh, L. PUBLIC Health Environment and Social Issue in India. *Diabetes: Causes, Sympt., Treat.* **2016,** 5; 56–67.
26. Li, W. L.; Zheng, H. C.; Bukuru, J.; Kimpe, N. D. Natural Medicines Used in the Traditional Chinese Medical System for Therapy of Diabetes Mellitus. *J. Ethnopharmacol.* **2004,** *92*, 1–21.
27. Brajendra, K. T.; Arvind, K. S. Diabetes Mellitus: Complications and Therapeutics. *Med. Sci. Monit.* **2006,** *12* (7), RA130–RA147.
28. World Health Organization. *Definition, Diagnosis and Classification of Diabetes Mellitus and its Complications*; World Health Organization: Geneva, 1999.
29. Loewen, S. L.; Haas, L. B. Complications of Diabetes: Acute and Chronic. *Nurse Pract. Forum* **1991,** *2* (3), 181–187.
30. Gillett, M. J. International Expert Committee Report on the Role of the A1c Assay in the Diagnosis of Diabetes. *Diabetes Care* **2009,** *32* (7), 1327–1334.
31. Guidance for Industry. *Diabetes Mellitus: Developing Drugs and Therapeutic Biologics for Treatment and Prevention*; US Department of Health and Human Services Food and Drug Administration Center for Drug Evaluation and Research (CDER), 2008, 3.
32. Suresh, B. L. Diabetes: Causes, Symptoms and Treatments. *Public Health Environment and Social Issues in India*, 1st ed., Serials Publications: New Delhi, Chapter 5, 2016; pp 55–67.
33. American Diabetes Association. Standards of Medical Care in Diabetes. *Diabetes Care* **2020,** *38* (1), pp. 1–29.
34. Puri, K. M.; Prabhu, P. S.; Dev, G.; Agarwal, S.; Murthy, P. S. Mechanism of Antidiabetic Action of Compound GII Purified from Fenugreek (*Trigonella foenum graecum*) Seeds. *Indian J. Clin. Biochem.* **2011,** *26* (4), 335–346.
35. Mishra, S. B.; Vijayakumar, M.; Ojha, S. K.; Verma, A. Antidiabetic Effect of *Jatropha curcas* L. Leaves Extract in Normal and Alloxan-Induced Diabetic Rats. *Int. J. Pharm. Sci. Rev. Res* **2010,** *2*, 482–487.
36. Milani, E.; Nikfar, S.; Khorasani, R. Zamani, M. J.; Abdollahi, M. Reduction of Diabetes-Induced Oxidative Stress by Phosphodiestrase Inhibitors in Rats. *Comp. Biochem. Physiol. C Toxicol. Pharmacol.* **2005,** *140*, 251–255.
37. Khan, R. M. M.; Chua, Z. J. Y; Tan, J. C.; Yang, Y.; Liao, Z.; Zhao, Y. From Pre-diabetes to Diabetes: Diagnosis, Treatments and Translational Research. *Medicina* **2019,** *55* (9), 546.
38. Singh, S. K.; Rai, P. K.; Jaiswal, D.; Watal, G. Evidence-based Critical Evaluation of Glycemic Potential of Cynodondactylon. *Evid. Based Complement Alternat. Med.* **2007,** *5* (4), 415–420.
39. Bharti, S. K.; Krishnan, S.; Gupta, A. K. *Herbal Formulation to Combat Type 2 Diabetes Mellitus*; LAMBERT Academic Publishing: Germany, 2013.
40. Rafiuddin, N. Plants Known as Antidiabetics from Aurangabad District, Maharashtra. *Ann. Pharm. Pharm. Sci.* **2010,** *1* (2), 85–87.
41. Hui, H.; Tang, G.; Go, V. L. Hypoglycemic Herbs and Their Action Mechanisms. *Chin. Med.* **2009,** *12*, 4–11.

42. Wylie-Rosett, J.; Delahanty, L. M. *Nutrition in the Prevention and Treatment of Disease*, 4th ed., Elsevier: Amsterdam, 2017; pp 691–707.
43. Forouhi, G. N.; Misra, A.; Mohan, V.; Taylor, R.; Yancy, W. Dietary and Nutritional Approaches for Prevention and Management of Type 2 Diabetes. *BMJ* **2018,** *361*, k2234.

CHAPTER 2

Natural Products for the Management of Diabetes: Achievements and Future Trends

KUNDAN SINGH BORA[1] and RICHA SHRI[2*]

[1]*University Institute of Pharmaceutical Sciences, Chandigarh University, Gharuan, Mohali 140413, Punjab, India*

[2]*Department of Pharmaceutical Sciences and Drug Research, Punjabi University, Patiala 147002, Punjab, India*

**Corresponding author. E-mail: richashri@pbi.ac.in*

ABSTRACT

Diabetes mellitus (DM) is a life-altering and debilitating syndrome marked by continued hyperglycemia due to flawed insulin production or insulin activity or both. Globally, healthcare professionals are working tirelessly to control this scourge. Management options include lifestyle modification and pharmacotherapy. The available drugs such as biguanides, thiazolidinediones, sulfonylureas, and meglitinides, though effective are limited by severe side effects especially on prolonged use. Therefore, newer approaches for the management of DM are highly desirable. Natural sources are a repertoire for drug discovery since they show immense diversity and novelty; are effective and are considered safer. Hence, development of antidiabetic drugs of natural origin is a viable option. The current review provides a scientific perspective on the usage and research of natural remedies for the management of diabetes. Literature survey

Therapeutic Mushrooms for Diabetes Mellitus: Current Evidences and Future Scope. Uzma Azeem, Khalid Rehman Hakeem, (Eds.)

reveals that numerous plants and mushrooms display potent antidiabetic actions (e.g., alpha-amylase inhibition, stimulation of insulin production and action, increased glucose uptake, management of free radicals) with minimal side effects in preclinical investigations. Detailed chemical investigations have led to the isolation of the compounds/fractions responsible for the activities. Moreover, bioactive plant/mushroom extracts/fractions act on different targets simultaneously thus showing effective control of experimental DM. But what is necessary is that authentication of plant or mushroom should be done, followed by standardization of extraction/isolation and characterization procedures along with detailed safety and efficacy studies. Preclinical studies should be followed by clinical evaluation thus generating scientifically validated natural antidiabetic therapies. The present review emphasizes the achievements and future trends of natural products in the effective management of DM.

2.1 INTRODUCTION: UNDERSTANDING DIABETES MELLITUS (DM)

Technological advancements and urbanization have revolutionized our lives. Our lifestyles have changed and, in many ways, become easier and more convenient. But the flipside of this is altered dietary patterns (intake of "fast food" and processed food) and lifestyle (reduced physical activities and sedentary living). This has led to ever-growing increase in noncommunicable ailments.[1] These impact quality of life, morbidity, and lifespan along with being an immense emotional and financial burden for the patient, caregivers, and society. Of these DM is a major scourge for the society. The International Diabetes Federation[2] states that more than 460 million adults have diabetes and by 2045 this figure will go up to 700 million. The number of people struggling with DM globally has been steadily escalating over the past few decades. Figure 2.1 gives a brief overview of DM.

The hallmark of DM is hyperglycemia. This is the result of:

- Absence or an inadequate production of insulin in the body (this is known as type 1 DM or insulin-dependent DM).
- Inability of body to utilize insulin (this is the more common form of DM-type 2 or noninsulin-dependent DM).

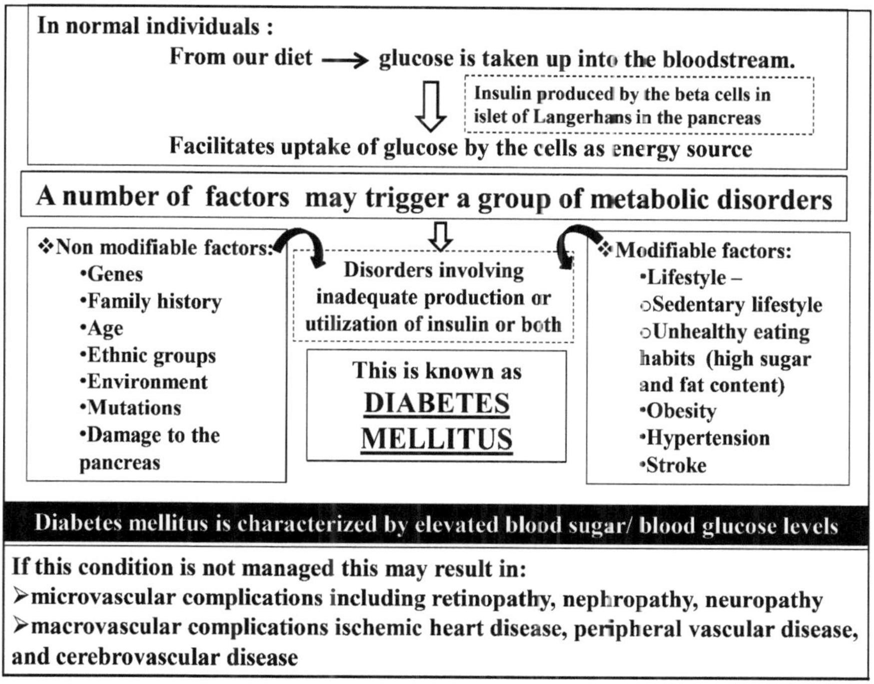

FIGURE 2.1 Diabetes mellitus: a brief overview.

Diabetics generally live with a wide range of symptoms ranging from mild to severe.[3–6] ***No country, no gender, no age group, and no economic social strata is insulated from this disorder***. Hence local, traditional as well as modern health practitioners are continuously striving to manage DM and alleviate the suffering caused by this.

Management of DM

- ✓**Lifestyle changes: Dietary alterations and increased physical activity**
- ✓**Pharmacotherapy**
- ✓**Combination of lifestyle changes and antidiabetic drug therapy**

Table 2.1 encapsulates the standard management of DM.[3,7]

TABLE 2.1 Conventional Management of DM.

What causes hyperglycaemia?	How to manage?	Available drug therapies
Little or no insulin production (i.e., type I DM)	• Insulin has to be used	• Insulin: • *Fast acting* • *Intermediate acting* • *Long acting* • *Continuous infusion pumps*
Type 2 DM—inadequate utilization of insulin		
Eating large quantities	• Reduce appetite	• Incretins; Guar gum
High carbohydrate intake	• Inhibit carbohydrate metabolism	• α-glucosidase inhibitors
Decreased insulin production	• Increase insulin production • Decrease glucagon secretion	• Sulfonylureas • Meglitinide/phenylalanine analogues • Glucagon-like peptide-1 (GLP-1) receptor agonists • Dipeptidyl peptidase-4 (DPP-4) inhibitors • Incretins
Decreased utilization of glucose by cells	• Increase glucose uptake by cells	• Biguanides • Thiazolidinediones (PPARγ activator)
Increased hepatic glucose output and gluconeogenesis	• Reduce hepatic glucose output	• Sulfonylureas • Thiazolidinediones
Neurotransmitter dysfunction	• Reduce hypothalamic drive to increase blood glucose levels	• Bromocriptine

The range of symptoms in patients with diabetes may be asymptomatic to lethal ketoacidosis, hence management has to be highly individualized. The objective is to maintain a normal blood glucose level (BGL) without producing hypoglycemia or influencing patient's routine.[8] *If not managed properly and in time, DM impacts every organ of the body leading to immense suffering and mortality!* ***Hence the importance of protecting the body from the consequences of hyperglycemia cannot be overemphasized.***

The available drug therapies are effective but are limited by severe side effects especially on prolonged use. Each class of antidiabetic drugs is constrained by undesirable effects—some of which are experienced immediately and some after longer use, which is essential for DM management. For example:

- Insulin therapy may cause hypoglycemia, along with central nervous system symptoms.
- The most frequent unwanted effect due to sulfonylureas is hypoglycemia, also may cause increase in weight, weakness, ataxia, disorientation, skin rashes, photosensitivity, and jaundice.
- The most commonly used biguanide—metformin causes adverse gastrointestinal symptoms in up to 20% of individuals taking the drug.
- Thiazolidinedione drugs may enhance the hypoglycaemia produced by concurrent use of sulfonylureas or insulin.
- Alpha-glucosidase inhibitors cause gastrointestinal disturbances.
- GLP-1 receptor antagonists result in GI disturbances, loss of appetite, and weight loss.
- Sodium-glucose co-transporter 2 inhibitors lead to increased risk of dehydration, genito-urinary tract infections.

2.2 QUEST FOR NEWER ANTIDIABETIC DRUGS

Since diabetic patients have to continue the drug therapy for long periods of time and often combination of different classes is being administered, they endure a number of side effects. Newer safer approaches for the management of DM are, thus, highly desirable.

Naturally derived products have been used for management of diseases and imparting health since the beginning of human life. Plants, mushrooms, minerals, and animal products have been employed in various traditional systems of medicine for management of DM. Traditionally Ayurveda, Traditional Chinese Medicine, Unani medicine, and African traditional medicine to name a few have turned to nature to assuage symptoms of DM. Their treatment regimen focussed on "Holistic approach" involving change in lifestyle along with the use of natural medicine. The drug therapies used were often combinations thus acting on various pathways of this complex disorder. Moreover, these therapies are cheaper, easily accessible, and people have faith that these are safer as compared with modern medicine. The medicines include:

- Crude drugs
- Powders and incinerated plants (ash/bhasma)

- Juice or decoctions
- Extracts/fractions

These show antihyperglycemic or hypoglycemic effects. Many traditional drugs have been investigated scientifically and there is evidence to support their use in DM patients. A scientifically tested poly-herbal formulation "BGR-34," was commercialized by Council of Scientific and Industrial Research, India in 2015 as the result of collective efforts of National Botanical Research Institute and Central Institute for Medicinal and Aromatic Plant and M/s Aimil Pharamaceuticals Pvt. Ltd., New Delhi. This is a combination of natural ingredients, based on Ayurvedic principles. This is used for control of type-II DM. However exhaustive pharmacological and clinical evidences are still required to strengthen and justify the application of traditional drugs for management of DM.

In addition to traditional uses, in modern medicine also natural sources (plants, mushrooms, animals, marine organisms, etc.) are valued as a repertoire for drug discovery since they show immense diversity and novelty; are effective and are considered safer. Natural products not only give useful drugs but also provide models based on which development of more effective compounds is envisaged. *Hence, development of antidiabetic drugs of natural origin is a viable option.*

This review aims to provide a scientific perspective on the usage and research of natural remedies for the management of diabetes. Detailed literature survey revealed that numerous plants and mushrooms have been investigated employing in vitro and in vivo experimental models. Many display potent antidiabetic actions, such as

- Stimulation of insulin production and action
- Increased uptake and peripheral utilization of glucose
- Decreased gluconeogenesis
- Alpha-amylase inhibition
- Retardation of carbohydrate absorption from the gut
- Control of free radicals and oxidative stress

Many plant extracts have ape insulin effects; lead to hypoglycaemic and antihyperglycemic effect; reduce postprandial spike in plasma glucose concentrations and prevent diabetic complications *with minimal side effects in preclinical investigations.* Some recent research work is presented in Table 2.2.

TABLE 2.2 Results of Some Experimental Studies on Antidiabetic Activity of Plants.

Family	Botanical name	Common name	Outcome	References
Acanthaceae	*Hygrophila auriculata*	Talmakhana	Chloride levels were managed thus cutting glucose uptake	[10,11]
	Strobilanthes crispus	Black face general	Glucose level declined	
Alliaceae	*Allium cepa*	Onion	Glucose level declined	[12–16]
	Allium sativum	Garlic	Reduced serum glucose and lipid levels and oxidative stress	
			Increased insulin	
Amaranthaceae	*Amaranthus esculentus*	–	Reduced glucose level, enhanced insulin	[17,18]
Anacardiaceae	*Mangifera indica*	Mango tree	Diminished glucose level	[10,19,20,32]
	Rhus coriaria	Sicilian Sumac	Reduction in glucose level	
Annonaceae	*Annona squamosa*	–	Reduced glucose, lipid levels, and lipid peroxidation	[21–24]
	Malmea depressa	–	Reduced glucose level	
Araliaceae	*Panax ginseng*	Ginseng	Reduced glucose level	[10]
Asphodelaceae	*Aloe barbadensis*	Barbados aloe	Reduced glucose, and lipid level, increased glucose tolerance	[10]
Asteraceae	*Chamaemelum nobile*	–	Reduced glucose level	[25–28]
	Eugenia jambolana	–	Reduced glucose, and lipid level, increased glucose tolerance	
	Artemisia sphaerocephala	Worm wood	Reduced glucose level	
Brassicaceae	*Lepidium sativum*	–	Decreased glucose levels	[29,30]
	Raphanus sativus	–	Decreased glucose and lipid levels	
Burseraceae	*Canarium schweinfurthi*	–	Decreased glucose level	[31]

TABLE 2.2 *(Continued)*

Family	Botanical name	Common name	Outcome	References
Cactaceae	*Opuntia dillenii*	Prickly pear	Diminished glucose level	[32]
Caricaceae	*Carica papaya*	Papaya	Diminished glucose and lipid levels	[32]
Caprifoliaceae	*Viburnum opulus*	Cranberry bush	Decreased glucose and lipid levels	[32]
Combretaceae	*Terminalia chebula*	Chebulic myrobalan	Decreased glucose level	[32–35]
	Terminalia superba	–	Decreased glucose level	
	Terminalia catappa	Indian almond	Decreased glucose and lipid levels	
	Tremella mesenterica	–	Decreased glucose level	
Crassulaceae	*Bryophyllum pinnatum*	–	Decreased glucose level	[36]
Ebenaceae	*Diospyros peregrine*	Gaub persimmon	Decreased glucose and lipid level	[32]
	Diospyros lotus	Date plum	Decreased glucose and lipid level	
Ericaceae	*Vaccinium myrtillus*	Bilberry	Decreased glucose and lipid level	[10,37]
	Vaccinium angustifolium	Wild blueberry	Decreased glucose level	
Euphorbiaceae	*Phyllanthus emblica*; *P. acidus*	Indian gooseberry	Decreased glucose and lipid level	[10,32]
Fabaceae	*Tamarindus indica*	Tatul tree	Decreased glucose level, prevents loss in body weight helps in revival of distorted hematological parameters	[10,32,38,39]
	Retama raetam	–	Decreased glucose levels	
Ganodermataceae	*Ganoderma lucidum*	Reishi mushroom	Decreased glucose level	[32]
Hypoxidaceae	*Hypoxis hemerocallidea*	–	Decreased glucose levels	[40]

TABLE 2.2 *(Continued)*

Family	Botanical name	Common name	Outcome	References
Lamiaceae	*Leonotis leonurus*	–	Decreased glucose level	[41,42]
	Salvia officinalis	–	Decrease glucose levels and gluconeogenesis	
Lauraceae	*Persea americana*	Avocado	Decreased glucose level	[10,32]
Lyophyllaceae	*Lyophyllum decastes*	Fried chicken mushroom	Decreased glucose level	[32]
Malvaceae	*Thespesia populnea*	Portia tree	Reduced glucose level	[32]
	Abelmoschus esculentus	Gumbo	Reduced glucose level	
Meliaceae	*Azadirachta indica*	Neem	Reduced glucose and lipid level	[10,32,43]
	Melia dubia	African mahogany	Reduced glucose level	
Menisper-maceae	*Coscinium fenestratum*	–	Reduced glucose level, HbA1C levels, glycogen, lipid, and oxidative stress	[28]
Meripilaceae	*Grifola frondosa*	Maitake	Reduced glucose level	[32]
Moraceae	*Egyptian Morus alba*		Reduced glucose and lipid peroxidation	[32,44,45]
	Artocarpus heterophyllus	Jackfruit	Decreased glucose and lipid levels	
Musaceae	*Musa sapientum*	Sweet banana	Decreased glucose level	[46]
Myrtaceae	*Psidium guajava*	Guava	Decreased glucose levels	[47–50]
	Eucalyptus globules	Blue gum	Decreased glucose level	
	Baccharis trimera	–	Reduced glucose levels	
	Syzygium cordatum	–	Reduced glucose, increased hepatic glycogen	
	Syzygium jambolanum	Jambolan	Reduced glucose level	
Nymphaeaceae	*Averrhoa bilimbi*	–	Reduced glucose and lipid levels	[51]

TABLE 2.2 *(Continued)*

Family	Botanical name	Common name	Outcome	References
Palmae	*Lodoicea sechellarum*	Sea coconut	Reduced glucose and lipid levels	[32]
Piperaceae	*Piper betle*	Pan	Reduced glucose levels and HbA1C	[52,53]
Punicaceae	*Punica granatum*	Pomegranate	Reduced glucose and lipid levels	[32]
Ranunculaceae	*Nigella sativa*	Roman coriander	Reduced glucose and lipid levels	[10,54]
Rhamnaceae	*Ziziphus spina-christi*	Christ thorn	Reduced glucose levels	[32,55]
Rutaceae	*Aegle marmelos*	Golden apple	Reduced glucose HbA1C levels, Increased C-peptide, glucose tolerance, and glycogen	[56–61]
	Citrus reticulata	Mandarin	Reduced glucose, lipid, and oxidative stress	
	Feronia elephantum	Wood apple	Reduced glucose level	
	Murraya koenigii	Curry-leaf tree	Reduced glucose, lipids and free radicals	
Rubiaceae	*Hintonia standleyana*	–	Reduced glucose level	[32,62]
	Morinda citrifolia	Indian mulberry	Reduced glucose level	
Scrophula-riaceae	*Scoparia dulcis*	–	Reduced glucose, lipid and oxidative stress, increased insulin	[63,64]
Solanaceae	*Withania somnifera*	Winter cherry	Reduced glucose level	[10,32,65–67]
	Lycium barbarum	Chirchita	Reduced glucose and oxidative stress, increase GLUT4, increase insulin	
	Withania coagulans	Vegetable rennet	Reduced glucose level	
	Physalis alkekengi	Strawberry tomato	Reduced oxidative stress	
Sterculiaceae	*Helicteres isora*	East Indian screw tree	Reduced glucose level	[32]
Zingiberaceae	*Curcuma longa*	Turmeric	Reduced glucose and lipid levels	[68]

Following numerous studies showing of significant antidiabetic activity in experimental models many plants were examined in clinical trials. Aegle marmelos,[69,70] *Allium cepa,*[71,72] *Gymnema sylvestre,*[73,74] *Momordica charantia,*[75–79] *Nigella sativa,*[80,81] *Ocimum sanctum,*[82,83] *Panax quinquefolius,*[84,85] *Salacia reticulata,*[86,87] *Silybum marianum, Trigonella foenumgraecum*, etc. have gone through the rigours of clinical trials with some favorable outcomes.

2.3 ROLE OF MUSHROOMS IN THE MANAGEMENT OF DM

Many species of mushrooms are used in our diet, also as dietary supplements as well as medicines in the management of DM. Antidiabetic potential of some species has been explored in various in vitro and in vivo models. For example *Catathelasma ventricosum* Peck (family: Tricholomataceae), a common mushroom found in southwest China. It is used in normal cuisine and for its health benefits. The Compendium of Materia Medica, states that this enhances immunity and reduces inflammation.[88] Extracts and polysaccharides (PLP) isolated from this species have shown reduction in experimental diabetes as oxidative stress; moreover these are documented to prevent secondary complications due to diabetes.[89–91] *Ganoderma lucidium* Lingzhi (family: Ganodermataceae) or reishi mushroom, which is revered for its diverse activities like immunity-enhancing and management of diabetes, cancer and inflammation since ancient times; has also demonstrated significant antidiabetic promise by α-glycosidase inhibition, aldose reductase suppression, free radical scavenging capacity as well as halting gene expression of phosphoenolpyruvate carboxykinase, which is involved in gluconeogenesis in diabetic mice.[92–95] Furthermore, *G. lucidium* PLP show potent activity.[96] *Hericium erinaceus* Bull. (family: Hericiaceaeis) is an edible and medicinal mushroom that has been studied a broadly. *Hericium erinaceus* (HE) well known in Chinese, as well as European and South American traditional medicine. Its extracts and PLP help normalize hyperglycemia, serum lipid levels, liver function, antioxidant enzyme actions probably due to phosphatidylinositol-3-kinase/protein kinase B (PI3K/Akt) signaling pathway triggering.[97–99]

Inonotus obliquus Ach. ex Pers. (family: Hymenochaetaceae) that is used traditionally in western Siberia and Russia, contains varied mycoconstituents, which exhibit diverse pharmacological activities. Reports show that dry matter, mushroom extracts, and triterpenoids with α,β-dimethyl, α,β-unsaturated δ-lactone side chains produced α-amylase and alpha-glucosidase inhibition, lipid lowering effects, reversal of injury of pancreatic tissues, mitigation of ROS and decline in BGL in diabetic rats. The effect may be due to stimulation of Akt and PI3K phosphorylation and translocation of GLUT4 in experimental animals.[100–104]

Another well-explored mushroom is *Phellinus linteus* Berk. (family: Aphylloporales) which is popular in Korea, China, and other Asian countries for management of a number of chronic ailments including diabetes.[105] Its extract and PLP show improved blood glucose profile and antioxidant status in experimental models.[106,107]

2.4 CLINICAL EVIDENCE OF ANTIDIABETIC POTENTIAL OF MUSHROOMS

Preclinical studies amply emphasize the antidiabetic capacity of mushrooms.[108] Mushrooms are considered safe dietary components for diabetics. These are rich in fiber, PLP, phenolic compounds, alkaloids and show gradual but marked blood glucose lowering along with lipid lowering and antioxidant effects. These also prevent postprandial spike in BGLs. Mushrooms are valued for their prebiotic effect due to which they modulate gut microflora and reduce insulin resistence.[109,110] Clinical trials, though not many or exhaustive, have demonstrated the blood glucose lowering capacity of mushroom species like *Agaricus*, *Coprinus*, *Ganoderma*, *Grifola*, and *Pleurotus*/mushrooms extracts/isolated PLP.[111–113] Clinical trials have been conducted with dietary mushrooms and certain mushroom extracts/preparations, e.g., extract of *Agaricus blazei* Murill, Vitamin D fortified with mushrooms, white button mushroom, oyster mushroom, ganopoly (PLP-rich fraction from *Ganoderma lucidum*) and Shitake extract.[114,115] Randomized, placebo-controlled double-blind clinical trials with extract of *Agaricus* species, ganopoly, *Pleurotus ostreatus* supplementation show drop in BBGL, enhanced glycemic control, and improved lipid profile.

The need of the hour is detailed pharmacological evaluation followed by clinical trials of the mushrooms that have demonstrated marked antidiabetic promise in experimental models.

2.5 FUTURE TRENDS

Since the beginning of life, human beings have turned to natural sources for all their needs including maintenance of well-being. From the above review, it is clearly evident that plants and mushrooms have strong anti-diabetic capacity. Figure 2.2 summarizes the fundamental steps for drug development from natural sources.

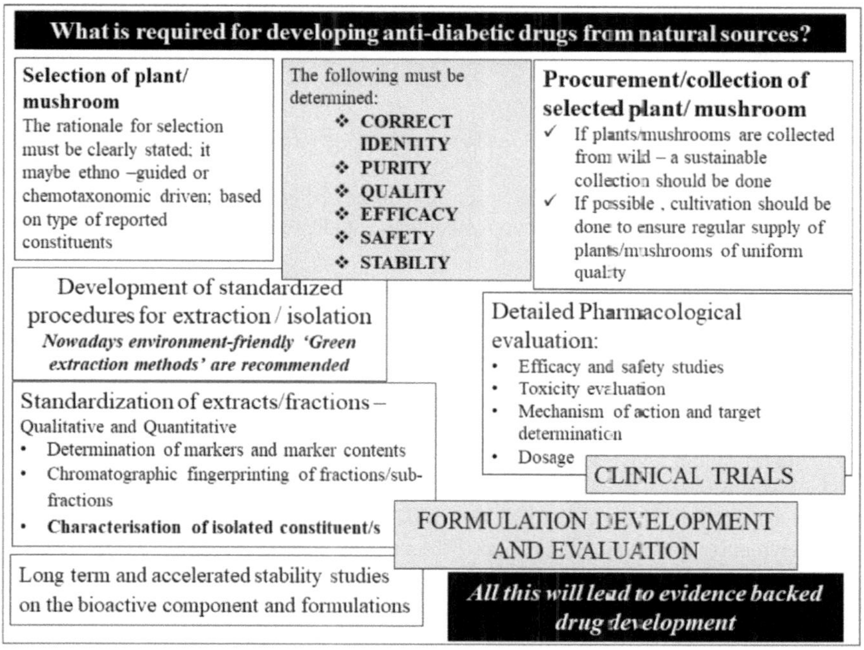

FIGURE 2.2 How to develop drugs from natural sources?

Thus, in order to translate the outcome of numerous experimental investigations into an antidiabetic drug a comprehensive and exhaustive study of natural products is required.

KEYWORDS

- **diabetes mellitus**
- **management**
- **mushrooms**
- **natural products**
- **plants**
- **prospects**

REFERENCES

1. https://www.who.int/health-topics/noncommunicable-diseases#tab=tab_1. Accessed on August 29th, 2021.
2. https://www.who.int/news-room/fact-sheets/detail/diabetes. Accessed on August 29th, 2021.
3. Tripathi, K. D. *Essentials of Medical Pharmacology*, 8th ed.; Jaypee Brothers Medical: New Delhi, India, 2018.
4. Katzung, B. G. *Basic & Clinical Pharmacology*; Lange Medical Books/McGraw Hill: New York, 2004.
5. https://www.cdc.gov/diabetes/index.html. Accessed on August 25th, 2021.
6. https://care.diabetesjournals.org/content/43/Supplement_1/S14. Accessed on August 25th, 2021.
7. Anonymous. *ICMR Guidelines for Management of Type 2 Diabetes*; Indian Council of Medical Research: Ansari Nagar, New Delhi, 2018.
8. Craig, C. R.; Stitzel, R. E. *Modern Pharmacology with Clinical Applications*; Lippincott Williams & Wilkins: Philadelphia, 2004.
9. https://www.thebetterindia.com/37127/anti-diabetes-herbal-drug-bgr-34/
10. Makheswari, M. U.; Sudarsanam, D. Database on Antidiabetic Indigenous Plants of Tamil Nadhu, India. *Int. J. Pharm. Sci. Res.* **2012,** *3* (2), 287–293.
11. Fadzelly, A. B.; Asmah, R.; Fauziah, O. Effects of *Strobilanthes crispus* Tea Aqueous Extracts on Glucose and Lipid Profile in Normal and Streptozotocin-induced Hyperglycemic Rats. *Plant Foods Human Nutr.* **2006,** *61*, 7–12.
12. Hattori, A.; Yamada, N.; Nishikawa, T.; Fukuda, H.; Fujino, T. Antidiabetic Effects of Ajoene in Genetically Diabetic KK-A(y) Mice. *J. Nutr. Sci. Vitaminol.* **2005,** *51* (5), 382–384.
13. Liu, C. T.; Wong, P. L.; Lii, C. K.; Hse, H.; Sheen, L. Y. Antidiabetic Effect of Garlic Oil But Not Diallyl Disulfide in Rats with Streptozotocin-induced Diabetes. *Food Chem. Toxicol.* **2006,** *44*, 1377–1384.
14. El-Demerdash, F. M.; Yousef, M. I.; El-Naga, N. I. Biochemical Study on the Hypoglycemic Effects of Onion and Garlic in Alloxan-induced Diabetic Rats. *Food Chem. Toxicol.* **2005,** *43*, 57–63.
15. Eidi, A.; Eidi, M.; Esmaeili, E. Antidiabetic Effect of Garlic (*Allium sativum* L.) in Normal and Streptozotocin Induced Diabetic Rats. *Phytomedicine* **2006,** *13*, 624–629.
16. Fetrow, C. W.; Avila, J. R. *Professional's Handbook of Complementary and Alternative Medicines*; Springhouse Corporation: Springhouse, PA, 1999.
17. Gupta, R. K.; Kesari, A. N.; Murthy, P. S.; Chandra, R.; Tandon, V.; Watal, G. Hypoglycemic and Antidiabetic Effect of Ethanolic Extract of Leaves of *Annona squamosa* L. in Experimental Animals. *J. Ethnopharmacol.* **2005,** *99*, 75–81.
18. Ojewole, J. A. Antiinflammatory, Analgesic and Hypoglycemic Effects of *Mangifera indica* Linn. (Anacardiaceae) Stem-bark Aqueous Extract. *Methods Find. Exp. Clin. Pharmacol.* **2005,** *27*, 547–554.
19. Prakash, P.; Gupta, N. Therapeutic Uses of *Ocimum sanctum* Linn. (Tulsi) with a Note on Eugenol and Its Pharmacological Actions: A Short Review. *Indian J. Physiol. Pharmacol.* **2005,** *49*, 125–131.

20. Gupta, R. K.; Kesari, A. N.; Watal, G.; Murthy, P. S.; Chandra, R.; Tandon, V. Nutritional and Hypoglycemic Effect of Fruit Pulp of *Annona squamosa* in Normal Healthy and Alloxan-induced Diabetic Rabbits. *Ann. Nutr. Metabol.* **2005,** *49,* 407–413.
21. Andrade-Cetto, A.; Martinez-Zurita, E.; Wiedenfeld, H. Hypoglycemic Effect of *Malmea depressa* Root on Streptozotocin Diabetic Rats. *J. Ethnopharmacol.* **2005,** *100*, 319–322.
22. Kaleem, M.; Asif, M.; Ahmed, Q. U.; Bano, B. Antidiabetic and Antioxidant Activity of *Annona squamosa* Extract in Streptozotocin-induced Diabetic Rats. *Singapore Med. J.* **2006,** *47*, 670–675.
23. Ojewole, J. A. Antinociceptive, Anti-inflammatory and Antidiabetic Effects of *Bryophyllum pinnatum* (Crassulaceae) Leaf Aqueous Extract. *J. Ethnopharmacol.* **2005,** *99*, 13–19.
24. Honda, S.; Aoki, F.; Tanaka, H.; Kishida, H.; Nishiyama, T.; Okada, S. M.; Abe, K.; Mae, T. Effects of Ingested Turmeric Oleoresin on Glucose and Lipid Metabolisms in Obese Diabetic Mice: A DNA Microarray Study. *J. Agric. Food Chem.* **2006,** *54* (24), 9055–9062.
25. Sharma, S. B.; Nasir, A.; Prabhu, K. M.; Murthy, P. S. Antihyperglycemic Effect of the Fruit-pulp of *Eugenia jambolana* in Experimental Diabetes Mellitus. *J. Ethnopharmacol.* **2006,** *104*, 367–373.
26. Ravi, K.; Rajasekaran, S.; Subramanian, S. Antihyperlipidemic Effect of *Eugenia jambolana* Seed Kernel on Streptozotocin-induced Diabetes in Rats. *Food Chem. Toxicol.* **2005,** *43*, 1433–1439.
27. Singh, L. W. Traditional Medicinal Plants of Manipur as Antidiabetics. *J. Med. Plant Res.* **2011,** *5* (5), 677–687.
28. Shirwaikar, A.; Rajendran, K.; Punitha, I. S. Antidiabetic Activity of Alcoholic Stem Extract of *Coscinium fenestratum* in Streptozotocin-nicotinamide Induced Type 2 Diabetic Rats. *J. Ethnopharmacol.* **2005,** *97*, 369–374.
29. Eddouks, M.; Maghrani, M.; Zeggwagh, N. A.; Michel, J. B. Study of the Hypoglycaemic Activity of *Lepidium sativum* L. Aqueous Extract in Normal and Diabetic Rats. *J. Ethnopharmacol.* **2005,** *97*, 391–395.
30. Taniguchi, H.; Kobayashi-Hattori, K.; Tenmyo, C.; Kamei, T.; Uda, Y. S.; Konshi, O. Y.; Takita, T. Effect of Japanese Radish (*Raphanus sativus*) Sprout (Kaiware-Daikon) on Carbohydrate and Lipid Metabolisms in Normal and Streptozotocin-induced Diabetic Rats. *Phytother. Res.* **2006,** *20* (4), 274–278.
31. Kamtchouing, P.; Kahpui, S. M.; Dzeufiet, P. D.; Tedong, L.; Asongalem, E. A.; Dimo, T. Anti-diabetic Activity of Methanol/Methylene Chloride Stem Bark Extracts of *Terminalia superba* and *Canarium schweinfurthii* on Streptozotocin-induced Diabetic Rats. *J. Ethnopharmacol.* **2005,** *104*, 306–309.
32. Vikrant, A.; Sharma, R. A Review on Fruits Having Antidiabetic Potential. *J. Chem. Pharm. Res.* **2011,** *3* (2), 204–212.
33. Lo, H. C.; Tsai, F. A.; Wasser, S. P.; Yang, J. G.; Huang, B. M. Effects of Ingested Fruiting Bodies, Submerged Culture Biomass, and Acidic Polysaccharide Lucuronoxylomannan of *Tremella mesenterica* Retz: Fr. on Glycemic Responses in Normal and Diabetic Rats. *J. Life Sci.* **2006,** *78*, 1957–1966.

34. Abdel-Zaher, A. O.; Salim, S. Y.; Assaf, M. H.; Abdel-Hady, R. H. Antidiabetic Activity and Toxicity of *Zizyphus spina-christi* Leaves. *J. Ethnopharmacol.* **2005,** *101*, 129–138.
35. Kim, H. K.; Kim, M. J.; Cho, H. Y.; Kim, E. K.; Shin, D. H. Antioxidative and Anti-diabetic Effects of Amaranth (*Amaranthus esculantus*) in Streptozotocin-induced Diabetic Rats. *Cell Biochem. Funct.* **2006,** *24*, 195–199.
36. Ojewole, J. A. Antinociceptive, Anti-inflammatory and Antidiabetic Effects of *Bryophyllum pinnatum* (Crassulaceae) Leaf Aqueous Extract. *J. Ethnopharmacol.* **2005,** *99*, 13–19.
37. Bhadoriya, S. S.; Ganeshpurkar, A.; Bhadoriya, R. P. S. Antidiabetic Potential of Polyphenolic-rich Fraction of *Tamarindus indica* Seed Coat in Alloxan-induced Diabetic Rats. *J. Basic Clin. Physiol. Pharmacol.* **2018,** *29* (1), 37–45.
38. Maghrani, M.; Michel, J. B.; Eddouks, M. Hypoglycaemic Activity of *Retama raetam* in Rats. *Phytother. Res.* **2005,** *19*, 125–128.
39. Louis, C. M.; Audrey, C.; Danielle S.; Ali, B. A.; Cory, H.; Bouchra, M.; Pierre, S. H. Anti-diabetic Properties of the Canadian Lowbush Blueberry *Vaccinium angustifolium* Ait. *Phytomedicine* **2006,** *13* (9–10), 612–623.
40. Ojewole, J. A. Antinociceptive, Anti-inflammatory and Antidiabetic Properties of *Hypoxis hemerocallidea* Fisch. and C. A. Mey. (Hypoxidaceae) Corm ["African Potato"] Aqueous Extract in Mice and Rats. *J. Ethnopharmacol.* **2006,** *103*, 126–134.
41. Ojewole, J. A. Antinociceptive, Antiinflammatory and Antidiabetic Effects of *Leonotis leonurus* (L.) R. Br. [Lamiaceae] Leaf Aqueous Extract in Mice and Rats. *Methods Find. Exp. Clin. Pharmacol.* **2005,** *27*, 257–264.
42. Lima, C. F.; Azevedo, M. F.; Araujo, R.; Fernandes-Ferreira, M.; Pereira-Wilson, C. Metformin-like Effect of *Salvia officinalis* (Common Sage): Is It Useful in Diabetes Prevention. *Br. J. Nutr.* **2006,** *96*, 326–233.
43. Schwab, U.; Louheranta, A.; Törrönen, A.; Uusitupa, M. Impact of Sugar Beet Pectin and Polydextrose on Fasting and Postprandial Glycemia and Fasting Concentrations of Serum Total and Lipoprotein Lipids in Middle-aged Subjects with Abnormal Glucose Metabolism. *Eur. J. Clin. Nutr.* **2006,** *60* (9), 1073–1080.
44. Singap, A. N.; El-Beshbishy, H. A.; Yonekawa, M.; Nomura, T.; Fukai, T. Hypoglycemic Effect of Egyptian *Morus alba* Root Bark Extract: Effect on Diabetes and Lipid Peroxidation of Streptozotocin-induced Diabetic Rats. *J. Ethnopharmacol.* **2005,** *100*, 333–338.
45. Omair, H. O.; Dhanasekar, S. S.; Senthil, K.; Ram, K. S.; Amit, R. In Vivo Antidiabetic Potential of Artocarpus Heterophyllus Plant Seeds in Streptozotocin-induced-diabetic Rats. *Biomed. Pharmacol. J.* **2009,** *2* (2), 339–343.
46. Dhanabal, S. P.; Suresh, K. M.; Ramanathan, M.; Suresh, B. Hypoglycemic Effect of Ethanolic Extract of *Musa sapientum* on Alloxan Induced Diabetes Mellitus in Rats and Its Relation with Antioxidant Potential. *J. Herb. Pharmacother.* **2005**, *5* (2), 7–19.
47. Ojewole, J. A. Hypoglycemic and Hypotensive Effects of *Psidium guajava* Linn. (Myrtaceae) Leaf Aqueous Extract. *Methods Find. Exp. Clin. Pharmacol.* **2005,** *27*, 689–695.
48. Musabayane, C. T.; Mahlalela, N.; Shode, F. O.; Ojewole, J. A. Effects of *Syzygium cordatum* (Hochst.) [Myrtaceae] Leaf Extract on Plasma Glucose and Hepatic

Glycogen in Streptozotocin-induced Diabetic Rats. *J. Ethnopharmacol.* **2005,** *97*, 485–490.
49. Chauhan, A.; Sharma, P. K.; Srivastava, P.; Kumar, N.; Duehe, R. Plants Having Potential Antidiabetic Activity: A Review. *Der Pharm. Lett.* **2010,** *2* (3), 369–387.
50. Cherian, S.; Augusti, K. T. Antidiabetic Effect of a Glycoside of Pelargonidin Isolated from the Bark of *Ficus bengalensis* Linn. *Indian J. Exp. Biol.* **1993,** *31* (1), 26–29.
51. Tan, B. K.; Tan, C. H.; Pushparaj, P. N. Anti-diabetic Activity of the Semi-purified Fractions of *Averrhoa bilimbi* in High Fat Diet Fed-streptozotocin-induced Diabetic Rats. *J. Life Sci.* **2005,** *76*, 2827–2839.
52. Arambewela, L. S.; Arawwawala, L. D.; Ratnasooriya, W. D Antidiabetic Activities of Aqueous and Ethanolic Extracts of Piper Betle Leaves in Rats. *J. Ethnopharmacol.* **2005,** *102*, 239–245.
53. Santhakumari, P.; Prakasam, A.; Pugalendi, K. V. Antihyperglycemic Activity of Piper Betle Leaf on Streptozotocin-induced Diabetic Rats. *J. Med. Food* **2006,** *9*, 108–112.
54. Kanter, M. Effects of *Nigella sativa* and Its Major Constituent, Thymoquinone on Sciatic Nerves in Experimental Diabetic Neuropathy. *Neurochem. Res.* **2008,** *33* (1), 87–96.
55. Mohamed, B.; Ziyyat, A.; Mekhfi, H.; Tahri, A.; Legssyer, A. Medicinal Plants with Potential Antidiabetic Activity—A Review of Ten Years of Herbal Medicine Research (1990–2000). *Int. J. Diabetes Metabol.* **2006,** *14*, 1–25.
56. Kamalakkannan, N.; Prince, P. S. The Effect of *Aegle marmelos* Fruit Extract in Streptozotocin Diabetes: A Histopathological Study. *J. Herb. Pharmacother.* **2005,** *5*, 87–96.
57. Adebajo, A. C.; Ayoola, O. F.; Iwalewa, E. O.; Akindahunsi, A. A.; Omisore, N. O.; Adewunmi, C O.; Adenowo, T. K. Anti-trichomonal, Biochemical and Toxicological Activities of Methanolic Extract and Some Carbazole Alkaloids Isolated from the Leaves of *Murraya koenigii* Growing in Nigeria. *Phytomedicine* **2006,** *13* (4), 246–254.
58. Kesari, A. N.; Gupta, R. K.; Singh, S. K.; Diwakar, S.; Watal, G. Hypo-glycemic and Antihyperglycemic Activity of *Aegle marmelos* Seed Extract in Normal and Diabetic Rats. *J. Ethnopharmacol.* **2006,** *107*, 374–379.
59. Narendhirakannan, R. T.; Subramanian, S.; Kandaswamy, M. Biochemical Evaluation of Antidiabetogenic Properties of Some Commonly Used Indian Plants on Streptozotocin-induced Diabetes in Experimental Rats. *Clin. Exp. Pharmacol. Physiol.* **2006,** *33*, 1150–1157.
60. Narender, T.; Shweta, S.; Tiwari, P.; Papi Reddy, K.; Khaliq, T.; Prathipati, P.; et al. Antihyperglycemic and Antidyslipidemic Agent from *Aegle marmelos*. *Bioorg. Med. Chem. Lett.* **2007,** *17* (6), 1808–1811.
61. Fröde, T. S.; Medeiros, Y. S. Animal Models to Test Drugs with Potential Antidiabetic Activity. *J. Ethnopharmacol.* **2008,** *115*, 173–183.
62. Navarrete, A.; Mata, R. Antihyperglycemic Effect of Constituents from *Hintonia standleyana* in Streptozotocin-induced Diabetic Rats. *Planta Medica* **2005,** *71*, 1099–1105.

63. Latha, M.; Pari, L. Effect of an Aqueous Extract of *Scoparia dulcis* on Plasma and Tissue Glycoproteins in Streptozotocin Induced Diabetic Rats. *Die Pharm.* **2005,** *60,* 151–154.
64. Pari, L.; Latha, M. Antihyperlipidemic Effect of *Scoparia dulcis* (Sweet Broomweed) in Streptozotocin Diabetic Rats. *J. Med. Food* **2006,** *9,* 102–107.
65. Zhao, R.; Li, Q.; Xiao, B. Effect of *Lycium barbarum* Polysaccharide on the Improvement of Insulin Resistance in NIDDM Rats. *Yakugaku Zasshi J. Pharm. Soc. Jpn.* **2005,** *125,* 981–988.
66. Wu, H.; Guo, H.; Zhao, R. Effect of *Lycium barbarum* Polysaccharide on the Improvement of Antioxidant Ability and DNA Damage in NIDDM rats. *Yakugaku Zasshi J Pharm Society Japan* **2006,** *126,* 365–3671.
67. Babu, P. S.; Prabuseenivasan, S.; Ignacimuthu, S. Cinnamaldehyde—A Potential Antidiabetic Agent. *Phytomedicine* **2007,** *14* (1), 15–22.
68. Honda, S.; Aoki, F.; Tanaka, H.; Kishida H.; Nishiyama, T.; Okada, S.; Matsumoto, I.; Abe, K.; Mae, T. Effects of Ingested Turmeric Oleoresin on Glucose and Lipid Metabolisms in Obese Diabetic Mice: A DNA Microarray Study. *J. Agric. Food Chem.* **2006,** *54* (24), 9055–9062.
69. Sankhla, A.; Sharma, S.; Sharma, N. Hypoglycemic Effect of Bael Patra (Aegle Marmelos) in NIDDM Patients. *J. Dairy. Food H. S.* **2009,** *28,* 233–236.
70. Ismail, M. Y. M. Clinical Evaluation of Antidiabetic Activity of *Trigonella* Seeds and *Aegle marmelos* Leaves. *World Appl. Sci. J.* **2009,** *7,* 1231–1234.
71. Imad, M. T. E.; Elhadi, M. A.; Abd, E. H. Preliminary Study of the Clinical Hypoglycemic Effects of *Allium cepa* (Red Onion) in Type 1 and Type 2 Diabetic Patients. *Environ. Health Insights* **2010,** *4,* 71–77.
72. Myint, Z.; Htun, H. L.; Thwin, T.; Mar, T. T.; New, M. M.; Oo, A. M.; Maw, L. Z.; Oo, T. K. K.; Kyaw, M. T. Acute Effect of Onion (*Allium cepa*) on Blood Glucose Level of Diabetic Patients. *Myanmar Health Sci. Res.* **2009,** *21,* 22–25.
73. Al-Romaiyan, A.; Al-Romaiyan, A.; Liu, B.; Asare-Anane, H.; Maity, C. R.; Chatterjee, S. K.; Koley, N.; Biswas, T.; Chatterji, A. K.; Huang, G. C.; Amiel, S. A.; Persaud, S. J.; Jones, P. M. A Novel *Gymnema sylvestre* Extract Stimulates Insulin Secretion from Human Islets in Vivo and in Vitro. *Phytother. Res.* **2010,** *24,* 1370–1376.
74. Paliwal, R.; Kathori, S.; Upadhyay, B. Effect of Gurmar (*Gymnema sylvestre*) Powder Intervention on the Blood Glucose Levels among Diabetics. *Ethno-Medicine* **2009,** *3,* 133–135.
75. Ahmad, N.; Hassan, M. R.; Halder, H.; Bennoor, K. S. Effect of *Momordica charantia* (Karolla) Extracts on Fasting and Postprandial Serum Glucose Levels in NIDDM Patients. *Bangla. Med. Res. Counc. Bull.* **1999,** *25,* 11–13.
76. Waheed, A.; Miana, G. A.; Sharafatullah, T.; Ahmad, S. I. Clinical Investigation of Hypoglycemic Effect of Unripe Fruit on *Momordica charantia* in Type 2 (NIDDM) Diabetes Mellitus. *Pak. J. Pharmacol.* **2008,** *25,* 7–12.
77. Rahman, I.; Malik, S. A.; Bashir, M.; Khan, R.; Iqbal, M. Serum Sialic Acid Changes in Non-insulin-dependant Diabetes Mellitus (NIDDM) Patients Following Bitter Melon (*Momordica charantia*) and Rosiglitazone (Avandia) Treatment. *Phytomedine* **2009,** *16,* 401–405.

78. Fuangchan, A.; Sonthisombat, P.; Seubnukarn, T.; Chanouan, T.; Chotchaisuwat, P.; Sirigulsatien, V.; Ingkaninan, K.; Plianbangchang, P.; Haines, S. T. Hypoglycemic Effect of Bitter Melon Compared with Metformin in Newly Diagnosed Type 2 Diabetes Patients. *J. Ethnopharmacol.* **2011,** *134*, 422–428.
79. Joseph, B.; Jini, D. Antidiabetic Effects of *Momordica charantia* (Bitter Melon) and Its Medicinal Potency. *Asian Pac. J. Trop. Dis.* **2013,** *3* (2), 93–102.
80. Bamosa, A. O.; Kaatabi, H.; Lebda, F. M.; Elq, A. M. A.; Al-Sultan, A. Effect of *Nigella sativa* Seeds on the Glycemic Control of Patients with Type 2 Diabetes Mellitus. *Indian J. Physiol. Pharmacol.* **2010,** *54*, 344–354.
81. El-Shamy, K. A.; Mosa, M. M.; El-Nabarawy, S. K.; El-Qattan, G. M. Effect of *Nigella sativa* Tea in Type 2 Diabetic Patients as Regards Glucose Homeostasis, Liver and Kidney Functions. *J. Appl. Sci. Res.* **2011,** *7*, 2524–2534.
82. Kochhar, A.; Sharma, N.; Schdeva, R. Effect of Supplementation of Tulsi (*Ocimum sanctum*) and Neem (*Azadirachta indica*) Leaf Powder on Diabetic Symptoms, Anthropometric Parameters and Blood Pressure of Non-insulin Dependent Male Diabetics. *Ethno-Medicine* **2009,** *3*, 5–9.
83. Agrawal, P.; Rai, V.; Singh, R. B. Randomized Placebo-controlled, Single Blind Trial of Holy Basil Leaves in Patients with Noninsulin-dependent Diabetes Mellitus. *Int. Clin. Pharmacol. Ther.* **1996,** *34*, 406–409.
84. Vuksan, V.; Sievenpiper, J. L.; Koo, V. Y. Y.; Francis, T.; Beljan-Zdravkovic, U.; Xu, Z.; Vidgen, E. American Ginseng (*Panax quinquefolius* L.) Reduces Postprandial Glycemia in Nondiabetic Subjects and Subjects with Type 2 Diabetes Mellitus. *Arch. Intern. Med.* **2000,** *160*, 1009–1013.
85. Vuksan, V.; Stavro, M. P.; Sievenpiper, J. L.; Beljan-Zdravkovic, U.; Leiter, L. A.; Josse, R. G.; Xu, Z. Similar Postprandial Glycemic Reductions with Escalation of Dose and Administration Time of American Ginseng in Type 2 Diabetes Mellitus. *Diabetes Care* **2000,** *23*, 1221–1226.
86. Jayawardena, M. H. S.; Alwis, N. M. W.; Hettigoda, V.; Fernando, D. J. S. A Double Blind Randomised Placebo Controlled Cross Over Study of a Herbal Preparation Containing *Salacia reticulata* in the Treatment of Type 2 Diabetes. *J. Ethnopharmacol.* **2005,** *97*, 215–218.
87. Radha, R.; Amrithaveni, M. Role of Medicinal Plant *Salacia reticulata* in the Management of Type II Diabetic Subjects. *Ancient Sci. Life* **2009,** *29*, 14–16.
88. Liu, Y.; Zeng, S.; Liu, Y.; Wu, W.; Shen, Y.; Zhang, L.; Li, C.; Chen, H.; Liu, A.; Shen, L.; Hu, B.; Wang, C. Synthesis and Antidiabetic Activity of Selenium Nanoparticles in the Presence of Polysaccharides from *Catathelasma ventricosum. Int. J. Biol. Macromol.* **2018,** *114*, 632–639.
89. Liu, Y.; Sun, J.; Rao, S.; Su, Y.; Yang, Y. Antihyperglycemic, Antihyperlipidemic and Antioxidant Activities of Polysaccharides from *Catathelasma ventricosum* in Streptozotocin-induced Diabetic Mice. *Food Chem. Toxicol.* **2013,** *57*, 39–45.
90. Liu, Y.; Sun, J.; Rao, S.; Su, Y.; Li, J.; Li, C.; Xu, S.; Yang, Y. Antidiabetic Activity of Mycelia Selenium-polysaccharide from *Catathelasma ventricosum* in STZ-induced Diabetic Mice. *Food Chem. Toxicol.* **2013,** *62*, 285–229.
91. Liu, Y.; Chen, D.; You, Y.; Zeng, S.; Hu, Y.; Duan, X.; Liu, A.; Chen, H.; Hu, X.; Chen, S.; Li, C.; Chen, D. Structural Characterization and Antidiabetic Activity

of a Glucopyranose-rich Heteropolysaccharide from *Catathelasma ventricosum*. *Carbohydr. Polym.* **2016,** *149*, 399–407.
92. Seto, S. W.; Lam, T. Y.; Tam, H. L.; Au, A. L. S.; Chan, S. W.; Wu, J. H.; Yu, P. H. F.; Leung, G. P. H.; Ngai, S. M.; Yeung, J. H. K.; Leung, P. S.; Lee, S. M. Y.; Kwan, Y. W. Novel Hypoglycemic Effects of Ganoderma lucidum Water-extract in Obese/Diabetic (+db/+db) Mice. *Phytomedicine* **2009,** *16* (5), 426–436.
93. Wu, T.; Xu, B. Antidiabetic and Antioxidant Activities of Eight Medicinal Mushroom Species from China. *Int. J. Med. Mushrooms* **2015,** *17* (2), 129–140.
94. Laurino, L. F.; Viroel, F. J. M.; Pickler, T. B.; Gerenutti, M. Functional Foods in Gestational Diabetes: Evaluation of the Oral Glucose Tolerance Test (OGTT) in Pregnant Rats Treated with Mushrooms. *Reprod. Toxicol.* **2017,** 72, 1–12.
95. Jia, J.; Zhang, X.; Hu, Y.-S.; Wu, Y.; Wang, Q.-Z.; Li, N.-N.; Guo, Q.-C.; Dong, X.-C. Evaluation of In Vivo Antioxidant Activities of *Ganoderma luicidum* Polysaccharides in STZ Diabetic Rats.. *Food Chem.* **2009,** *115* (1), 32–36.
96. Li, F.; Zhang, Y.; Zhong, Z. Antihyperglycemic Effect of *Ganoderma lucidum* Polysaccharides on Streptozotocin-induced Diabetic Mice. *Int. J. Mol. Sci.* **2011,** *12* (9), 6135–6145.
97. Wang, J. C.; Hu, S. H.; Wang, J. T.; Chen, K. S.; Chia, Y. C. Hypoglycemic Effect of Extract of *Hericium erinaceus*. *J. Sci. Food Agric.* **2005,** *85* (4), 641–646.
98. Liang, B.; Guo, Z.; Xie, F.; Zhao, A. Antihyperglycemic and Antihyperlipidemic Activities of Aqueous Extract of *Hericium erinaceus* in Experimental Diabetic Rats. *B.M.C. Complement. Altern. Med.* **2013,** *13* (1), 253.
99. Cai, W. D.; Ding, Z. C.; Wang, Y. Y.; Yang, Y.; Zhang, H.-N.; Yan, J. K. Hypoglycemic Benefit and Potential Mechanism of a Polysaccharide from *Hericium erinaceus* in Streptozotoxin-induced Diabetic Rats. *Process Biochem.* **2020,** *88*, 180–188.
100. Sun, J. E.; Ao, Z. H.; Lu, Z. M.; Xu, H. Y.; Zhang, X. M.; Dou, W. F.; Xu, Z. H. Antihyperglycemic and Antilipidperoxidative Effects of Dry Matter of Culture Broth of *Inonotus obliquus* in Submerged Culture on Normal and Alloxan-diabetes Mice. *J. Ethnopharmacol.* **2008,** *118* (1), 7–13.
101. Wang, C.; Gao, X.; Santhanam, R. K.; Chen, Z.; Chen, Y.; Xu, L.; Wang, C.; Ferri, N.; Chen, H. Effects of Polysaccharides from *Inonotus obliquus* and Its Chromium(III) Complex on Advanced Glycation End-products Formation, α-Amylase, α-Glucosidase Activity and H_2O_2-induced Oxidative Damage in Hepatic L02 Cells. *Food Chem. Toxicol.* **2018,** *116* (B), 335–345.
102. Wang, J.; Wang, C.; Li, S.; Li, W.; Yuan, G.; Pan, Y.; Chen, H. Anti-diabetic Effect If *Inontous obliquus* Polysaccharides in Streptozotocine-induced Type-2 Diabetic Ice and Potential Mechanism Via PI3K-Akt Signal Pathway. *Biomed. Pharmacother.* **2017,** *95,* 1669–1677.
103. Ying, Y. M.; Zhang, L. Y.; Zhang, X.; Bai, H. B.; Liang, D. E.; Ma, L. F.; Shan, W. G.; Zhan, Z. J. Terpenoids with Alpha-glucosidase Inhibitory Activity from the Submerged Culture of *Inonotus obliquus*. *Phytochemistry* **2014,** *108,* 171–176.
104. Stojkovic, D.; Smiljkovic, M.; Ciric, A.; Glamoclija, J.; Van Griensven, L.; Ferreira, I. C. F. R.; Sokovic, M. An Insight into Antidiabetic Properties of Six Medicinal and Edible Mushrooms: Inhibition of α-Amylase and α-Glucosidase Linked to Type-2 Diabetes. *S. Afr. J. Bot.* **2019,** *120*, 100–103.

105. Chen, H.; Tian, T.; Miao, H.; Zhao, Y. Y. Traditional Uses, Fermentation, Phytochemistry and Pharmacology of *Phellinus linteus*: A Review. *Fitoterapia* **2016,** *113*, 6–26.
106. Feng, H.; Zhang, S.; Wan, J. M. F.; Gui, L.; Ruan, M.; Li, N.; Zhang, H.; Liu, Z.; Wang, H. Polysaccharides Extracted from *Phellinus linteus* Ameliorate High-fat High-fructose Diet Induced Insulin Resistance in Mice. *Carbohydr. Polym.* **2018,** *200*, 144–153.
107. Kim, H. M.; Kang, J. S.; Kim, J. Y.; Park, S. K.; Kim, H. S.; Lee, Y. J.; Yun, J.; Hong, J. T.; Kim, Y.; Han, S B. Evaluation of Antidiabetic Activity of Polysaccharide Isolated from *Phellinus linteus* in Non-obese Diabetic Mouse. *Int. Immunopharmacol.* **2010,** *10* (1), 72–78.
108. Ganesan, K.; Xu, B. Anti-diabetic Effects and Mechanisms of Dietary Polysaccharides. *Molecules* **2019,** *24*, 2556. doi: 10.3390/molecules24142556.
109. Yusuke, O.; Tomoya, M.; Takeshi, O. Relationship between Dietary Patterns and Risk Factors for Cardiovascular Disease in Patients with Type 2 Diabetes Mellitus: A Cross-sectional Study. *Nutr. J.* **2016,** *15*, 15. doi: 10.1186/s12937-016-0132-6.
110. Khursheed, R.; Sachin, K. S.; Sheetu, W.; Monica, G.; Ankit, A. Therapeutic Potential of Mushrooms in Diabetes Mellitus: Role of Polysaccharides. *Int. J. Biol. Macromol.* **2020,** *164*, 1194–1205.
111. Katarzyna, W.; Wanda, M.; Klaudia, G.; Małgorzata, G. Mushrooms of the Genus *Ganoderma* Used to Treat Diabetes and Insulin Resistance. *Molecule* **2019,** *24*, 4075.
112. Venturella, G.; Ferraro, V.; Fortunato, C.; Maria, L. G. Medicinal Mushrooms: Bioactive Compounds, Use, and Clinical Trials. *Int. J. Mol. Sci.* **2021,** *22*, 634. https://doi.org/10.3390/ijms22020634
113. Lindequist, U.; Haertel, B. Medicinal Mushrooms for Treatment of Type 2 Diabetes: An Update on Clinical Trials. *Int. J. Med. Mushrooms* **2020,** *22* (9), 845–854.
114. https://clinicaltrials.gov/ct2/results?cond=Diabetes+Mellitus&term=Mushrooms&cntry=&state=&city=&dist=. Accessed on March 2nd, 2020.
115. https://clinicaltrials.gov/ct2/results?cond=Obesity&term=Mushrooms&cntry=&state=&city=&dist=. Accessed on March 4th, 2020.

CHAPTER 3

Human Medicinal Mushroom Use

MARIANO TORRES-GÓMEZ[1,2*]

[1]*Interdisciplinary Group for the Development of Ethnomycology in Mesoamerica A.C. (GIDEM), Coyoacan, Mexico*

[2]*Research Institute in Ecosystems and Sustainability (IIES), National Autonomous University of Mexico (UNAM), Antigua Carretera a Patzcuaro No. 8701, Ex Hacienda de San Jose de la Huerta, 58190 Morelia, Michoacan, Mexico*
E-mail: mtorres@cieco.unam.mx

ABSTRACT

Despite the differences, fungi and animals share a common ancestry more than 460 million years ago and these evolutionary relationships had developed in several fungal compounds that are active against many diseases that afflict human beings. Macroscopic fungi were already well established and playing a fundamental role in most ecosystems on the planet, when hominids appeared. In different contexts and circumstances, humans and other hominids gradually appropriated and incorporated fungi in their cultures, generating cognitive, and perceptual systems around these organisms. In these learning processes, humans learned the existence of some fungi with edible, hallucinogenic, deadly or highly toxic, and also medicinal properties, thus emerging mycophilic and mycophobic civilizations or worldwide. Many indigenous people discovered that some macroscopic mushrooms, like some polypores are effective at preventing

Therapeutic Mushrooms for Diabetes Mellitus: Current Evidences and Future Scope. Uzma Azeem, Khalid Rehman Hakeem, (Eds.)

and curing several diseases and infections. Humans have traditionally used some mushrooms as powerful medicines for millennia. Mushrooms have deep roots in humanity, especially in Africa, America, Asia, Europe, and Siberia. In Asia, especially in China, the use of medicinal mushrooms has been performed at least for 5000 years. A good example is the Pen Ts'ao document where 16 medicinal mushrooms species are described, among those stand out a few highly effective in preventing and combating cases of diabetes mellitus. Traditional knowledge and scientific validation should lead us to better understanding of different human illness and diseases and therefore the production of better medicine.

3.1 INTRODUCTION

As fungi and animals are more likely to each other than with plants, protozoans, and bacteria, due to we share a common ancestry, is hypothesized that we have some common enemies, so within fungal compounds we had find medicinal properties that are active against many diseases that afflict humans.[1] Fungi as we know them today, were already well established, diversified, and playing a fundamental role in different ecosystems on the planet, when humans appeared, more than 300,000 years ago.[2,3] Although some cultures consider fungi as organisms that cause disease, some others acknowledge that fungi are fundamental to human life. They influence most aspects of human well-being. Fungi are fundamental in an incredible range of ways: (1) like recycling nutrients, mushrooms are responsible for most of nutrient and organic matter recycling, returning them to the soil so it can be reused for other plants, mushrooms, and microorganisms;[4] (2) in the establish and growth of terrestrial plants, first by helping and guiding semiaquatic plants to colonize terrestrial landscapes around 600 million years ago, by mutualistic associations between plants and fungi, before roots evolved, therefore, terrestrial fungi colonized landscapes long before plants.[5] Then by been vital for the growth and health of most plants (80–90% worldwide) including all kinds of crops, through mycorrhizal associations.[6] These relationships between plants and fungi are essential for forests, jungles, and farmland productivity. Without mycorrhizal associations, trees, plants, and grasses would not survive.[7] Nowadays, mycorrhizal inoculants are available in many countries in gardening supply stores as soil amendments by organic agriculture growers, making improvements to crops, because if agriculture growth were reduced, human life (among others) would be seriously damaged through starvation due to plants are at the base of most food chains;[8] (3) food for humans and other organisms, many mushrooms are edible (with more than 3000 species known and used) and many of these species can be cultivated in small scale (home) or industrial and be sold worldwide which include also economical topics.[9] Eating wild and cultivated mushrooms still are a small proportion of actual human food, nevertheless, other kind of fungi are used in the elaboration of many of our daily foods like bread, cheeses, soya bean products, and also in common drinks like wine, beer, traditional beverages, just to mention a few;[10] (4) While many wild fungi are edible, some others are toxic, some of them deadly if they are consumed, like the famous "Destroying Angel" and "Death Cap" (Images 3.1–3.3).

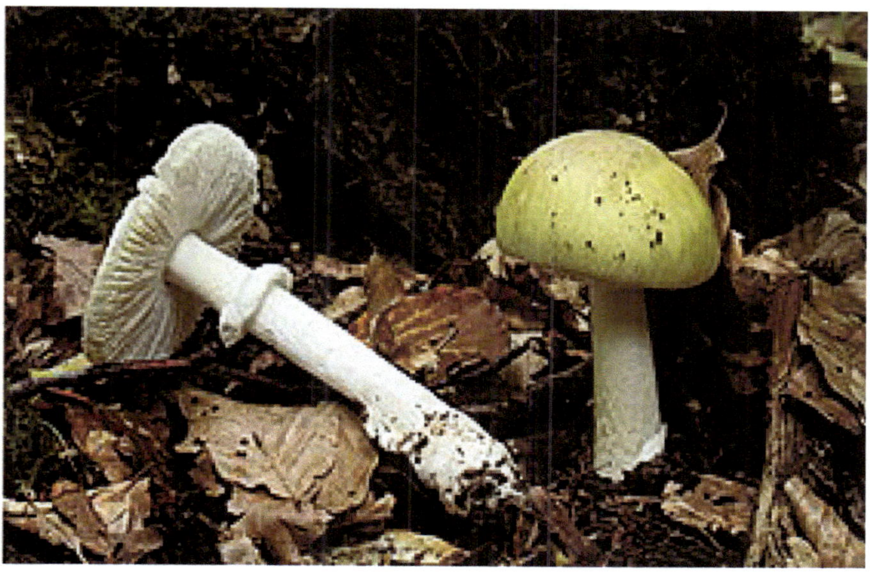

IMAGE 3.1 Death cap mushroom. *Amanita phalloides* (Vaill. ex Fr.) Link.

Source: Holger Krisp. https://commons.wikimedia.org/wiki/File:Gr%C3%BCner_Knollenbl%C3%A4tterpilz_Amanita_phalloides.jpg https://creativecommons.org/licenses/by/3.0/deed.en

(5) In medicine, most of the natural-based antibiotics are developed or isolated from fungal compounds, like penicillin, most known antibiotic is isolated from a fungus called *Penicillium* (Image 3.4) and so many others; antibiotics discovery revolutionized human health worldwide. Important medicine like immunosuppressant cyclosporine, which reduces

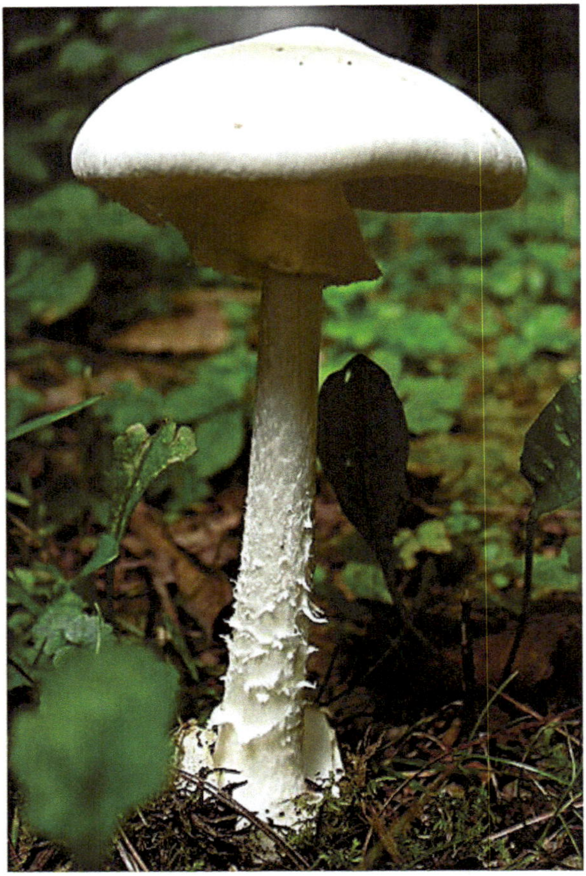

IMAGE 3.2 European destroying angel. *Amanita virosa* (Fr.) Bertillon.

Source: Jason Hollinger. https://commons.wikimedia.org/wiki/File:European_Destroying_Angel.jpg https://creativecommons.org/licenses/by/2.0/deed.en

the risk of rejection after organ transplant is isolated from fungi;[11] (6) as "nature's" biological control, a natural phenomenon that regulates, in this case, insects' populations (biotic mortality agents) by parasitizing them. This group of fungi (*Cordyceps*) is extremely diverse and host specific that some species can be used or preventing and controlling crop insect pests (Image 3.5), by spreading the spores on the crop pests or in urban landscapes. It is speculated that this method would be low cost and less damaging to ecosystems than the chemicals that we have been applying

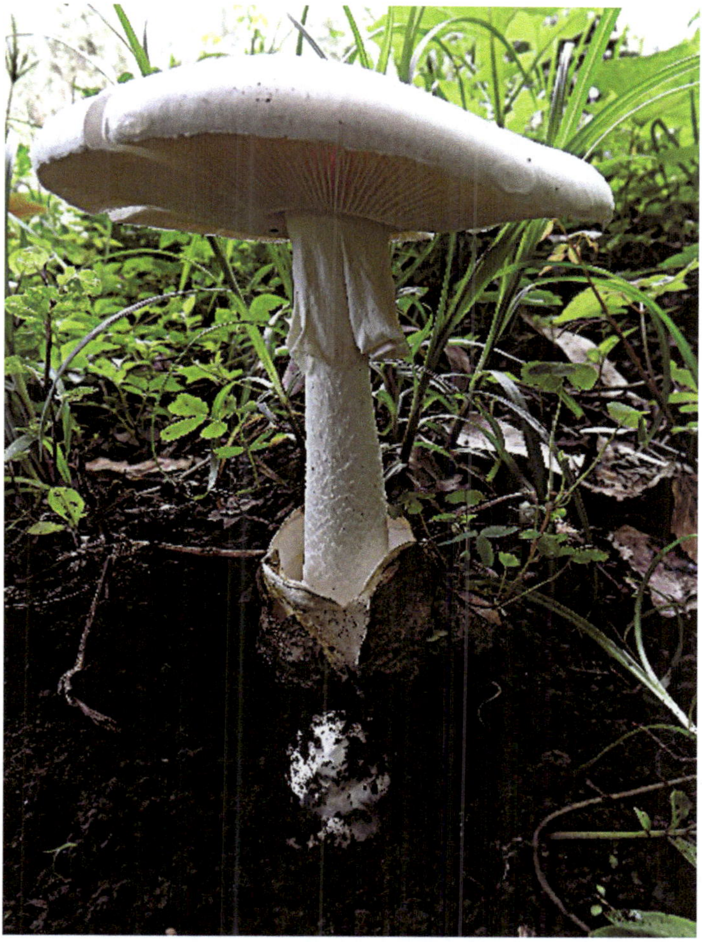

IMAGE 3.3 *Amanita bisporigera* G.F. Atk., American "Destroying angel."
Source: Mariano Torres-Gómez.

for decades.[12] (7) Some other fungi are plant parasites and have important negative consequences in crops and food production around the world, it is been estimated that approximately 80% of crops infections are caused by this kind of fungi.[13]

These are only some of the fundamental importance of fungi in Earth history.

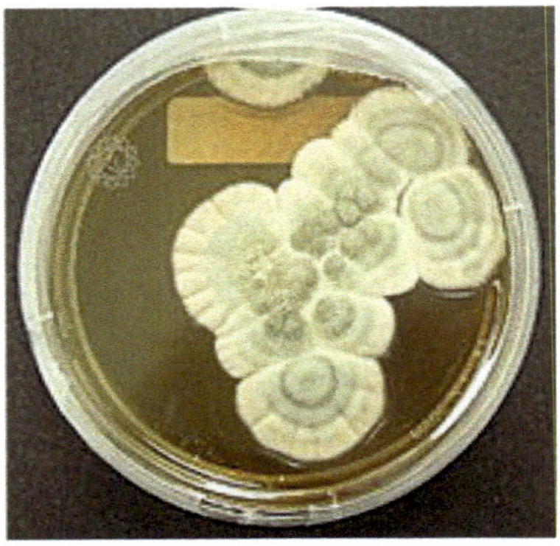

IMAGE 3.4 *Penicillium chrysogenum* Thom, syn. *Penicillium notatum.*

Source: Crulina 98. https://commons.wikimedia.org/wiki/File:Penicillium_notatum.jpg https://creativecommons.org/licenses/by-sa/3.0/deed.en

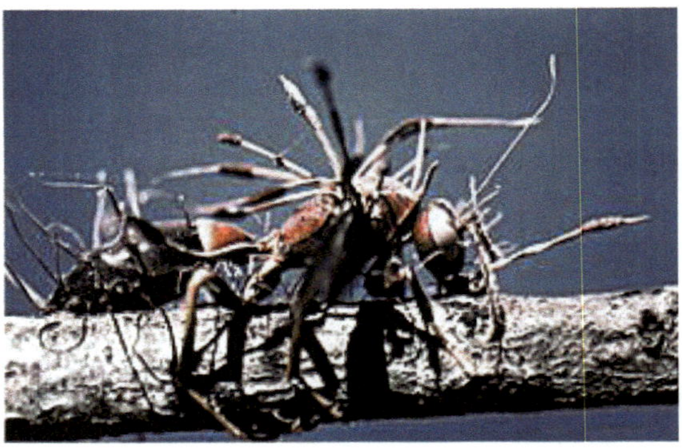

IMAGE 3.5 Wasp is parasitized by the fungus *Cordyceps.*

Source: Erich G. Vallery. https://commons.wikimedia.org/wiki/File:Cordyceps.jpg https://commons.wikimedia.org/wiki/File:Cordyceps.jpg

3.2 USE OF MUSHROOMS

The use of fungi (including microscopic species) by mankind (*Homo sapiens sapiens*) extends up to 20,000 years ago with fermented fruit drinks to produce different types of wine used by several primitive people in Africa, Middle East, and Asia,[14] or fermented grain to produce beer and bread in Mesopotamia in 6000 BCE (Before the Common Era) with native and wild yeast species (*Saccharomyces cerevisiae* and other similar species) used to ferment and brewing. These fermentation methods are ancient and most human cultures have practiced for millennia.[15]

However, with the beginning of civilizations, approximately (or at least) 10,000 years ago, based from different anthropological, ethnological, and archeological record and representations we have been able to know the importance that mushrooms (mostly macroscopic) have in several ancient civilizations.[16] For example, edible species used in Chile, 13,000 years ago[87] or the case of the cave paintings in the Tassili n Ajjer plateau in the Sahara, Algeria, Africa, that date from the year 5000 BCE, where several anthropomorphic figures with mushroom heads or mushrooms above their heads are dancing all together as a whole are shown, as well as the "mushroom-man" representing the "shaman" (traditional spiritual guide) with a body covered with mushrooms that resemblances hallucinogenic species and a bee head, which testifies the use of mushrooms as an essential part of ancient cultures and rituals.[17]

Then is the amazing finding of Ötzi, a Neolithic man (3000 BCE) who was found by two alpinist in the border between Austria and Italy in 1991 in a melting glacier, who had in his leather bag, among many interesting objects, two species of mushrooms (Images 3.6 and 3.7), both polypores (crusty mushrooms with pores and tubes on the underside), used for two different purposes, one used to start (ignite) and transport fire (*Fomes fomentarius* "tinder fungus") and another one edible and medicinal (*Fomitopsis betulina* "birch polypore"), which are still used in native communities around the territory. This species is used to alleviate gastrointestinal symptoms.[18] These uses mentioned above show us that mushrooms have been useful for more than just food.

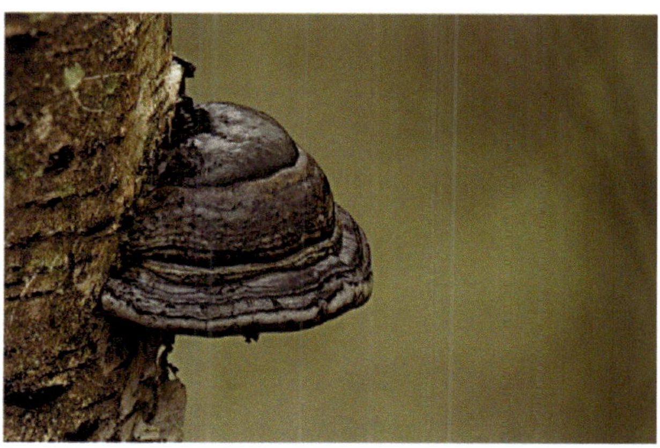

IMAGE 3.6 "Tinder fungus." *Fomes fomentarius* (L.) Fr.

Source: Richard Bartz. https://commons.wikimedia.org/wiki/File:Fomes_fomentarius_Zunderschwamm.jpg https://creativecommons.org/licenses/by-sa/2.5/deed.en

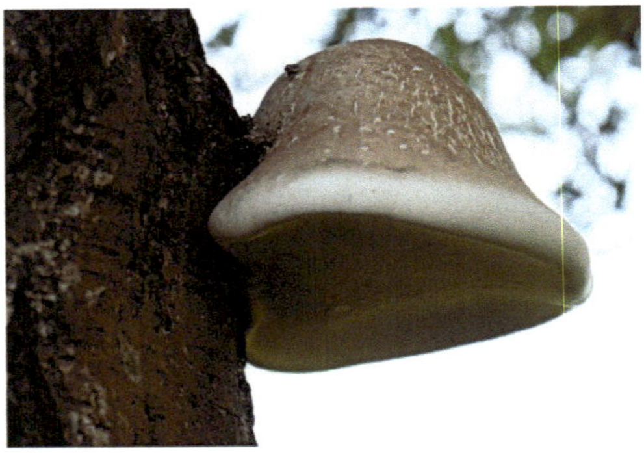

IMAGE 3.7 "Birch polypore." *Fomitopsis betulina* (Bull.) B.K. Cui, M.L. Han & Y.C. Dai.

Source: Captainpixel. https://commons.wikimedia.org/wiki/File:Piptoporus_betulinus_55.jpg Public domain.

Other mushroom uses beside food, medicine, and firestarter by humans are the ritualistic or divine, like the case of "Soma" the divine narcotic from India (3500 years ago) that for more than 2000 years the active compound was not known until fairly recently; it was discovered that *Amanita muscaria* (Image 3.8) was the mushroom used and called "Soma." This is one of the oldest hallucinogens used by mankind (and other animals) in both hemispheres[19] and it's the most iconic and known mushroom species worldwide.

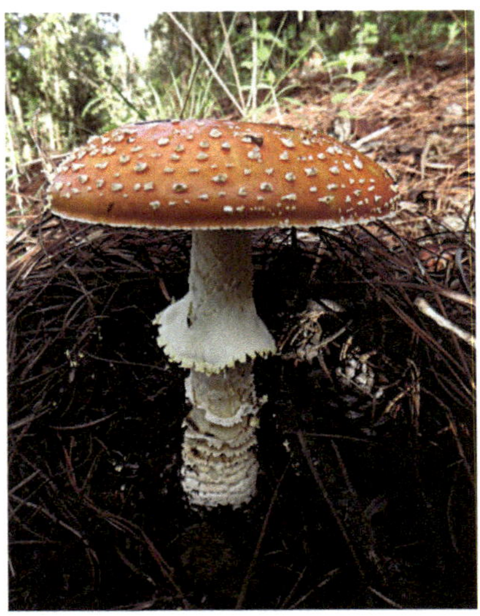

IMAGE 3.8 "Fly agaric," "Fly amanita." *Amanita muscaria* (L.) Lam.

Source: Mariano Torres-Gómez.

However, the consumption of mushrooms predates the human species, since our closest extinct relatives, the Neanderthals, already used wild mushroom species,[3] such as *Schizophyllum commune* (Image 3.9), an edible and medicinal species that it's present throughout the world and possibly is the most consumed mushroom worldwide nowadays.[20] These important discoveries were the result of an investigation on the behavior, diseases, and diet that different groups of Neanderthals had at least 48,000 years ago (Image 3.10), using DNA and other methods of regional differences. Neanderthal diet on Belgium zone was primarily meat based (woolly rhinoceros and wild sheep) and in Spain zone no meat was detected in their diet, but mushrooms, nuts, and moss were detected, for gathering and self-medication.[3]

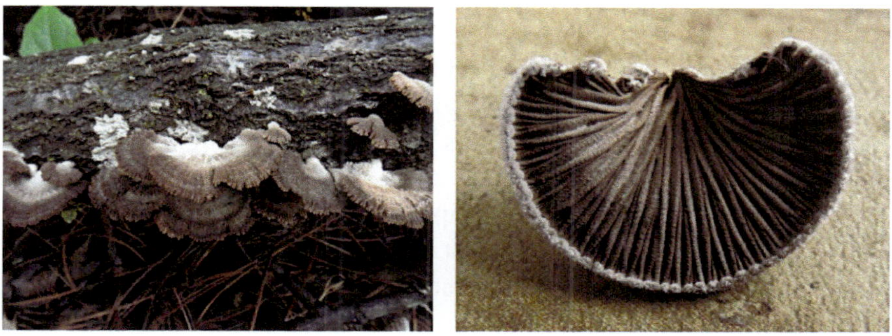

IMAGE 3.9 Left: Caps of *Schizophyllum commune* Fr. on a log. Right: Underside (Hymenium).

Source: Mariano Torres-Gómez.

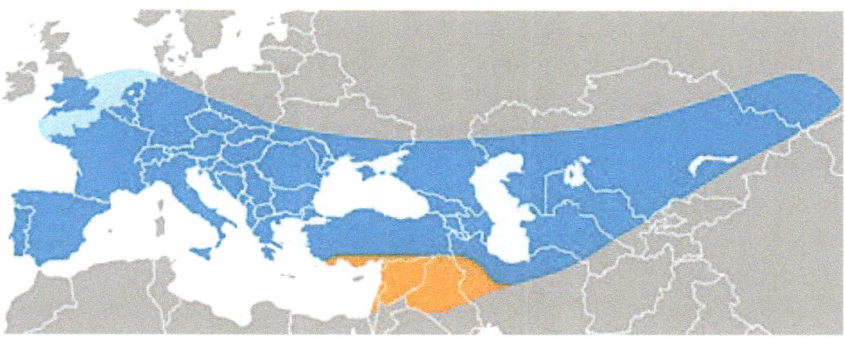

IMAGE 3.10 Range of Neanderthals in the Levant (orange) and elsewhere (blue).

Source: Modified from Nilenbert. https://commons.wikimedia.org/wiki/File:Range_of_Neanderthals.png https://creativecommons.org/licenses/by-sa/3.0/deed.en

In fact, it has been speculated or hypothesized that the increase of human brain size and therefore a more complex and creative thinking (among other impressive characteristics), the prerequisite for the evolution of modern humans, occurred when our ancestors began to intentionally and regularly consume psychoactive plants and mushrooms 1.5 million years ago.[16,21]

Today humans know and understand that for several millennia humans and other hominids, in different contexts and circumstances, gradually appropriated these organisms, incorporating them into different cultures and thus generating cognitive, perceptual, attitudinal, and pragmatic systems around them.[22] In these learning processes, humans learned the existence of some fungi with edible, hallucinogenic, deadly or highly toxic, and also medicinal properties, thus emerging mycophilic and mycophobic civilizations or worldwide.[1,10,23] In mycophilic cultures, mushrooms are highly valued as food, medicine, and ceremonial and there is a strong and long tradition of popular use, cataloging, and naming, while in mycophobic societies, a minor regard for fungi is held and they are often feared or seen as bad, dangerous, and to be avoid at any cost.[88] Most known mushroom species contain different active components that can affect different illness in humans, so it is not surprising that they have played an extremely important role in most ancient cultures and religions worldwide, like Egyptian, Greek, Roman, Mithraism, Judaism, Christianity, and many others.[16,24–27] It is believed that Vikings used to eat hallucinogenic mushrooms before battle to become ferocious fighters without fear. Buddhist and Taoist monks were the principal actors in spreading the medicinal effects of some mushroom species used in different ceremonies and rituals from several places. For example, it is believed that Buddha died intoxicated from eating a poisonous mushroom.[28] Some Egyptian hieroglyphics show some mushrooms species, some of them as food, some of them as medicine, and some other found in tombs and vessels as part of their rituals, they called them "sons of the gods," sent to Earth on lightning bolts by the gods and were eaten only by nobles and pharaohs (as in many other cultures around the world). The Aztecs also used several mushrooms species, for food, medicine, and for spiritual purposes, like the sacred mushroom called "the flesh of the gods" which they ingest in special ceremonies, and many Spanish documents described these and other mushrooms uses by the locals 500 years ago. And it is undeniable that many mushroom species, edibles, medicinal, and psychoactive played a crucial part in the development of

Mesoamerican cultures such as the Olmecs, Maya, Aztecs, and also Inca in the south.[28] Because this and more, humans understood the fundamental role of fungi in civilizations and began to study this relationship between mushrooms, culture, and mankind.

Ethnomycology is a biological/mycological/social discipline that studies the relationship between people, culture, and fungi and is an area of academic interest due to the importance of biocultural heritage of different people worldwide. One of the firsts publications about this topic is "Mushrooms, Russia, and history" by the Wasson couple, where they analyzed several differences between cultures that appreciate mushrooms and other that dislike them (mycophilic and mycophobic), among other interesting discoveries.[88] In fact, Mexico is the birthplace of ethnomycology discipline thanks to Robert Gordon Wasson around 1957.[29] The merit of pointed out the persistence of ritual ceremonies associated with the sacred mushrooms by the Mazatec people corresponds to the ethnobotanist Richard Evans Schultes and the ethnologist Robert Weitlaner. During a trip to Oaxaca, Mexico. Schultes discovered that local communities of Mazatec's, Chinantec's, and Zapotecs used some mushrooms with psychoactive properties, leading him to conclude that the Aztec mushroom called "teonanácatl" (sacred mushroom) consisted in one or more *Panaeolus* species.[30] Schultes in 1939 published a note regarding the use of sacred mushrooms, revealing the determination of the fungus used in rituals was *Panaeolus sphinctrinus*, a specie that later was found not to be the one that Mesoamerican people used in their rituals, revealing that the real species used as "teonanacatl" were *Psilocybe* species (Image 3.11) like *Psilocybe caerulescens* Murr. var. *mazatecorum* Heim. Indigenous people of Oaxaca collected these mushrooms and dry them before consuming them for ceremonial, prophetic, and divine purposes. Wasson and his wife Valentina Pavlovna in 1957, wrote an article on their fungal discoveries in Mexico, especially in the part of the Mazatec mountain range in a small Oaxacan town. They describe their encounter with priestess María Sabina and their experience with the sacred mushrooms and the discovery of the sculpture of the god (or prince) of the entheogens "Xochipilli"; (Image 3.12). Wasson distinguishes that in the sculpture of "Xochipilli" ("Prince of flowers" in Nahuatl or "God of art, games, beauty, dance, flowers, and song" for Aztecs) there are mushrooms that resemble *Psilocybe* species, like *Psilocybe aztecorum*, and other plants some with psycoactive properties and the tobacco flower. One year later Heim and Wasson published

"Les Champignons Hallucinogénes du Mexique" where they incorporate the use and knowledge of various species of mushrooms like *Psilocybe* (among others) in different rites and ceremonies, and they mention that they were exclusively Mexican.[31] Mexico holds the largest number of *Psilocybe* species (40% of the world).[32]

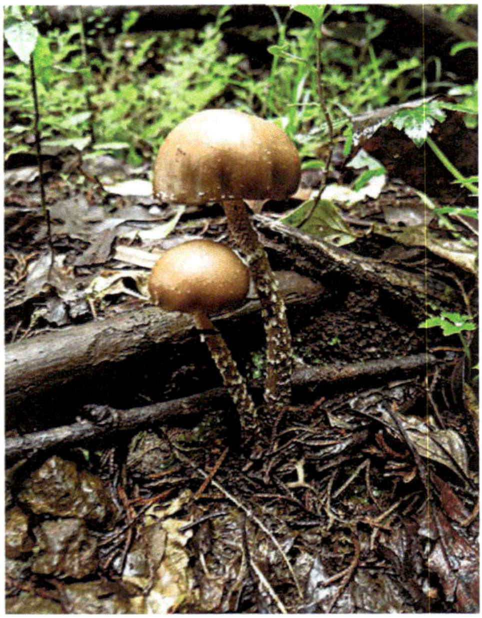

IMAGE 3.11 *Psilocybe zapotecorum* R. Heim.

Credit: Fabs1009. https://commons. wikimedia.org/wiki/File:Psilocybe_caerulescens_var._Bosque_-_Costa_Rica_(1).jpg https://creativecommons.org/licenses/by-sa/4.0/deed.en

Although ethnomycology began with a clear interest in hallucinogenic mushrooms, later turned to wild edible and medicinal fungi, and their cultural significance. During the last half century, researchers have increased worlds knowledge of local mushrooms traditions in Africa, Asia, and Mesoamerica mainly.[88]

The historical influence of Swedish culture in Finland did little to enthuse local interest in mushrooms in that mycophobic society, inversely, Karelian people who came from Russia to Finland brought a much stronger tradition and liking for wild edible fungi because they came from a mycophilic culture. Russians are worldwide known for their general (though not universal) love of wild edible fungi, so much so that in some parts of the

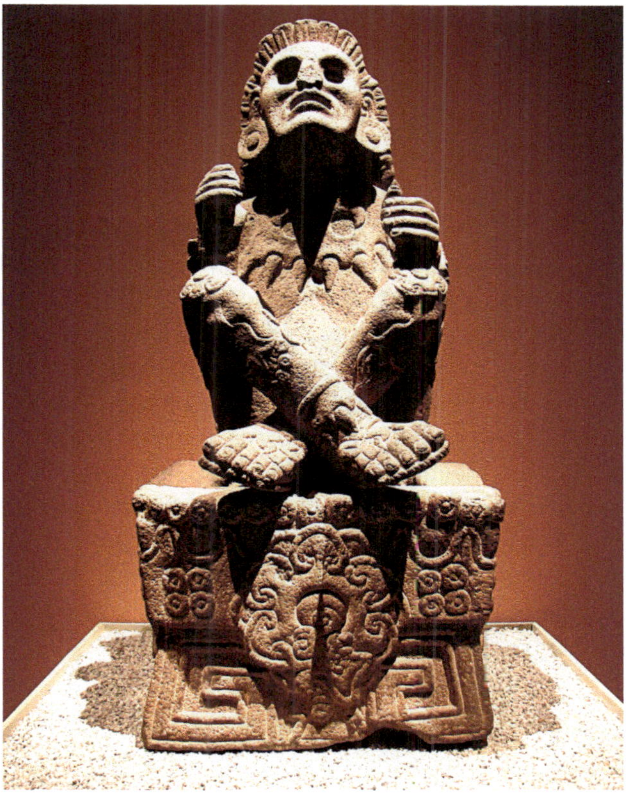

IMAGE 3.12 Xochipilli.

Source: Antony Stanley - https://www.flickr.com/photos/antonystanley/2105549511/ https://creativecommons.org/licenses/by-sa/2.0/

world, like Estonia, where they are not fond to mushrooms, have a saying that describes the Russian mushroom passion, they say: "Where there is a mushroom popping, there is always a Russian waiting for it." Another example of this contrasting point of view, is in Finland, where they used to say "Shouting like Russians in a mushroom forest."[89]

Since ethnomycological studies arise worldwide mankind began to realize and understand the importance of biocultural richness of ancient cultures, specially of Africa, America, Asia, Europe, and Siberia.[42] Countries like China and Mexico are especially rich in edible mushroom species used traditionally, with more than 1000 and 400, respectively.[9] Mexico, India, China, and Nigeria are the countries with more published ethnomycological studies in the last decades.[42,43] Within these studies and gathered information, there are thousands of functional mushroom species described and used worldwide, and in this learning process, humans acknowledge the lack of information specially of medicinal ones (mushrooms and lichens).[35]

3.3 MEDICINAL USE

Mushrooms and some plants have been used in indigenous traditional medicine since the beginning of civilizations. Mushroom species used are different among locations and cultures; nevertheless, in Asia, especially China and Japan more species have been used than in Europe and America cultures.[33]

The Greek, father of medicine Hippocrates around 450 BCE described that some fungi were useful to cure diseases, like the species *F. fomentarius* or "amadou" as an excellent anti-inflammatory and also for cauterizing wounds and alleviating chronic problems associated with the kidneys.[34] In China, the "chaga" fungus (*Inonotus obliquus*; Image 3.13) played a fundamental role in medicine, considered the elixir of life for 7000 years at least and it has been used also in Siberia and North America for centuries for the same purposes.[28]

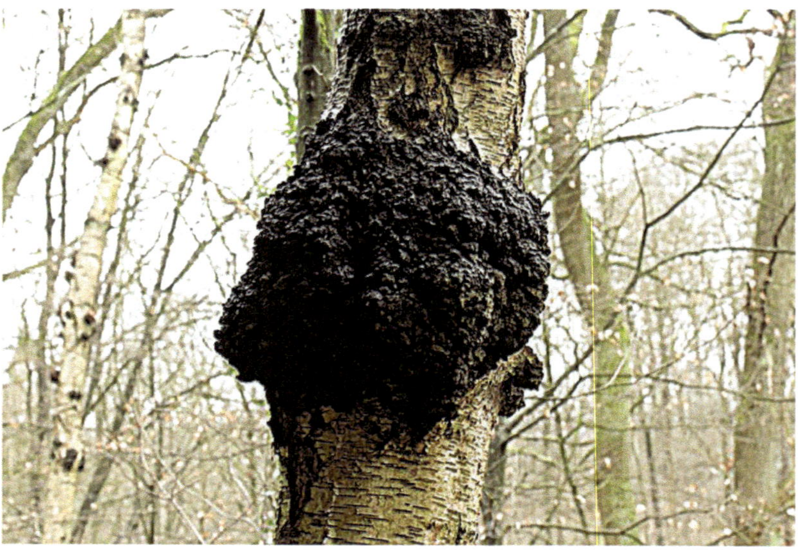

IMAGE 3.13 "Chaga" fungus (*Inonotus obliquus*).

Source: Björn S... https://commons.wikimedia.org/wiki/File:Chaga_Mushroom_Inonotus_obliquus_(40358524662).jpg https://creativecommons.org/licenses/by-sa/2.0/deed.en

Chinese emperors once decreed that "reishi" mushrooms be handed over to them. The Emperor Ti ordered his fleet of boats to set sail in search of this mushroom species of *Ganoderma lucidum sensu lato* (Image 3.14) by the seas of East China due to the fact that this species is considered the fungus of immortality since it is attributed medicinal properties such as improving memory, relaxing, strengthening the heart, lungs, and liver among others. In the *Pen Ts'ao* document 16 species of medicinal mushrooms are described, among those standout *G. lucidum* and *Grifola frondosa* for their antidiabetic properties.[35]

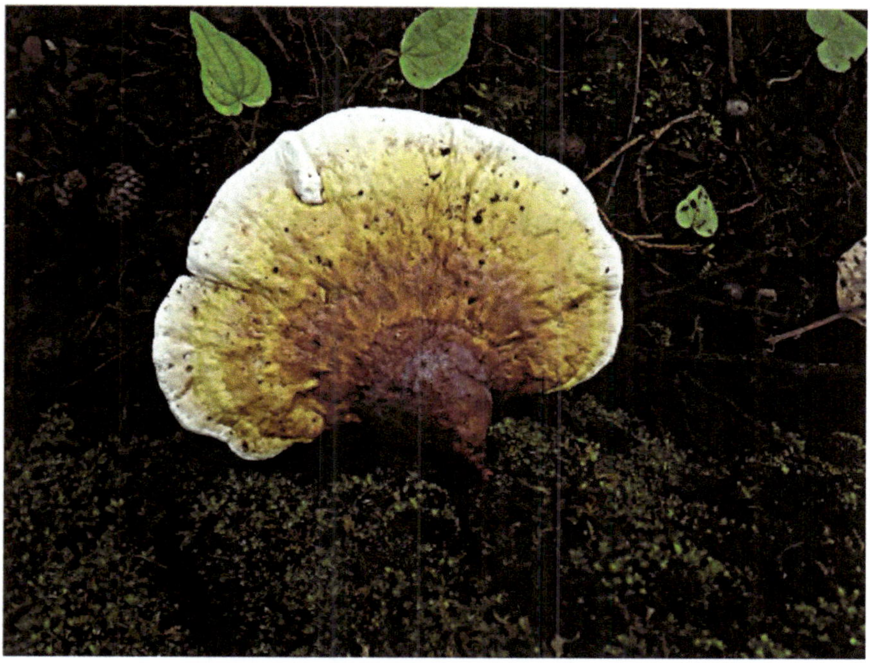

IMAGE 3.14 "Reishi" *Ganoderma lucidum sensu lato.*

Source: Mariano Torres-Gómez.

Chinese have for millennia used, described and valued many species, some for food, some for ceremonial, and others also healing properties. These traditions are as strong today as they were centuries ago due the biocultural importance of this relationship between mushrooms and people, and nowadays China is the leading exporter of cultivated edible and medicinal mushrooms.[34]

Native American traditions also have different mushrooms species used for several purposes, like curing several diseases, like smallpox introduced with the discovery of America by Europeans. Curiously most of them are the same species used or their taxonomical similars (American, Asian or European) like "Agarikon" (*Fomitopsis officinalis*), "Birch polypore" (*F. betulina*), "Chaga" (*I. obliquus*), "Reishi" (*Ganoderma* spp.) and "Turkey tail" (*Trametes versicolor*).[36] Indigenous people discovered that some mushrooms (principally polypores) are exceptionally effective at preventing and curing infections. Whether or not our ancestors understood that many diseases were caused by microbes, humans have traditionally viewed some mushrooms species as powerful medicines for centuries and share in common the practice by doctors today.[1] Countries such as Mexico, Turkey, India, and Africa also have a ancient tradition of using wild edible and medicinal fungi.

In Chignahuapan, Puebla, Mexico there is a church that was dedicated to the cult of a mushroom, unique in its type, it holds a small petrified polypore fungus (*Ganoderma lobatum*), which is revered by the locals. Legend says that in 1880, a peasant found the image of Christ crucified with a sun and a moon in the underside of the mushroom (in the pores), so in that place the church of "Our Lord of the mushroom" was built; after a few years it was renamed to "The Lord of Health," which was later changed again to "Our Lady of the Sacred Heart of Jesus." According to Ramón Kuri Camacho, there are two important aspects in the founding of this temple and its veneration: One is the mystical tradition of the use of mushrooms by the locals, and second, the evangelization strategies of the Mercedarian friars.[37] It is worth mentioning that this mushroom revered is a lignin polypore that grows on oak wood (*Quercus* sp.) and is distinguished by its reddish-brown color and has medicinal properties not psychoactive. Today there are still few indigenous people who when visit the temple go directly to the place where the mushroom is (aside of the altar) to perform proper prayers.[37]

The actual beginning of scientific research on medicinal mushrooms was in the 1950 decade, after the gathering of information thanks to ethnomycology studies. It started mostly for treating cancer, then antiviral studies increased dramatically in the 1980s, since AIDS epidemic. Scientific reports on medicinal mushrooms come mainly from China, Japan, Germany, the United States, and Europe.[1] Medicinal fungi metabolites and active compounds include some antibiotics, others with anticancer properties, cholesterol inhibitors, to name a few.[33]

3.4 MUSHROOMS AS ANTIDIABETIC

Today, modern medicine and scientific research are investigating the evidence with this long history of fungi use and knowledge, trying to determine and corroborate the effects of this compounds to human health. Mycologists and others are looking and focusing on the potential uses using formal and scientific studies to confirm the clinical applications on human health.[1]

Approximately 95,000 species of fungi have been described in the world, of those 22,000 are macroscopic where the most of species used by mankind are. Worldwide fungal diversity estimations go from 1,500,000 to 5,000,000,[38,39] these differences are basically due to differences between northern and tropic diversity; but some other experts estimate a greater number, they estimate 13,500,000 species if entomopathogenic fungi (fungi that infects or parasites insects, like *Cordyceps*) are included (Fig. 3.1).[40,41]

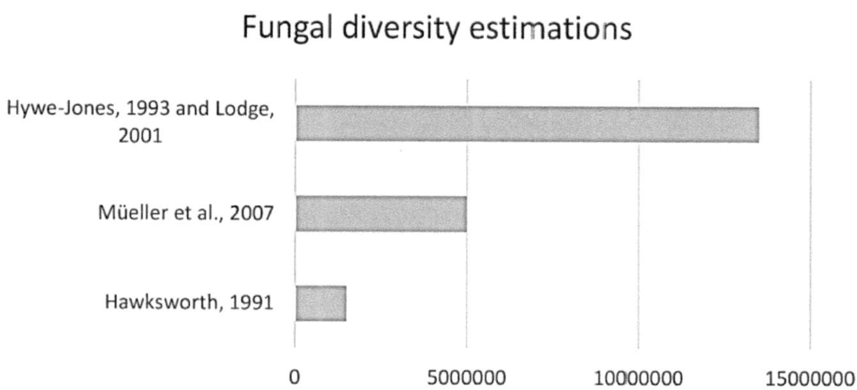

	Hawksworth, 1991	Müeller et al., 2007	Hywe-Jones, 1993 and Lodge, 2001
Species estimated	1500000	5000000	13500000

FIGURE 3.1 Worldwide fungal diversity estimations.

Humans have described and used about 850 medicinal mushroom species worldwide, but only a small portion of these species has ever been formally and scientifically tested. Even the total number of fungal species is unknown (Fig. 3.2) and most are still undiscovered.[38] Some scientists estimate it might take us about 4000 years until we understand the whole of mushroom medicinal properties. Moreover, mushrooms have been proved some abilities of reducing some illness associated by obesity and aging.[76]

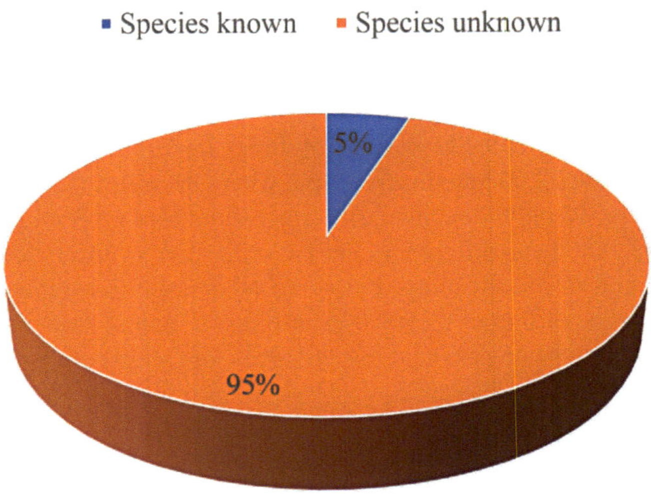

FIGURE 3.2 Percentage of fungal species known *vs* the estimated unknown worldwide.

For millennia, mushrooms were valued by mankind as edible and medicinal with properties like anti-inflammatory, analgesic, blood coagulating, sugar reducing, and wound healing resources.[1] Most of the traditional knowledge about medicinal properties of mushrooms comes from the east and have long been recognized in China, Korea, Japan, and Africa, as well as in central and north America. Several cultures, especially in Mexico, used psychoactive mushrooms like *Amanita* and *Psilocybe* species in ancient religious and medical practices.[77] Modern western countries recently began to consider the enormous potential of medicinal mushrooms. Some mushroom species are capable to decrease high glucose and lipid levels in blood and are recommended as neurotonics, vasotonics, hepatoprotectives, and thrombolytic agents. Many of the polysaccharides, terpenes, and steroids found in mushrooms are active compounds effective in fighting infections, expiratory problems, heart problems, AIDS, and diabetes.[78]

Diabetes mellitus is a chronic disease/metabolic disorder that happens when insulin is not produced or not enough, this illness affects millions of individuals worldwide, and when it is not treated properly, it can lead to organ failure and death.[79] A study in 2014 found that around 8.5% of 18 years and older in world's population have diabetes, and by 2016, this disease was the cause of 1.6 million deaths. There were 108 million people with diabetes in 1980 and increased to 422 million by 2014, that's like four times in only 30 years.[80] Now we know that American Indians and Alaskan Natives are more than two times more likely to have diabetes as white people,[83,91] while New Zealand people have about three times higher probability of have diabetes, and their mortality rates in the 40–65 age group are close than ten times higher than for people in Europe. Australian aboriginal people experience four times higher this illness than general population.[76,92] At this rate the number of diabetic people worldwide will double in the next years.[80] Now we know that diabetes has been rising more rapidly in developing countries than in developed countries. Data shows the danger that indigenous people have because most of ethnic groups worldwide reside in developing countries, their mycological (among others) traditional knowledge is higher than the rest of developed countries, nevertheless they are more prone to be diabetic or related illness. This illness can lead to loss of sight, heart attacks, kidney failure, strokes, and even limb amputation,[80] and worst, the problem generally remain undiagnosed for years without notorious symptoms and this can end up with untreatable complications or even death. Evidence shows that diabetes can be prevented by following a healthy lifestyle which includes a healthy diet and frequent exercise.[34] There are many synthetic medicine available for controlling diabetes, but usually their long-term use can lead to other side effects. That's why today research has turned toward natural compounds found in plants and mushrooms, and so far these compounds are considered to be comparatively safe.[81] It does not matter where the communities are located, their traditions and culture, the increasing diabetes rate among indigenous people, is caused mostly by unhealthy diets, scarce or null physical activity, tobacco use, among others,[90] and its speculated that these reasons are related to decreasing ethnomycological knowledge worldwide.[43,107] Therefore, effective health programs and early diagnosis around the world are fundamental to reducing or preventing the risk to suffer diabetes or related complications.

Plants and fungi are the main sources of natural compounds used for medicine, that's one of the reason that nowadays we can observe the increasing interest of bioactive metabolites found in fungi.[93] Scientific corroboration of traditional knowledge can hold enough evidence of positive effects of consuming wild edible mushrooms on human health. Today we have identified a wide variety of bioactive compounds isolated from many species of mushrooms, wild and cultivated, that can help humanity to reduce and control diabetes among other illness.[94] Edible mushrooms are becoming one of the most used potential antidiabetic alternative medicine. They hold natural compounds rich in fibers, polysaccharides, phenolics, and alkaloids, known for antidiabetic effects.[34,71] In numerous communities from China, India, Japan, Korea, and Mexico mushrooms have been used as health boosters in traditional medicine to alleviate many illness and diseases.[34,36,60,70,73,82,83]

Healthy diets can incorporate many mushrooms species as supplemental foods for diabetes patients and similar illness[84] along with regular physical activity and avoiding tobacco to prevent diabetes.[81,82] Many edible and medicinal mushrooms appear to be effective for controlling glucose levels in the bloodstream. Several examples of medicinal mushrooms species with antidiabetic properties are described in specialized literature worldwide,[85] such as some button mushrooms species like *Agaricus bisporus*, *A. subrufescens*, or Hitler's ink mushroom *Coprinus comatus*, many bracket species as *G. lucidum*, *I. obliquus*, or insect parasites like *Ophiocordyceps sinensis*, the velvety *Phellinus linteus*, several species of *Pleurotus*, the cauliflower mushroom *Sparassis crispa* and *Wolfiporia cocos* (to mention a few) have been reported to be used for diabetes issues.[49–73] Although these mushrooms have been used by several cultures since ancient times, only recently has modern science rediscovered that mushrooms can be powerful medicines for several human illnesses like diabetes.[33]

For example, possibly the most iconic and popular medicinal mushrooms in the world, the bracket fungus called lingzhi or reishi (in China and Japan, respectively) has a long history of use in Asia, along with shiitake mushroom (*Lentinula edodes*), both principally used for their medicinal properties. These *Ganoderma* species are mentioned in a poem from the Han dynasty that is at least 2000 years old, and it is described as the mushroom of Immortality,[101] this species is believed to have a wide range of properties and is used in several cultures around the world to treat different types of cancer, stress, some seizures, virus, cardiovascular problems, and also diabetes.[86] Nowadays we know that *G. lucidum* has at least 200,000 compounds of which 400 are active constituents.[33] Some molecules identified and isolated from lion's mane mushroom (*Hericium erinaceus*) (Image 3.15) have become associated with neurological health and growth, which attracts attention of older people populations for the compounds that eventually can control, prevent or even cure Alzheimer's disease.[101] It has been tested and supported that active compounds stimulate nerve and neuron growth in some experiments with rats and human cultured nerve cells.[102] These compounds and effects are now summited additional experiments and analysis.[101]

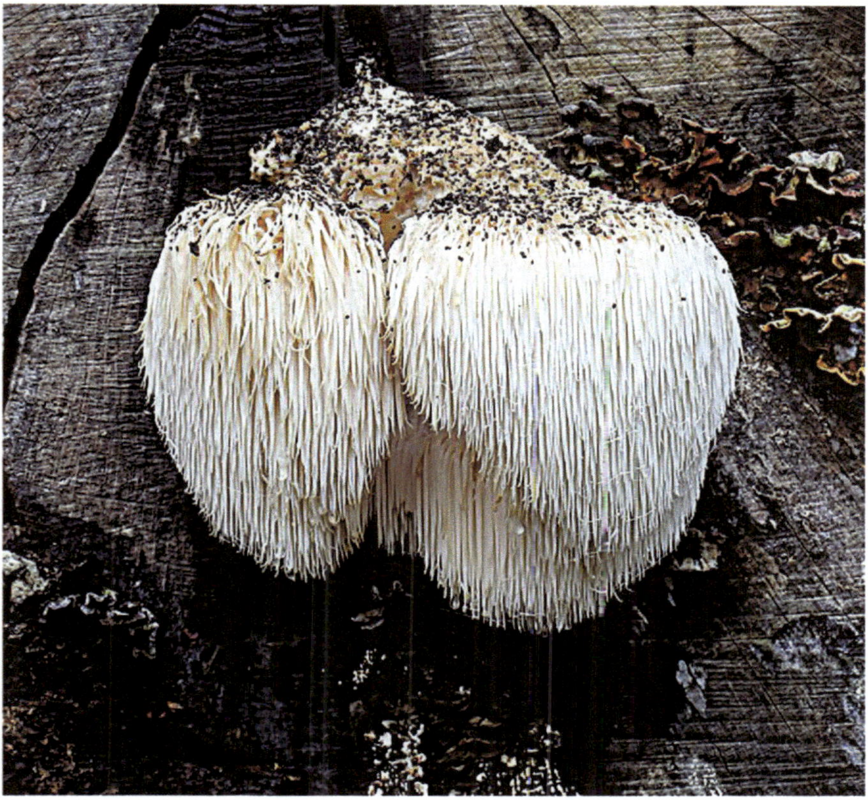

IMAGE 3.15 *Hericium erinaceus* (Bull.) Pers. the Lion's mane mushroom.

Source: gailhampshire. https://commons.wikimedia.org/wiki/File:Lion%27s_Mane_Fungi._Hericium_erinaceus.jpg https://creativecommons.org/licenses/by/2.0/deed.en

Today, there are 370 million indigenous people around the world across at least 90 countries, belonging to more than 5000 different ethnic groups and speaking more than 4000 languages. They represent about 5% of the world's population.[103] Most of these ethnic groups have traditionally used an incredible number of forest products, goods, and services, among those are several mushrooms' species. Some used for food and for economic income by selling them in local markets,[104] for medicine, toxins ,and psychoactive properties[106] and some other uses like firestarter[18] and for playing and toying like *Cookeina sulcipes* and *Cookeina tricholoma* species in south Mexico.[105] In these processes cultures factually and empirically learned the edibility, toxicity, and an amazing range of medicinal properties of thousands of mushrooms species, some of them specifically for treating diabetes.[34] Here we present a list of several mushrooms' species used traditionally around the world by different cultures and people to treat diabetes and also the ones that have been tested in scientific/clinical research/studies (Table 3.1).

TABLE 3.1 Mushroom species with Antidiabetic properties traditionally used worldwide.[35,44–75,94–100]

Species	Used in (reported)
Agaricus bisporus (J.E. Lange) Imbach	America, Asia, Europe*
Agaricus blazei Murrill	America, Asia, Europe*
Agaricus campestris L.	Africa, America, Asia, Europe, Oceania*
Agaricus subrufescens Peck	Africa, America, Asia, Europe, Oceania*
Agaricus sylvaticus Schaeff	Africa, America, Europe*
Amanita tullossii Guzmán & Ram.-Guill.	America
Armillaria aff. gallica Marxm. & Romagn.	America, Asia, Europe
Auricularia auricula-judae (Bull.) Quél.	Africa, America, Asia, Europe, Oceania*
Boletus aff. luridiformis var. *discolor* (Quél.) Krieglst	America, Europe
Boletus edulis Bull. s.l.	America, Asia, Europe
Boletus reticulatus Schaeff.	America, Europe
Catathelasma sp.	America
Cerrena unicolor (Bull.) Murrill	America, Asia, Europe*
Coprinus comatus (O.F. Müll.) Pers.	Africa, America, Europe, Oceania*
Cordyceps militaris (L.) Fr.	Asia, Europe*
Crepidotus parvulus Murrill	America
Daldinia fissa Loyd	America, Europe
Fomitopsis officinalis (Vill.) Bondartsev & Singer	America, Asia, Europe
Fulvifomes merrillii (Murrill) Baltazar & Gibertoni	Asia*
Ganoderma lucidum s.l. (Curtis) P. Karst.	America, Asia, Europe*

TABLE 3.1 *(Continued)*

Species	Used in (reported)
Grifola frondosa (Dicks.) Gray	America, Asia, Europe*
Gyroporus castaneus (Bull.) Quél.	America, Asia, Europe, Oceania
Hericium erinaceus (Bull.) Pers.	Asia, Europe*
Hypomyces lactifluorum (Schwein.) Tul.	America
Hypomyces luteovirens (Fr.) Tul.	America
Hypsizygus marmoreus (Peck) H.E. Bigelow	Asia, Europe*
Infundibulicybe gibba (Pers.) Harmaja	America, Asia, Europe
Inonotus baumii (Pilát) T. Wagner & M. Fisch.	Africa*
Lactarius deliciosus (L.) Gray	America, Europe, Oceania
Lactarius indigo (Schwein.) Fr.	America, Asia, Europe
Laetiporus sulphureus var. *miniatus* (P. Karst.) Imazeki	America, Europe*
Leccinum rugocipes (Peck) Singer.	America, Asia
Lentinula edodes (Berk.) Pegler	Asia*
Lentinus strigosus Fr.	America*
Lepista nuda (Bull.) Cooke	America, Europe, Oceania
Lycoperdon peckii Morgan	America
Lycoperdon perlatum Pers.	Africa, America, Asia, Europe, Oceania
Lycoperdon pusillum Fr.	America
Lyophyllum decastes (Fr.) Singer	America
Lyophyllum shimeji (Kawam.) Hongo	Asia, Europe
Morchella conica Pers.	Africa, America, Europe*
Ophiocordyceps sinensis (Berk.) G.H. Sung, J.M. Sung, Hywel-Jones & Spatafora	Asia*
Phellinus linteus (Berk. & M.A. Curtis)	Africa, Asia
Phylloporia ribis (Schumach.) Ryvarden	Asia*
Pleurotus cornucopiae (Paulet) Rolland	America, Asia, Europe*
Pleurotus eryngii (DC.) Quél.	Asia, Europe*
Pleurotus floridanus Singer	Africa, Asia, Oceania*
Pleurotus pulmonarius (Fr.) Quél.	America, Asia, Europe*
Polyporus umbellatus (Pers.) Fr.	America, Asia, Europe
Ramaria spp.	America
Russula brevipes Peck	America, Europe
Sparassis crispa (Wulfen) Fr.	America, Europe*
Sanghuangporus baumii (Pilát) L.W. Zhou & Y.C. Dai	Asia*

TABLE 3.1 *(Continued)*

Species	Used in (reported)
Taiwanofungus camphoratus (M. Zang & C.H. Su) Sheng H. Wu, Z.H. Yu, Y.C. Dai & C.H. Su	America, Asia*
Tremella aurantia Schwein.	America
Tremella fuciformis Berk.	America, Asia, Oceania*
Tremella mesenterica Schumach.	Africa, America, Asia, Europe, Oceania*
Tuber indicum Cooke & Massee	Europe
Ustilago maydis (DC.) Corda	America
Wolfiporia cocos (F.A. Wolf) Ryvarden & Gilb.	Asia*
Wolfiporia extensa (Peck) Ginns	Asia*

**Species been summited for clinical studies.*

3.5 CONCLUSIONS

Mushrooms have been fundamental for the planet and for humanity in many ways. Our ancestors found out incredible opportunities by making them part of their diet, cosmovision, religions, tales, cults, and folklore; then in modern time, science brought them into industry and medicine. Many clinically medicine have been isolated directly or indirectly from plants and fungi. In the last 20 years, the recognition of mushrooms in human immune system for maintaining good health has been significantly increased do research studies results. Mushrooms contain many molecules and compounds that can be incredibly useful in controlling, treating, preventing, and curing several human illnesses. Diseases such as diabetes (among many others) are increasingly affecting people worldwide, especially indigenous communities, and therefore being given special attention from medical researchers and clinicians alike. But also, had generated a global appetite for herbal and fungal medicines in the pursuit of better-quality life.

It's imperative to protect the biocultural heritage of ethnic groups around the world, to keep investigating the relationship of different cultures with mushrooms and other organisms. The list of functional mushrooms used, and its purposes needs to be increased continually in each continent, in each ethnic group. Nevertheless, we also must use modern science and medicine to put them to the test with formal investigation, with the only goal of finding and generating new effective medicine that could help mankind fight against many terrible diseases like diabetes. Clearly, mushrooms hold compounds worthy of medical investigations and wide open for scientific exploration.

KEYWORDS

- **mushroom traditional use**
- **ethnomycological knowledge**
- **diabetes mellitus**
- **ethnic groups**

REFERENCES

1. Stamets, P. *Mycomedicinals. An Informational Treatise on Mushrooms*; Colorcraft Ltd.: Hong Kong, 2002; p 96. ISBN: 096379719-0.
2. Moreno-Fuentes, A. Un recurso alimentario de los grupos originarios y mestizos de México: los hongos silvestres. *Anal. Antropol.* **2014,** *48* (1), 241–272. https://doi.org/10.1016/S0185-1225(14)70496-5
3. Weyrich, L.; Duchene, S.; Soubrier, J.; Arriola, L.; Llamas, B.; Breen, J.; Morris, A. G.; Alt, K. W.; Caramelli, D.; Dresely, V.; Farrell, M.; Farrer, A. G.; Francken, M.; Gully, N.; Haak, W.; Hardy, K.; Harvati, K.; Held, P.; Holmes, E. C.; Kaidonis, J.; Lalueza-Fox, C.; de la Rasilla, M.; Rosas, A.; Semal, P.; Soltysiak, A.; Townsend, G.; Usai, D.; Wahl, J.; Huson, D. H.; Dobney, K.; Cooper, A. Neanderthal Behavior, Diet, and Disease Inferred from Ancient DNA in Dental Calculus. *Nature* **2017,** *544* (7650), 357–361. doi: 10.1038/nature21674. PMID: 28273061.
4. Smith, S. E.; Read, D. J. *Mycorrhizal Symbiosis*; Academic Press: Amsterdam, 2008; 787 p. ISBN 978-0-12-370526-6. https://doi.org/10.1016/B978-0-12-370526-6.X5001-6
5. Brundrett, M. C. Coevolution of Roots and Mycorrhizas of Land Plants. *New Phytol.* **2002**. https://doi.org/10.1046/j.1469-8137.2002.00397.x
6. Brundrett, M. C. Mycorrhizal Associations and Other Means of Nutrition of Vascular Plants: Understanding the Global Diversity of Host Plants by Resolving Conflicting Information and Developing Reliable Means of Diagnosis. *Plant Soil* **2009,** *320* (1–2), 37–77. https://doi.org/10.1007/s11104-008-9877-9
7. Molina, R.; Massicotte, H.; Trappe, J. M. Specificity Phenomena in Mycorrhizal Symbiosis: Community-Ecological Consequences and Practical Implications. In *Mycorrhizal Functioning. An Integrative Plant-Fungal Process*; Allen, M., Ed.; Chapman and Hall: New York, 1992; pp 357–423.

8. Komonen, A.; Ikävalko, J.; Weiying, W. Diversity Patterns of Fungivorous Insects: Comparison between Glaciated vs. Refugial Boreal Forests. *J. Biogeogr.* **2003,** *30* (12), 1873–1881. http://www.jstor.org/stable/3554639
9. Pérez-Moreno, J.; Guerin-Laguette, A.; Arzú, R. F.; Yu, F. Mushrooms, Humans and Nature in a Changing World: Perspectives from Ecological, Agricultural and Social Sciences. *Mushrooms, Humans and Nature in a Changing World*, 2020. doi: 10.1007/978-3-030-37378-8. ISBN: 978-3-030-37377-1.
10. Stamets, P. Notes on Nutritional Properties of Culinary-Medicinal Mushrooms. *Int. J. Med. Mushrooms* **2005,** *7*, 109–116. doi: 10.1615/IntJMedMushr.v7.i12.100.
11. Quirke, V. M. History of Penicillin. *Encyclopedia of Life Sciences*, 2001. https://doi.org/10.1038/npg.els.0003626
12. Winkler, D. Yartsa Gunbu (*Cordyceps sinensis*) and the Fungal Commodification of Tibet's Rural Economy. *Econ. Bot.* **2008,** *62* (3), 291–305. https://doi.org/10.1007/s12231-008-9038-3
13. Agrios, G. Plant Diseases Caused by Fungi. *Plant Pathol.* **2005**. doi: 10.1016/B978-0-08-047378-9.50017-8.
14. Englund, R. Grain Accounting Practices in Archaic Mesopotamia. In *Changing Views on Ancient Near Eastern Mathematics. BBVO 19*; Høyrup, J., Damerow, P., Eds.; Reimer Verlag: Berlin, 2001; pp 1–36.
15. Damerow, P. Sumerian Beer: The Origins of Brewing Technology in Ancient Mesopotamia. *Cuneiform Digital Library Initiative*, 2012. ID: 16699235.
16. Ruck, C. A. P.; Hoffman, M. A.; González, J. A. *Mushrooms, Myth & Mithras: The Drug Cult That Civilized Europe*; City Lights: San Francisco, 2011. ISBN-10 0872864707. ISBN-13 9780872864702.
17. Lajoux, J. D. *Merveilles du Tassili n'Ajjer*; Thames and Hudson: London, 1963; p 6. ASIN: B000I9PZLM.
18. Peintner, U.; Pöder, R.; Pümpel, T. The Iceman's Fungi. *Mycol. Res.* **1998,** *102* (10), 1153–1162. https://doi.org/10.1017/S0953756298006546
19. Schultes, R. E.; Hofmann, A. *Plants of the Gods: Origins of Hallucinogenic Use*; McGraw-Hill: New York, 1979.
20. Kuo, M. *100 Edible Mushrooms*; University of Michigan Press: Ann Arbor, 2007. doi: 10.3998/mpub.157982.
21. McKenna, T. K. *Food of the Gods: The Search for the Original Tree of Knowledge: A Radical History of Plants, Drugs, and Human Evolution.* Bantam Books: New York, 1992. ISBN-10: 0553371304 ISBN-13: 978-0553371307.
22. Moreno-Fuentes, A. Estudio etnomicológico comparativo entre comunidades rarámuris de la Alta Tarahumara, en el estado de Chihuahua. *Tesis de Doctorado. Facultad de Ciencias*, Universidad Nacional Autónoma de México, México, D.F., 2002.
23. Ruán-Soto, F. Micofilia y micofobia: revisión de los conceptos, su reinterpretación e indicadores para su evaluación. In *La etnomicología en México. Estado del Arte*; Moreno-Fuentes, A., Garibay-Orijel, R., Eds.; Red de Etnoecología y Patrimonio Biocultural (CONACyT), Universidad Autónoma del Estado de Hidalgo, Instituto de Biología (UNAM), Sociedad Mexicana de Micología, Asociación Etnobiológica Mexicana, AC Grupo Interdisciplinario para el Desarrollo de la Etnomicología

en México, Sociedad Latinoamericana de Etnobiología: México, 2014. ISBN: 9786074823691.

24. González, J. A. Hombres, dioses y hongos. *EDAF ENSAYO*, 2002. ISBN: 9788441410459.
25. Stamets, P. *Mycelium Running: How Mushrooms Can Help Save the World*; Ten Speed Press: Berkeley, CA, 2005. ISBN-10: 1580085792ISBN-13: 978-1580085793.
26. Irvin, J. R.; Herer, J. *The Holy Mushroom: Evidence of Mushrooms in Judeo-Christianity*. Place of Publication Not Identified: Gnostic Media Research & Pub, 2008. doi: 10.1111/j.1556-3537.2010.01023.x.
27. Atkinson, T. Sacred Mushroom/Holy Grail: The Long-lost Origin of Our Most Intriguing Legend. Jorvik Press, Portland, OR, 2013. ISBN: 9780988412248.
28. Halpern, G. *Healing Mushrooms*; Square One Publishers, Inc.: Garden City, NY, 2007. ISBN 0757001963, 9780757001963.
29. Guzmán, G. La micología en México. Una Reseña de Sus Tradiciones, Inicios y Avances. *Rev. Mex. Micol.* **1990,** *6*, 11–28. https://doi.org/10.33885/sf.1990.3.756
30. Aguilar, M. Etnomedicina en Mesoamérica. *Arqueol. Mex.* VIII, **2003,** *59*, 26–37. http://raices.com.mx/tienda/revistas-alucinogenos-prehispanicos-AM059
31. Heim, R.; Wasson, R. G. Les champignons hallúcinogenes du Mexique. *Arch. Museo Nac. Hist. Nat. París* **1958,** *7*, 100–122.
32. Guzmán, G. Los hongos en México. *Supl. Mens. Ecol.* **1999,** *6*, 79–85.
33. Stamets, P. E.; Zwickey, H. Medicinal Mushrooms: Ancient Remedies Meet Modern Science. *Integr. Med.* **2014,** *13* (1), 46–47. PMCID: PMC4684114. PMID: 26770081.
34. Hobbs, C. *Medicinal Mushrooms: An Exploration of Tradition, Healing, and Culture*; Botanica Press: New Zealand, 2002; p 251. ISBN: 1570671435, 9781570671432.
35. Bautista-González J.; Moreno-Fuentes, A. Los Hongos Medicinales en México. En *La Etnomicología en México*; Moreno-Fuentes, A., Garibay-Orijel, R., Eds.; Estado del Arte. Red de Etnoecología y Patrimonio Biocultural (CONACYT), Universidad Autónoma del Estado de Hidalgo, Instituto de Biología UNAM, Sociedad Mexicana de Micología, Asociación Etnobiológica Mexicana A.C., Grupo Interdisciplinario para el Desarrollo de la Etnomicología en México, Sociedad Latinoamericana de Etnobiología: México, D.F., 2014; pp 145–176. ISBN: 9786074823691.
36. Hobbs, C. *Kombucha: Tea Mushroom: The Essential Guide*; Botanical Press: New Zealand, 1995. ISBN-10: 188436005X, ISBN-13: 978-1884360053.
37. Guzmán, G.; Wasson, R. G.; Herrera, T. Una iglesia dedicada al culto de un hongo, Nuestro Señor del honguito en Chignahuapan, Puebla. *Bol Sociedad Mex. Micol.* **1975,** *9*, 137–147.
38. Hawksworth, D. L. The Fungal Dimension of Biodiversity: Magnitude, Significance, and Conservation. *Mycol. Res.* **1991,** *95*, 641–655. https://doi.org/10.1016/S0953-7562(09)80810-1
39. Mueller, G. M.; Schmit, J. P. Fungal Biodiversity: What Do We Know? What Can We Predict? *Biodivers. Conserv.* **2007,** *16*, 1–5. https://doi.org/10.1007/s10531-006-9117-7
40. Hywel-Jones, N. L. *Torrubiella luteorostrata* a Pathogen of Scale Insects and Its Association with *Paecilomyces cinnamomeus* with a Note on *Torrubiella tenuis*. *Mycol. Res.* **1993**, *97*, 1126–1130. https://doi.org/10.1016/S0953-7562(09)80514-5

41. Lodge, D. J. Implications for Nitrogen Additions from Air Pollutants on Litter Decay Fungi and Ecosystem Processes. *Mycol. Res.* **2001,** *105*, 898–899.
42. Moreno-Fuentes, A.; Garibay-Orijel. R. La etnomicología en México. Una introducción al estado del arte. In *La etnomicología en México. Estado del Arte*; Moreno-Fuentes, A.; Garibay-Orijel, R., Eds.; Red de Etnoecología y Patrimonio Biocultural (CONACyT), Universidad Autónoma del Estado de Hidalgo, Instituto de Biología (UNAM), Sociedad Mexicana de Micología, Asociación Etnobiológica Mexicana, AC-Grupo Interdisciplinario para el Desarrollo de la Etnomicología en México, Sociedad Latinoamericana de Etnobiología: México, 2014; pp 3–14. ISBN: 9786074823691.
43. Moreno-Fuentes, A.; Garibay-Orijel, R.; Tovar, V.; Cifuentes, J. Situación Actual de la Etnomicología en México y el en el Mundo. *Etnobiología* **2001,** *1*, 75–84. ISSN: 1665-2703.
44. Bautista-González, J. A. Conocimiento tradicional de hongos medicinales en seis localidades diferentes del país. *Tesis de licenciatura, Facultad de Ciencias*; UNAM: Mexico, 2013.
45. Guzmán, G. Diversity and Use of Traditional Mexican Fungi. A Review. *Int. J. Med. Mushrooms* **2008,** *10*, 209–217. doi: 10.1615/IntJMedMushr.v10.i3.20.
46. Martínez-Alfaro, M. A.; Pérez-Silva, E.; Aguirre-Acosta, E. Etnomicología y exploraciones micológicas en la Sierra Norte de puebla. *Bol. Soc. Mex. Mic.* **1983,** *18*, 51–63. ISSN: 0085-6223.
47. Lampman, A. M. Ethnomycology: Medicinal and Edible Mushrooms of Tzeltal Maya of Chiapas, Mexico. *Int. J. Med. Mushrooms* **2007,** *9*, 1–5. doi: 10.1615/IntJMedMushr.v9.i1.10.
48. Estrada-Torres, E.; Aroche, R. M. Acervo etnomicológico en tres localidades del municipio de Acambay, estado de México. *Rev. Mex. Mic.* **1987,** *3*, 109–131. ISSN: 0187-3180.
49. Zolla, C.; Argueta, A. *Biblioteca Digital de la Medicina Tradicional Mexicana*; UNAM, 2009. http://www.medicinatradicionalmexicana.unam.mx/
50. Jeong, S. C.; Jeong, Y. T.; Yang, B. K.; Islam, R.; Koyyalamudi, S. R.; Pang, G.; Cho, K. Y.; Song, C. H. White button mushroom (*Agaricus bisporus*) lowers blood glucose and cholesterol levels in diabetic and hypercholesterolemic rats. *Nutr. Res.* **2010,** *30*, 49–56. doi: 10.1016/j.nutres.2009.12.003.
51. Kim, Y. W.; Kim, K. H.; Choi, H. J.; Lee, D. S. Anti-diabetic Activity of Beta-glucans and Their Enzymatically Hydrolyzed Oligosaccharides from *Agaricus blazei*. *Biotechnol. Lett.* **2005,** *27*, 483–487. doi: 10.1007/s10529-005-2225-8.
52. Orsine, J. V. C.; Novaes, M. R. C. G.; Asquieri, E. R. Nutritional Value of *Agaricus sylvaticus*; Mushroom Grown in Brazil. *Nutr. Hosp.* **2012,** *27* (2), 449–455. doi: 10.1590/S0212-16112012000200015.
53. Kim, S. K.; Hong, U. P.; Kim, J. S.; Kim, C. H.; Lee, K.W.; Choi, S. E.; Park, K. H.; Lee, M. W. Antidiabetic Effect of *Auricularia auricula* Mycelia in Streptozotocin-Induced Diabetic Rats. *Nat. Prod. Sci.* **2007**, *13*, 390–393. 1226-3907 (pISSN)/2288-9027 (eISSN).
54. Yamac, M.; Zeytinoglu, M.; Kanbak, G.; Bayramoglu, G.; Senturk, H. Hypoglycemic Effect of Crude Exopolysaccharides Produced by *Cerrena unicolor*, *Coprinus*

comatus, and *Lenzites betulina* Isolates in Streptozotocin-Induced Diabetic Rats. *Pharm Biol.* **2009,** *47*, 168–174. https://doi.org/10.1080/13880200802436950.

55. Yun, Y. H., Han, S. H.; Lee, S. J.; Ko, S. K.; Lee, C. K.; Ha, N. J.; Kim, K. J. Anti-diabetic Effects of CCCA, CMKSS and Cordycepin from *Cordyceps militaris* and the Immune Responses in Streptozotocin-Induced Diabetic Mice. *Nat. Prod. Sci.* **2003,** *9*, 291–298. 1226-3907 (pISSN)/2288-9027 (eISSN).
56. Hwang, H. S.; Yun, J. W. Hypoglycemic Effect of Polysaccharides Produced by Submerged Mycelial Culture of *Laetiporus sulphureus* on Streptozotocin-induced Diabetic Rats. *Biotechnol. Bioprocess. Eng.* **2010,** *15*, 173–181. https://doi.org/10.1007/s12257-009-0160-6
57. Yamac, M.; Kanbak, G.; Zeytinoglu, M.; Bayramoglu, G.; Senturk, H.; Uyanoglu, M. Hypoglycemic Effect of *Lentinus strigosus* (Schwein.) Fr. Crude Exopolysaccharide in Streptozotocin-induced Diabetic Rats. *J. Med. Food* **2008,** *11*, 513–517. doi: 10.1089/jmf.2007.0551.
58. Hwang, H. J.; Kim, S. W.; Lim, J. M.; Joo, J. H.; Kim, H. O.; Kim, H. M.; Yun, J. W. Hypoglycemic Effect of Crude Exopolysaccharides Produced by a Medicinal Mushroom *Phellinus baumii* in Streptozotocin-induced Diabetic Rats. *Life Sci.* **2005,** *76*, 3069–3080. doi: 10.1016/j.lfs.2004.12.019.
59. Huang, G. J.; Hsieh, W. T.; Chang, H. Y.; Huang, S. S.; Lin, Y. C.; Kuo, Y. H. α-Glucosidase and Aldose Reductase Inhibitory Activities from the Fruiting Body of *Phellinus merrillii*. *J. Agric. Food Chem.* **2011,** *59*, 5702–5706. doi: 10.1021/jf2003943.
60. Lee, I. K.; Lee, J. H.; Yun, B. S. Polychlorinated Compounds with PPAR-gamma Agonistic Effect from the Medicinal Fungus *Phellinus ribis*. *Bioorg. Med. Chem. Lett.* **2008,** *18* (16), 4566–4568. doi: 10.1016/j.bmcl.2008.07.034.
61. Kim, J. I.; Kang, M. J.; Im, J.; Seo, Y. J.; Lee, Y. M.; Song, J. H.; Lee, J. H.; Kim, M. E. Effect of King Oyster Mushroom (*Pleurotus eryngii*) on Insulin Resistance and Dyslipidemia in db/db Mice. *Food Sci. Biotechnol.* **2010,** *19*, 239–242. doi: 10.1007/s10068-010-0033-y.
62. Badole, S. L.; Shah, S. N.; Patel, N. M.; Thakurdesai, P. A.; Bodhankar, S. L. Hypoglycemic Activity of Aqueous Extract of *Pleurotus pulmonarius* in Alloxan-Induced Diabetic Mice. *Pharm. Biol.* **2006,** *44*, 421–425. https://doi.org/10.1080/13880200600794196
63. Kwon, A. H.; Qiu, Z.; Hashimoto, M.; Yamamoto, K.; Kimura, T. Effects of Medicinal Mushroom (*Sparassis crispa*) on Wound Healing in Streptozotocin-induced Diabetic Rats. *Am. J. Surg.* **2008,** *197* (4), 503–509. doi: 10.1016/j.amjsurg.2007.11.021.
64. Kiho, T.; Kochi, M.; Usui, S.; Hirano, K.; Aizawa, K.; Inakuma, T. Antidiabetic Effect of an Acidic Polysaccharide (TAP) from *Tremella aurantia* and Its Degradation Product (TAP-H). *Biol. Pharm. Bull.* **2001,** *24*, 1400–1403. doi: 10.1248/bpb.24.1400.
65. Lo, H. C.; Tsai, F. A.; Wasser, S. P.; Yang, J. G.; Huang, B. M. Effects of Ingested Fruiting Bodies, Submerged Culture Biomass, and Acidic Polysaccharide Glucuronoxylomannan of *Tremella mesenterica* Retz.: Fr. on Glycemic Responses in Normal and Diabetic Rats. *Life Sci.* **2006,** *78* (17), 1957–1966. doi: 10.1016/j.lfs.2005.08.033.
66. Li, N.; Li, L.; Fang, J. C.; Wong, J. H.; Ng, T. B.; Jiang, Y.; Wang, C. R.; Zhang, N. Y.; Wen, T. Y.; Qu, L. Y.; Lv, P. Y.; Zhao, R.; Shi, B.; Wang, Y. P.; Wang, X.

Y.; Liu, F. Isolation and Identification of a Novel Polysaccharide Peptide Complex with Antioxidant, Antiproliferative and Hypoglycaemic Activities from the Abalone Mushroom. *Biosci. Rep.* **2011,** *32* (3), 221–228. doi: 10.1042/BSR20110012.

67. Stojkovic, D.; Smiljkovic, M.; Ciric, A.; Glamoclija, J.; Van Griensven, L.; Ferreira, I. C. F. R.; Sokovic, M. An Insight into Antidiabetic Properties of Six Medicinal and Edible Mushrooms: Inhibition of α-Amylase and α-Glucosidase Linked to Type-2 Diabetes. *S. Afr. J. Bot.* **2019,** *120*, 100–103, ISSN 0254-6299. https://doi.org/10.1016/j.sajb.2018.01.007
68. Maa, A. Y.; Feuer, W. J.; Davis, C. Q.; Pillow, E. K.; Brown, T. D.; Caywood, R. M.; Chasan, J. E.; Fransen, S. R. A Novel Device for Accurate and Efficient Testing for Vision-threatening Diabetic Retinopathy. *J. Diabetes Compl.* **2016,** *30*, 524–532. doi: 10.1016/j.jdiacomp.2015.12.005.
69. Wu, Q. X.; Mueller, G. M. Biogeographic Relationships between the Macrofungi of Temperate Eastern Asia and Eastern North America. *Can. J. Bot.* **1997,** *75*, 2108–2116. https://doi.org/10.1139/b97-922
70. Chang, S. T.; Mshigeni, K. E. *Ganoderma lucidum*-Paramount among Medicinal Mushrooms. *Discov. Innov.* **2000,** *12*, 97–101. doi: 10.4314/dai.v12i3.15574.
71. Khursheed, R.; Singh, S. K.; Wadhwa, S.; Gulati, M.; Awasthi, A. Therapeutic Potential of Mushrooms in Diabetes Mellitus: Role of Polysaccharides. *Int. J. Biol. Macromol.* **2020,** *164*, 1194–1205. ISSN 0141-8130. https://doi.org/10.1016/j.ijbiomac.2020.07.145
72. Valverde, M. E.; Hernández-Pérez, T.; Paredes-López, O. Edible Mushrooms: Improving Human Health and Promoting Quality Life. *Int. J. Microbiol.* **2015,** 376–387. doi: 10.1155/2015/376387.2015.1–14.
73. Lee, K.; Morris, S. L.; Yang, X.; Huang, R.; Zhou, T.; Wu, S.; Shi, Q.; Itokawa, H. Recent Progress of Research on Medicinal Mushrooms, Foods, and Other Herbal Products Used in Traditional Chinese Medicine. *J. Trad. Complement. Med.* **2012,** *2*, 1–12. https://doi.org/10.1016/S2225-4110(16)30081-5
74. Yang, B. K.; Dong Kim, D. H.; Jeong, S. C.; Das, S.; Choi, Y. S.; Shin, J. S.; Lee, S. C.; Song, C. H. Hypoglycemic Effect of a *Lentinus edodes* Exo-polymer Produced from a Submerged Mycelial Culture. *Biosci., Biotechnol. Biochem.* **2002,** *66* (5), 937–42. https://doi.org/10.1271/bbb.66.937
75. Milani, C.; Ferrario, C.; Turroni, F.; et al. The Human Gut Microbiota and Its Interactive Connections to Diet. *J. Hum. Nutr. Diet.* **2016,** *29*, 539–546. doi: 10.1111/jhn.12371.
76. Paterson, R. R.; Lima, N. Biomedical Effects of Mushrooms with Emphasis on Pure Compounds. *Biomed. J.* **2014,** *37*, 357–368. doi: 10.4103/2319-4170.143502.
77. Pérez-Moreno, J.; Lorenzana-Fernández, A.; Carrasco-Hernández, V.; Yescas-Pérez, A. *Los hongos comestibles silvestres del parque nacional Izta-Popo, Zoquiapan y anexos*. Colegio de Postgraduados, SEMARNAT, CONACyT: Montecillo, Texcoco, Estado de México, 2010; pp 167. ISSN 0187-7380.
78. Lindequist, U. Structure and Biological Activity of Triterpenes, Polysaccharides and Other Constituents of *Ganoderma lucidum*. In *Proceedings of the 6th International Symposium on Recent Advances in Ganoderma lucidum Research*, Kim, B. K., Kim, I. H., Kim, Y. S., Eds.; The Pharmaceutical Society of Korea: Seoul, 1995; pp 61–91.

79. Shobana S.; Sreerama, Y. N.; Malleshi, N. G. Composition and Enzyme Inhibitory Properties of Finger Millet (*Eleusine coracana* L.) Seed Coat Phenolics: Mode of Inhibition of α-Glucosidase and Pancreatic Amylase *Food Chem.* **2009,** *115*, 1268–1273. https://doi.org/10.1016/j.foodchem.2009.01.042
80. WHO (World Health Organization). *Diabetes Program*, 2021. https://www.who.int/news-room/fact-sheets/detail/diabetes
81. Oritz, A. R. R.; Garcia, J. S.; Castillo, E. P.; Ramirez, A. G.; Villalobos, M. R.; Estrada, S. S. Alpha-glucosidase Inhibitory Activity of the Methanolic Extract from *Tournefortia hartwegiana*: An Anti-hyperglycemic Agent. *J. Ethnopharmacol.* **2017,** *109*, 48–53. doi: 10.1016/j.jep.2006.07.002.
82. Halpern, G. M. Medicinal Mushrooms. *Prog. Nutr.* **2010,** *12*, 29–36. ISBN-13: 978-0871319814
83. De Silva, D.; Rapior, S.; Hyde, K. D.; Bahkali, A. H. Medicinal Mushrooms in Prevention and Control of Diabetes Mellitus. *Fung. Divers.* **2012,** *56*, 1–29. doi: 10.1007/s13225-012-0187-4.
84. Ulziijargal, E.; Mau, J. L. Nutrient Compositions of Culinary-Medicinal Mushroom Fruiting Bodies and Mycelia. *Int. J. Med. Mushrooms* **2011,** *13* (4), 343–349. doi: 10.1615/IntJMedMushr.v13.i4.40.
85. Gray, A. M.; Flatt, P. R. Insulin-releasing and Insulin-like Activity of *Agaricus campestris* (Mushroom). *J. Endocrinol.* **1998,** *157*, 259–266. doi: 10.1677/joe.0.1570259.
86. Wachtel-Galor, S.; Yuen, J.; Buswell, J. A.; Benzie, I. F. F. *Ganoderma lucidum* (Lingzhi or Reishi): A Medicinal Mushroom. In: *Herbal Medicine: Biomolecular and Clinical Aspects*, 2nd ed.; Benzie, I. F., Wachtel-Galor, S., Eds.; CRC Press: Boca Raton, FL, 2011; pp 175–199. ISBN-13: 978-1-4398-0713-2.
87. Rojas, C.; Mansur, E. Ecuador: Informaciones Generales Sobre Productos Non Madereros en Ecuador. In *Memoria, Consulta De Expertos Sobre Productos Forestales no Madereros Para America Latina y el Caribe. Serie Forestal 1*, Santiago, FAO, Oficina Regional para America Latina y el Caribe, 1995; pp 208–223.
88. Wasson, V. P.; Wasson, R. G. *Mushrooms, Russia, and History*; Pantheon Books: New York, 1957. https://doi.org/10.2307/4113701
89. Härkönen, M. An Ethnomycological Approach to Tanzanian Species of Amanita. *Acta Univ. Ups. Symb. Bot. Ups.* **1995,** *30*, 145–151. http://hdl.handle.net/123456789/11878
90. Gracey, M.; King, M. Indigenous Health Part 1: Determinants and Disease Patterns. *Lancet* **2009,** *374*, 65–75. doi: 10.1016/S0140-6736(09)60914-4.
91. CDC: *National Diabetes Fact Sheet, United States*, 2003. http://www.cdc.gov/diabetes/pubs/pdf/ndfs_2003.pdf
92. Couzos, S.; Murray, R. Aboriginal Primary Health Care: An Evidence-based Approach. Oxford University Press: Melbourne, 2003 https://doi.org/10.18773/austprescr.2004.006
93. Cragg, G. M.; Newmann, D. J.; Snader, K. M. Natural Products in Drug Discovery and Development. *J. Nat. Prod.* **1997,** *60*, 52–60. https://doi.org/10.1021/np9604893
94. Wong, S. P.; Naidu, M.; David, P.; Bakar, R.; Vikineswary, S. Neurogenerative Potential of Lion's Mane Mushroom, *Hericium erinaceus* (Bull.: Fr.) Pers., (Higher Basidiomycetes), in the Treatment of Peripheral Nerve Injury. *Int. J. Med. Mushrooms* **2012,** *14*, 427–446. doi: 10.1615/intjmedmushr.v14.i5.10.

95. Prabu, M.; Kumuthakalavalli, R. Antioxidant Activity of Oyster Mushroom (*Pleurotus florida* [Mont.] Singer) and Milky Mushroom (*Calocybe indica* P and C). *Int. J. Curr. Pharm. Res.* **2016,** *8* (3), 48–51. ISSN: 0975-7066.
96. Henkel, T.; Aime, W. M.; Chin, M.; Andrew, C. Edible Mushrooms from Guyana. *Mycologist* **2004,** *18* (3), 104–111. https://doi.org/10.1017/S0269915X04003027
97. Mandeel, Q A.; Al-Laith, A. A. A. Ethnomycological Aspects of the Desert Truffle among Native Bahraini and Non-Bahraini Peoples of the Kingdom of Bahrain. *J. Ethnopharmacol.* **2007**, *110* (1), 118–129. https://doi.org/10.1016/j.jep.2006.09.014
98. Paterson, M.; Russell, R. *Ganoderma*—A Therapeutic Fungal Biofactory. *Phytochemistry* **2006,** 1985–2001. https://doi.org/10.1016/j.phytochem.2006.07.004
99. Lee, S. S.; Chang, Y. S.; Noraswati, M. N. R. Utilization of Macrofungi by Some Indigenous Communities for Food and Medicine in Peninsular Malaysia. *For. Ecol. Manage.* **2009**, *257* (10), 2062–2065. https://doi.org/10.1016/j.foreco.2008.09.044
100. Piearce, G. D. Zambian Mushrooms—Customs and Folklore. *Bull. Br. Mycol. Soc.* **1981,** *15* (2), 139–142. https://doi.org/10.1016/s0007-1528(81)80013-2
101. Money, N. P. Are Mushrooms Medicinal? *Fungal Biology*; Elsevier Ltd.: Amsterdam, 2016; pp 1–5. https://doi.org/10.1016/j.funbio.2016.01.006
102. Ma, B. J.; Shen, J. W.; Yu, H. Y.; Ruan, Y.; Wu, T. T.; Zhao, X. Hericenones and Erinacines: Stimulators of Nerve Growth Factor (NGF) Biosynthesis in *Hericium erinaceus. Mycology* **2010**, *1*, 92–98. https://doi.org/10.1080/21501201003735556
103. Kipuri, N. "Kenya." In The *Indigenous World 2007*; Stidsen, S. Ed.; *The Indigenous World. International Work Group for Indigenous Affairs Yearbooks*; Jensen, M. W. (Horn of Africa and East Africa Regional ed.), Ed.; IWGIA, Transaction Publishers: Copenhagen, 2007; pp 468–476. ISBN 978-87-91563-23-2. ISSN 1024-0217. OCLC 30981676.
104. Torres-Gómez, M.; Garibay-Orijel, R.; Casas, A.; Pérez-Salicrup, D. R. Ectomycorrhizal Trees Intermingled within *Cupressus lusitanica* Plantations Sustain the Diversity and Availability of Edible Mushrooms. *Agrofor. Syst.* **2018,** *92* (2), 575–588. doi: 10.1007/s10457-017-0081-x.
105. Ruan-Soto, F.; Cifuentes, J.; Mariaca, R.; Limón, F.; Pérez-Ramírez, L.; Sierra, S. Uso y manejo de hongos silvestres en dos comunidades de la Selva Lacandona, Chiapas, México. *Rev. Mex. Micol.* **2009**, *29*, 61–72. ISSN 0187-3180.
106. Rubel, W.; Arora, D. A Study of Cultural Bias in Field Guide Determinations of Mushroom Edibility Using the Iconic Mushroom, *Amanita muscaria*, as an Example. *Econ. Bot.* **2008**, *62* (3), 223–243. doi: 10.1007/s12231-008-9040-9.
107. Torres-Gómez, M. Conocimiento y uso popular de macromicetos silvestres en la comunidad de Arantepacua, Municipio de Nahuátzen, Michoacán, México. *Tesis de licenciatura*, UMSNH, 2008; p 92.

CHAPTER 4

Bioactive Constituents from Mushrooms for Management of Diabetes: A Scientific Corroboration

VARINDER SINGH[1], SHIVEENA BHATIA[1], AND RICHA SHRI[2*]

[1]*Chitkara College of Pharmacy, Chitkara University, Punjab, India*

[2]*Department of Pharmaceutical Sciences and Drug Research, Punjabi University, Patiala 147002, Punjab, India*

**Corresponding author. E-mail: rshri587@hotmail.com*

ABSTRACT

Mushrooms are popular as food, dietary supplements, traditional medicine, nutraceuticals, and pharmaceuticals. Mushrooms are valued in traditional as well as modern medicine since they show an array of activities in in-vitro, in-vivo as well as clinical studies. One key effect is their antidiabetic activity. Mushrooms are considered as an ideal food for diabetics since they are rich in minerals, vitamins, amino acids, fiber, antioxidants and at the same time are low in fat and sugar content. In traditional systems of medicines, mushrooms have been used for a multitude of health-promoting activities including lowering blood sugar levels. Scientific reports corroborate many health benefits of mushrooms. Studies on mushroom powder, extracts as well as mycoconstituents of many mushrooms like *Agaricus*, *Cordyceps*, *Ganoderma*, *Inonotus*, *Phellinus*, *Pleurotus*, *Morchella*, *Rigidoporus*, *Tremella* species show that these show distinct hypoglycemic and antihyperglycemic activities. Different

Therapeutic Mushrooms for Diabetes Mellitus: Current Evidences and Future Scope. Uzma Azeem, Khalid Rehman Hakeem, (Eds.)

studies highlight the diverse mechanisms by which mushrooms produce antidiabetic effects—these include inhibition of carbohydrate metabolism, enhanced beta-cell activity, increased insulin production, sensitivity and release, and augmented antioxidant defense. This chapter summarizes results on investigations on mushroom constituents. Mushrooms contain a wide range of constituents including high molecular weight components (oligosaccharides, polysaccharides, lipopolysaccharides, glucoproteins, polysaccharide–protein complexes) and low molecular weight metabolites (alkaloids, flavonoids, lectins, phenolic acids, polyphenols, terpenoids). Many of these bioactive constituents have been isolated, characterized and their antidiabetic potential has been evaluated. Some facilitate proper functioning of the liver, pancreas and other endocrinal glands, promote formation of insulin thus ensure robust metabolic functions. For example, the extensively examined—beta-glucans restore the function of pancreas, increase insulin output by β-cells, thereby lowering blood glucose levels. It has also resulted in improved sensitivity of peripheral tissues to insulin. The need of the hour is a detailed study of bioactive mycoconstituents, their isolation, characterization along with toxicity and pharmacological assessment in order to determine their mechanism of action and dose so that these unique mushroom constituents may be developed into reliable antidiabetic nutraceuticals or drugs.

4.1 INTRODUCTION

Mushrooms or macrofungi have been known as the "Food of Gods" and "Elixirs for life" and rightly so! Mushrooms are structurally unique, nutritionally rich, chemically diverse, and biologically immensely valuable. These are beneficial for the environment, for human health, and are economically lucrative (Fig. 4.1). In nature, these help to maintain equilibrium in the ecosystems they exist in. Some of the species of mushrooms live in a symbiotic mycorrhizal relationship with certain plants and trees while some saprophytic mushrooms help in the breakdown of organic waste.[1] Human beings have, since beginning of life, turned to plants and mushrooms for nutrition as well as for curing illnesses. In the contemporary world, mushrooms occupy a position of pride in the culinary and remedial world—these are varied, have distinct flavor and are valued for their nutritive content—amino acids, proteins, vitamins [A, C,

D and B complex vitamins B1 (Thiamine), B2 (Riboflavin), B3 (Niacin), B5 (Pantothenic acid)], fiber, minerals (calcium, phosphorus, iron, copper, chlorine, sodium, zinc, manganese, and bromine) and oligosaccharides.[2,3] These have low or no fat and sugar content; thus are desirable food for diabetics and people suffering from high cholesterol. Mushrooms are considered safe for all age groups. Mushroom teas, extracts, and isolated mycoconstituents are popular as nutraceuticals and health supplements.[4] However, when these are cultivated for food or preparation of nutraceuticals, mushroom farming gives good economic returns to the cultivators. Moreover, the spent mushroom substrate can be used for manure, biofuel, and biogas production.[5,6] Along with the above advantages, mushrooms are displaying good outcomes in bio-remedial programs since these can be used for lignin degradation of agricultural waste. Above all, mushrooms have always fascinated folk and traditional medicine practitioners!

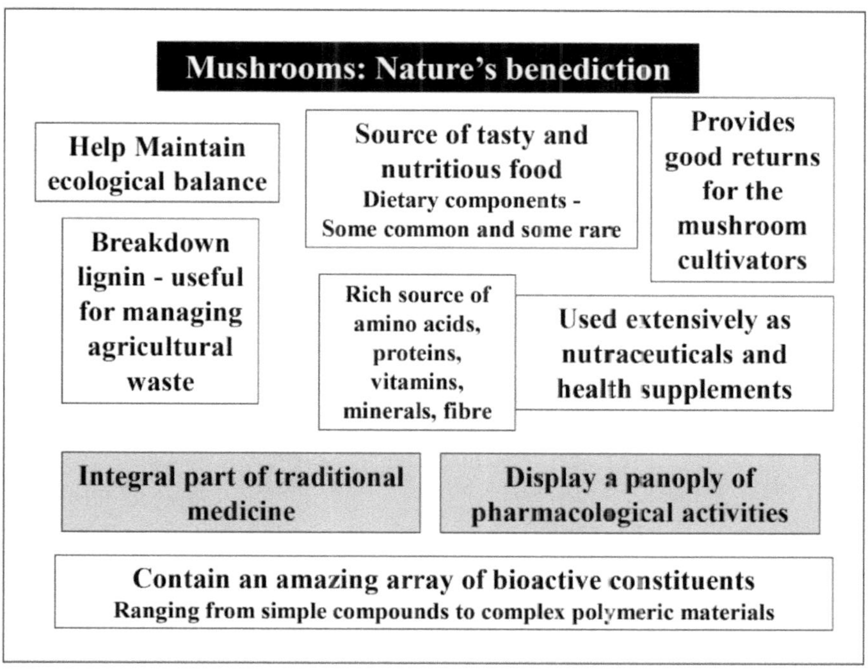

FIGURE 4.1 Advantages of mushrooms.

Edible and medicinal mushrooms have displayed a wide array of therapeutic activities in complementary and alternative medicine. This inspired researchers to carry out in depth investigations on these exceptional natural resources. Systematic scientific investigations have shown that mushrooms contain diverse bioactive compounds ranging from oligosaccharides, beta glucans, glucoproteins, lipopolysaccharides to low-molecular weight metabolites like alkaloids, lectins, phenolic compounds, flavonoids, terpenoids to name a few.[7–9] Biological evaluations have highlighted the medicinal potential of mushrooms—in-vitro, in-vivo, and some clinical studies show that different mushroom species have anxiolytic, antidepressant, antimicrobial, antioxidant, antidiabetic, antiviral, lipid lowering, immunomodulatory, hepatoprotective, and neuroprotective activities.[9–12] In traditional systems of medicine, mushrooms have been widely used for lowering blood sugar levels. Scientific reports show that powders, extracts as well as mycoconstituents of many mushrooms show distinct hypoglycemic and antihyperglycemic activities.[4,13] Different studies highlight the diverse mechanisms by which mushrooms produce antidiabetic effects (Fig. 4.2).

Mushrooms: The perfect antidiabetics!

Contain negligible or no fats and sugars hence are perfect dietary components for diabetics.

Mushroom teas, powders, extracts, oligosaccharides, polysaccharides are used nutraceuticals for managing blood sugar

Basic research and pre-clinical studies have highlighted the antidiabetic potential of many mushrooms and derived powders/ extracts/ constituents.

These produce antihyperglycemic or hypoglycemic effects by:

- **✓Inhibition of carbohydrate metabolism,**
- **✓Enhanced beta-cell activity, insulin production, sensitivity and release**
- **✓ Augmented antioxidant defence**
- **✓Facilitating glucose consumption and uptake in peripheral cells,**
- **✓ Increased GLUT4 translocation,**
- **✓Increasing hepatic glycogenesis and reduction of gluconeogenesis**

FIGURE 4.2 Mushrooms for managing diabetes.

The objective of this review is to compile scientific results of pharmacological and chemical investigations on the antidiabetic promise of mushrooms, to highlight the success stories, and to share future perspectives for developing safe and effective antidiabetic drugs from mushrooms.

4.2 USE OF MEDICINAL MUSHROOM FOR MANAGEMENT OF DIABETES: A CRITICAL APPRAISAL

During the past few decades, knowledge of medicinal value and bioactive components of mushrooms has grown significantly. Scientific investigations aiming to reveal the therapeutic value of mushrooms and derived components have shown their wide range of bioactivities including antidiabetic effect. Mushrooms possess diverse classes of secondary metabolites such as polysaccharides, phenols, alkaloids, sterols, terpenoids, and lactones which have been reported to be associated with their biological effects.[9] These compounds have been found to interact and modulate the key metabolic pathways of diabetes and thus help in reducing blood glucose levels (BGL) and maintaining normal insulin levels. Often, mushrooms and their components show antidiabetic effects via stimulating insulin secretion, improving insulin sensitivity (activate AMPK), inhibiting dietary carbohydrate metabolizing enzymes (α-amylase and α-glucosidase), facilitating glucose consumption and uptake in peripheral cells, increasing GLUT4 translocation, increasing hepatic glycogenesis, and reducing oxidative stress.[13,14] Table 4.1 lists extracts of various mushroom species demonstrating antidiabetic activity.

In the following section, the reported antidiabetic effects and associated mechanism of action of few selected mushroom extracts and constituents are discussed in detail.

4.3 ANTIDIABETIC EFFECTS OF MUSHROOM-DERIVED EXTRACTS

4.3.1 *AGARICUS SPECIES*

Agaricus L.: Fr. Emend Karst. is an important genus of the family Agariaceae and its species are characterized by white, yellow, or brown pileus.

TABLE 4.1 In-Vitro and In-Vivo Evidences Showing Antidiabetic Effects of Mushrooms.

Mushroom	Extract	In-vitro/In-vivo assay	Dose	Result	Reference
Agaricus blazei	Methanol	In-vitro α-amylase and α-glycosidase inhibition	IC_{50} =1719.20 ± 89.53 μg/mL; IC_{50} = 357.23 ± 20.11 μg/mL	Inhibited enzyme activity	[15]
Agrocybe aegerita	70% ethanol	In-vitro α-glycosidase inhibition	IC_{50} > 500 mg/mL	Inhibited enzyme activity	[16]
Auricularia auriculajudae	70% ethanol	In-vitro α-glycosidase inhibition	IC_{50} > 500 mg/mL	Inhibited enzyme activity	[16]
Calvatia gigantea	Methanol	In-vitro α-amylase inhibition	IC_{50} = 0.46 μg/mL	Inhibited enzyme activity	[17]
Calvatia gigantea	Methanol	Alloxan-induced diabetes in rats	100, 200, and 400 mg/kg dose administered.	Reduced BGL	[17]
Coprinus comatus	Methanol	In-vitro α-amylase and α-glycosidase inhibition	IC_{50} = 714.45 ± 44.44 μg/mL; IC_{50} = 322.74 ± 11.21 μg/mL	Inhibited enzyme activity	[15]
Cordyceps militaris	Methanol	In-vitro α-amylase and α-glycosidase inhibition	Not active; IC_{50} = 415.66 ± 36.12 μg/mL	Inhibited enzyme activity	[15]
C. militaris	Aqueous	90% pancreatectomized rats	0.5 g/kg, p.o.	Reduced fasting BGL, increased glucose utilization in skeletal muscles, GLUT4 content increases	[18]
C. militaris	Aqueous	High fat diet and STZ-induced diabetes in rats	0.5, 1.0 and 2.0 g/kg, p.o.	Reduced BGL	[19]
Ganoderma lucidum	Total triterpene fraction	In-vitro α-glucosidase inhibition	IC_{50} 10.02 ± 0.95 μg/mL	Inhibited enzyme activity	[20]
G. lucidum	Total triterpene fraction	In-vitro α-glucosidase inhibition	IC_{50} 31.82 ± 4.30 μg/mL	Inhibited enzyme activity	[20]

TABLE 4.1 *(Continued)*

Mushroom	Extract	In-vitro/In-vivo assay	Dose	Result	Reference
G. lucidum	Petroleum ether	Alloxan-induced diabetes in rats	200–800 mg/kg, p.o., for 7 days	Reduced plasma glucose levels, HbA1c, total cholesterol, triglyceride and low-density lipoprotein-cholesterol and increased plasma insulin and high-density lipoprotein cholesterol levels	[21]
G. lucidum	Methanol	Alloxan-induced diabetes in rats	200–800 mg/kg, p.o. for 7 days	Reduced plasma glucose levels, HbA1c, total cholesterol, triglyceride and low-density lipoprotein-cholesterol and increased plasma insulin and high-density lipoprotein cholesterol levels	[21]
G. lucidum	Aqueous	Lean (+db/+m) and the obese/diabetic (+db/+db) mice	0.3 g/kg, p.o. for 4 weeks	Lowered serum glucose and insulin levels and suppressed hepatic phosphoenol pyruvate carboxykinase expression	[22]
G. lucidum	Ethanol	Alloxan-induced diabetes in rats	250, 500, 1000 mg/kg for 14 days	Dose dependently reduced BGL	[23]
G. lucidum	70% ethanol	STZ-induced diabetes in rats	1 ml/kg for 30 days	Reduced BGL and protected pancreatic cells	[24]
G. lucidum	70% ethanol	In-vitro α-glycosidase inhibition	IC_{50} 4.88 mg/mL	Inhibited enzyme activity	[16]
Grifola frondosa	70% ethanol	In-vitro α-glycosidase inhibition	$IC_{50} > 500$ mg/mL	Inhibited enzyme activity	[16]
Hericium erinaceus	70% ethanol	In-vitro α-glycosidase inhibition	$IC_{50} > 500$ mg/mL	Inhibited enzyme activity	[16]

TABLE 4.1 *(Continued)*

Mushroom	Extract	In-vitro/In-vivo assay	Dose	Result	Reference
Inonotus obliquus	Methanol	In-vitro α-amylase and α-glycosidase inhibition	IC_{50} 830.32 ± 28.24 μg/mL; IC_{50} 220.31 ± 7.37 μg/mL	Inhibited enzyme activity	[15]
Lentinus edodes	70% ethanol	In-vitro α-glycosidase inhibition	IC_{50} > 500 mg/mL	Inhibited enzyme activity	[16]
Lignosus rhinocerotis	Powder	STZ-induced diabetes in rats	100, 250 and 500 mg/kg twice daily for 2 months	Reduced BGL; restored endogenous antioxidants (glutathione, catalase and superoxide dismutase)	[25]
Morchella conica	Methanol	In-vitro α-amylase and α-glycosidase inhibition	Not active; IC_{50} 521.12 μg/mL ± 16.45 μg/mL	Inhibited enzyme activity	[15]
Phellinus igniarius	Polyphenol-rich extract	In-vitro L6 cell lines	10, 20, 30 μg/mL	Increased glucose uptake, GLUT4 expression	[26]
Phellinus igniarius	Polyphenol rich Extract	KK-Ay mice with spontaneous type 2 diabetes mellitus	40, 80 and 160 mg/kg/day, p.o. for 4 weeks	Reduced body weight, BGL, insulin resistance, serum triglyceride, free fatty acid, LDL-C; increased serum HDL-C GLUT4 expression in skeletal muscle; reduced hepatic steatosis and protected pancreatic beta-cells	[26]
Phellinus linteus	Aqueous	High fat diet and STZ-induced diabetes in rats	300 and 600 mg/kg/daily for 8 weeks	Reduced BGL by inhibiting gluconeogenesis and glycogen degradation enzymes	[27]
P. linteus	Methanol	In-vitro α-amylase and α-glycosidase inhibition	IC_{50} = 1479.46 ± 92.86 μg/mL; IC_{50} = 477.33 ± 17.55 μg/mL	Inhibited enzyme activity	[27]
Pleurotus fossulatus	Aqueous	STZ-induced diabetes in rats	250 and 500 mg/kg	Increased animal body weight; reduced BGL, blood urea nitrogen, creatinine, uric acid and improved blood lipid profile	[28]

TABLE 4.1 *(Continued)*

Mushroom	Extract	In-vitro/In-vivo assay	Dose	Result	Reference
Russula sanguinea	70% ethanol	In-vitro α-amylase and α-glycosidase inhibition	$IC_{50} > 500$ mg/mL	Inhibited enzyme activity	[16]
Tremella fuciformis	70% ethanol	In-vitro α-glycosidase inhibition	$IC_{50} > 500$ mg/mL	Inhibited enzyme activity	[16]
Calocybe indica	Aqueous	In-vitro α-amylase inhibition, glucose uptake by yeast cells, and oral starch tolerance test in mice	8–40 mg/mL for in-vitro studies and 200 and 400 mg/kg, p.o. for in-vivo studies	Inhibited enzyme in-vitro (IC_{50} =18.07 mg/mL; inhibited glucose transport across yeast cells and reduced BGL in mice	[29]
Calocybe indica	Aqueous	In-vitro α-amylase inhibition, glucose uptake by yeast cells, and oral starch tolerance test in mice	200 and 400 mg/kg, p.o.	Inhibited enzyme in-vitro (IC_{50} =18.07 mg/mL; inhibited glucose transport across yeast cells and reduced BGL in mice	[29]
Ganoderma philippii	70% Methanol	In-vitro α-amylase and α-glycosidase inhibition	1–100 mg/mL	Inhibited enzymes concentration dependently with maximum inhibition of 40.22%	[30]
Lenzites elegans	70% Methanol	In-vitro α-amylase and α-glycosidase inhibition	1–100 mg/mL	Inhibited enzymes concentration dependently with maximum inhibition of 26.57%	[30]
Rigidoporus ulmarius	70% Methanol	In-vitro α-amylase and α-glycosidase inhibition	1–100 mg/mL	Inhibited enzymes concentration dependently with maximum inhibition of 65.54%	[30]

The genus has more than 400 edible and poisonous species[31]; however, *Agaricus bisporus* Imbach (known as button mushroom) and *Agaricus blazei* Murrill (known as Cogumelo do Sol) are the two prominent species because of their high nutritional and medicinal value. *A. bisporus* is one of the most cultivated (around 38% of the total mushroom production) edible mushrooms in the world. It is native to North America and Europe. It has luscious taste and flavor and is highly nutritious as it includes vitamins, proteins, minerals, unsaturated fatty acids, and fibers.[32] Besides functional food, it is consumed for its health-promoting effects and is used in pharmaceutical and cosmetic industry. Conventionally, it is recommended in brain and heart disorders, to boost immunity and in diabetes and cancer.[33] Scientific studies have shown its possible use in diabetes. In streptozotocin (STZ)-induced diabetic rats, the aqueous extract normalized the increased BGL, restored liver alanine aminotransferase, and aspartate aminotransferase. Jeong et al.[34] showed that administration of mushroom powder (200 mg/kg) for 3 weeks to STZ-induced diabetic rats bought BGL and triglycerides levels to normal value along with liver enzymes.[34] Also, *A. bisporus* powder enhanced the insulin secretion and repaired the pancreatic β-cell.[35] In alloxan-induced diabetic rats, ethanolic basidiocarp extract (500 and 750 mg/kg) was effective in reducing the elevated glucose levels and lipid peroxidation and restoring endogenous antioxidant levels in blood.[36] *A. blazei* Murrill is an edible mushroom native to Brazil and is now widely cultivated and consumed in Japan and the United States as a functional medicinal food. Traditionally it has been employed in the management of diabetes, atherosclerosis, cancer, hepatitis, dermatitis, hyperlipidemia, and cardiac disorders.[37] It is a rich source of polysaccharides, protein and fibers.[38] The antidiabetic activity of *A. blazei* lies in its aqueous extract due to the presence of β-glucan-derived oligosaccharides. In STZ-induced diabetic rats, administration of *A. blazei* oligosaccharides (2% in water) for 6 weeks showed decrease in BGL by stimulating the release of insulin from pancreas.[39] The ethyl acetate (EA) fraction (200 mg/kg) obtained from aqueous extract of fruiting bodies of *A. blazei* was effective in normalizing BGL in oral glucose tolerance test in rats. Moreover, the fraction (200 and 400 mg/kg) suppressed the rise in BGL by stimulating insulin secretion in STZ-induced diabetic rats.[40] Recently, it was reported that the ethanol extract (EE) and its EA fraction inhibited α-glucosidase activity in a concentration dependent manner. In HepG2 cells, both EE and EA enhanced the glucose consumption, thereby reducing the increased BGL.[41] *A. campestris* L. is another medicinal mushroom, which is traditionally used as an antidiabetic drug. The aqueous extract (1 mg/mL) of this mushroom lowered BGL in rats by its insulin releasing and insulin-like effects. Moreover, the extract facilitated glucose uptake, glucose transporter activity, and convert glucose to glycogen in rat abdominal muscles.[42]

4.3.2 *CORDYCEPS* SPECIES

Cordyceps genus (L.) Fr. (Clavicipitaceae family) is one of the most diversified genus containing more than 680 parasitic fungi that are well documented as traditional Chinese medicine (TCM).[43,44] The species are widely distributed in India, China, Nepal, Bhutan, and Tibet.[44] Many *Cordyceps* sp. are used in traditional medicines in China, Japan, Korea, Taiwan, and other eastern Asian countries. *Cordyceps sinensis* (Berk) Sacc. syn. *Ophiocordyceps sinensis* (known as caterpillar fungus) is a rare, exotic, and the most documented species since late 1400 by Tibetan doctors. In 1964, it was given a status of drug and included in the Chinese Pharmacopoeia.[43] In TCM, it is used in cardiovascular, metabolic, and nervous disorders and as lung and kidney tonic. In 2003, during SARS outbreak a sharp increase in the demand and thus, medicinal value, of caterpillar fungus was observed in China.[43] *C. sinensis* is also known for its BGL lowering and potential in treating both type 1 and type 2 diabetes. The antidiabetic effects of fruiting body (1 g/day for 4 weeks, p.o.) of *C. sinensis* were determined in diabetic rats induced by nicotinamide and STZ. The treatment was reported to be effective in lowering BGL in oral glucose tolerance test along with decreasing water intake and increasing insulin levels and body weight in diabetic rats.[45] The same research group in their another study, compared the antidiabetic effect of fermented mycelia (1 g/day, 4 weeks, p.o.) with fruiting body (1 g/day, 4 weeks, p.o.) of *C. sinensis* in nicotinamide and STZ-diabetic rats. The study revealed that both fermented mycelia and fruiting bodies had similar antidiabetic efficacy.[46] Pretreatment of rats with crude extract (100 mg/kg) and polysaccharide- rich fraction (10 mg/kg) obtained from fruiting bodies and mycelia for 13 days showed marked decrease BGL in STZ-diabetic rats.[47] The fermented mycelia EE (four consecutive weeks) showed gain in body weight and increased HDL/LDL ratio in high fat diet induced KK/HIJ diabetic mice.[48] The MTT assay revealed the fermented alcoholic extract had protective and regenerative effects on pancreatic beta cells against STZ. However, the study showed no significant effect on BGL in KK/HIJ diabetic mice.[48] These reported antidiabetic effects of *C. sinensis* could be related to its polysaccharides. The crude polysaccharides when injected to STZ rats significantly lowered the BGL.[49] The hypoglycemic effects of caterpillar fungus could be related to its ability to increase the sensitivity of cells toward insulin. The fermented mycelia when administered to rats at 2 g/kg daily for 30 days showed increased insulin sensitivity of whole body cells and were able to reduce BGL.[50] *C. militaris* (L.) Link (northern worm grass), an anamorph of *C. sinensis*, is another valuable Chinese medicine used in various metabolic, cardiovascular, and immune disorders.[51] The aqueous extract of *C. militaris* reduced the glucose induced increase in reactive oxygen species generation and caspase-3 activity in human umbilical vein endothelial cells.[52] The polysaccharide-rich extract administered at the dose of 10 mg/kg to STZ rats showed marked decrease in BGL.[47] Cheng et al.[53] reported that *C. militaris* fruiting body aqueous extract (10 mg/kg) had hypoglycemic effects and lowered the BGL via enhancing insulin secretion and cholinergic activation (increased the insulin receptor substrate 1 and glucose transporter 4) in normal rats.[53] In high fat-induced diabetic rat, the whole mushroom extract of *C. militaris* showed fall in BGL and increased insulin sensitivity without altering the body weight of the animals.[54] Similarly, alcoholic (0.05 g/kg) and aqueous (2 g/kg) extracts showed decrease in BGL by facilitating glucose metabolism in diet-STZ-induced diabetic rats.[55] Also, the aqueous extract exhibited α-glucosidase along and increased GLUT2 activity, thereby increasing the glucose uptake in HepG2 cells.[56]

4.3.3 GANODERMA SPECIES

Ganoderma is a polypore mushroom genus of family Ganodermataceae that contains more than 80 species. *Ganoderma* species have been used since centuries in Asian countries to promote general well-being and longevity. These species are valuable source of micro- and macro-nutrients, vitamins, minerals, fibers, and biomolecules. They can be found wildly in the tropical regions of the world. *G. lucidum* (Fr.) Krast popularly known as "Ling-Zhi" in China and "Reishi" in Japan, is a white rot fungus which is valued for its nutritional and medicinal properties. Ethnically, it is used to prolong vitality, longevity, good health, and used as general tonic. Over the past few years, extensive research established Reishi as antidiabetic, neuro-protective, anti-inflammatory, cardioprotective, and immunomodulatory drug. Reishi was explored for its antidiabetic effects using various in-vitro and in-vivo assays.[57] Oral administration of water soluble mycelia extract (1 g/kg daily for 9 weeks) reduced BGL, triglyceride levels, lipid peroxide levels, and increased antioxidant status (catalase, superoxide dismutase, and glutathione peroxidase) in STZ-diabetic mice.[58] Polysaccharides (50 and 150 mg/kg/day for 28 days) rich fraction from *G. lucidum* resulted in increase in animal body weight and insulin levels in STZ-diabetic mice.[59] This fraction had hypoglycemic effects as it reduced the fasting BGLs.[59] To reveal the antidiabetic mechanism of action, Teng et al.[60] determined the effects of proteoglycan extract from *G. lucidum* fruiting bodies on plasma glucose levels, insulin levels, expression of protein tyrosine phosphatase 1B (PTP) and the tyrosine phosphorylation level of the insulin receptor (IR) β-subunit in the liver and skeletal muscles of STZ-diabetic rats.[60] The study showed that proteoglycan extract (40 and 120 mg/kg dose for 30 days) had antihyperglycemic effects by virtue of its ability to reduce fasting plasma glucose levels, enhance serum insulin levels, inhibit PTP and reduce free fatty acid, triglyceride, and LDL levels.[60] The ethanolic extract showed strong α-glucosidase inhibitory effects.[61] The overall antidiabetic effects of *G. lucidum* may be attributed to its polysaccharides (50 mg/kg/day for 5 days, i.p.) as they were effective in reducing fasting BGLs, downregulating liver glucose regulatory enzymes via AMPK activation (increased GLUT4 levels, decreased fatty acid synthase) and improving insulin resistance in STZ-diabetic mice.[62] Besides, having blood glucose lowering effects, *G. lucidum* has antihyperlipidemic effects (reduced triglyceride, total cholesterol and LDL and increased HDL levels). Therefore, Reishi may have beneficial effects in diabetes-related comorbidities.[59] *Ganoderma applanatum* (Pers.) Pat is another revered Chinese mushroom that is known to have strong anticancer effects.[63] Jung et al.[64] indicated the possible use of *G. applanatum* in diabetic complications. The authors determined the antidiabetic and inhibitory effects of methanol and aqueous extracts (200 mg/kg/day, 2 weeks) of mushroom in STZ-diabetic rats and rat lens aldose reductase enzyme. The extracts reduced the potent enzyme inhibition activity and lowered the BGL in diabetic rats.[64] Other *Ganoderma* species such as *Ganoderma lipsiense*

(Batsch) G.F. Atk. and *Ganoderma resinaceum* Boud have also shown antihyperglycemic effects. The extract of *G. lipsiense* grown in red rice medium and synthetic medium inhibited α-glucosidase activity with IC_{50} of 0.269 mg/mL and 0.218 mg/mL, respectively.[65] In alloxan-induced diabetic rats, administration of alcoholic and water extracts of *G. resinaceum* fruiting bodies for 5 days showed decrease in BGL in oral glucose tolerance test and increase in Langerhans islets.[66]

4.3.4 *INONOTUS OBLIQUUS*

Inonotus obliquus (Fr.) Pilat (family Hymenochaetaceae, popularly called as Chaga mushroom) is a white parasitic fungus that is commonly found at Birche plant (Betula species) and other hard wood species. It is distributed in Japan, Russia, Europe, and northeastern China.[67] It is a Russian traditional medicine and is employed as antidiabetic, cardioprotectant, diuretic, anticancer, and in gastrointestinal disorder since 16th century.[39,68–71] In Siberia, it is used as liver tonic, blood purifier, to treat worms, stomach disorders, tuberculosis, and pain.[70,72,73] It is consumed as food in the form of tea, concentrate, and syrup.[74] Systematic investigations identified more than 200 bioactive compounds and majority of the bioactivities have been related to the presence of polysaccharides.[75] Various preclinical studies have shown the beneficial effects of Chaga mushroom in the both type 1 and 2 diabetes. Diet supplemented with fermented (50 g/kg/day, p.o. for 8 weeks) *I. obliquus* powder showed reduced water intake, serum triglyceride levels, and total cholesterol levels in genetically diabetic Otsuka Long-Evans Tokushima fatty rats which indicated its possible role in managing obesity-related noninsulin-dependent diabetes mellitus.[76] The BGL lowering ability of dry matter of culture broth of *I. obliquus* (500 and 1000 mg/kg/day, p.o. for 21 days) was evaluated in normal and glucose and alloxan-induced hyperglycemic mice by Sun et al.[77] The treatment lowered the BGL in normal mice (hypoglycemic effect) and in alloxan diabetic mice. Also, administration of culture broth to alloxan-diabetic mice showed reduction in serum low-density lipoprotein-cholesterol free fatty acid, triglyceride, and total cholesterol; elevation in high-density lipoprotein-cholesterol, hepatic glycogen content, insulin level, superoxide dismutase, glutathione peroxidase; regenerated pancreatic tissue. However, the culture broth failed to lowered the BGL in glucose-diabetic mice.[77] Besides having potential antidiabetic effects, Chaga mushrooms are safe and devoid of any potential side effect. Therefore, these results are of suggestive that *I. obliquus* could be developed as functional food for treating both type 1 and 2 diabetes.

4.3.5 PHELLINUS SPECIES

P. linteus (Berkeley & M.A. Curtis) is a horseshoe-shaped mushroom whose medicinal properties were recognized for more than 2000 years ago.[78] It can be found growing on the trunk of *Populus* Linn, Betula, and *Morus alba* L.[78] It is abundant in Korea, China, and Japan and widely distributed in Africa and America.[79] It plays a crucial role in traditional Chinese system of medicine as it is believed to be beneficial in maintaining body's homeostasis, abdominal pain, liver disorders, chronic diarrhea, diabetes, gastrointestinal ailments, and as blood purifier.[79,80] Scientific evidences have shown the antidiabetic effects of *P. linteus* in various in-vitro and in-vivo assays (Table 4.1). In STZ-diabetic rats, the aqueous extract (300 and 600 mg/kg/day, p.o. for 8 weeks) obtained from solid state culture of *P. linteus* reduced BGL and improved insulin resistance. The extract was found to inhibit hepatic glucose production via reducing the expression of FBPase and G6Pase that aid gluconeogenesis.[27] *Phellinus baumii* Pilát is a hoof-shaped bitter mushroom that is often found on mulberry tree. It is frequently used in Asian folk medicine. The ethanol and ethylacetate extracts (100, 200, and 400 mg/kg/day, p.o., for 16 days) ameliorated the rise in BGL in STZ-diabetic rats by stimulating the insulin secretion.[68] The antidiabetic effects of *Phellinus* have been largely attributed to the presence of polysaccharides.[80]

4.3.6 PLEUROTUS SPECIES

Genus *Pleurotus* (family Pleurotaceae, popularly known as Oyster mushrooms) comprise of more than 40 species that can be found across all regions of the world particularly in forests.[81,82] These are world's third largest cultivated mushroom after genus *Agaricus* and *Lentinul*.[83] These are the type of gilled mushrooms. A few of the prominent species of this genus are *Pleurotus ostreatus* (tree oyster), *Pleurotus sajor-caju* (Indian oyster), *Pleurotus pulmonarius* (grey oyster), *Pleurotus platypus*,

Pleurotus sapidus, Pleurotus cornucopiae, *Pleurotus florida* (white oyster) and *Pleurotus eryngii* (King oyster).[6] These species have pleasant taste and have great nutritional value as these are rich in vitamins, minerals, amino acids, and fibers with low sugar and cholesterol content.[82,84] *Pleurotus* species have been documented to possess a wide array of biological effects. The antidiabetic effects of *P. ostreatus* f. carpathicus (Kalchbr.) Pilát are described using rodent model of STZ and alloxan-induced diabetes. The ethanolic extract (250 mg/kg, i.p.) of *P. ostreatus* showed antidiabetic and hypolipidemic effects in alloxan-diabetic mice. The post-treatment of animals resulted in decrease in BGL, serum triglycerides, cholesterol, and LDL levels.[85,86] In STZ-diabetic rats, the methanol and ethylacetate extract (200 mg/kg/day for 30 days) of *P. ostreatus* lowered the BGL along with serum triglycerides and LDL.[87] The extract was also reported to be effective in protecting pancreas from the deleterious effects of STZ.[87] Besides lowering BGL in diabetic animals, the extract (200 and 400 mg/kg/day, p.o. for 30 days) reduced liver DNA fragmentation and sperm abnormalities, thereby indicating the possible use of *P. ostreatus* in diabetic-related comorbidities.[88] Data from our lab determined the mechanisms associated with BGL effects of *P. ostreatus* using in-vitro assays. The aqueous extract of *P. ostreatus* inhibited in-vitro α-amylase activity, prevented glucose update by yeast cells and showed marked glucose adsorption capacity.[29] In oral starch tolerance test, the extract (200 and 400 mg/kg) was found to be effective in lowering the BGL.[29] Similarly aqueous and acetone extracts (200 and 400 mg/kg/day, p.o. for 2 weeks) of *P. pulmonarius* (Fr.) Quél showed decrease in BGL, and improved serum lipid profile. The in-vitro analyses showed that aqueous extract had better α-amylase (an intestinal carbohydrate metabolising enzyme) inhibitory effects (99.23% inhibition) at 1000 μg/mL.[89] In line with these studies, *Pleurotus sajor-caju* (Fr.) Singer extract is reported to have hypoglycaemic effects in normal rats and antidiabetic activity in STZ-induced diabetic rats. In oral glucose tolerance test, the aqueous extract at 500, 750, and 1000 mg/kg reduced BGL in normal animals with maximum decrease at 750 mg/kg. The administration of extract at dose of 750 mg/kg/day, p.o. for 21 days resulted in decrease in BGL, HbA1c, serum triglycerides, cholesterol and LDL levels, and increased HDL levels.[90] Methanol extract of *P. florida* Singer is reported to have strong in-vitro α-amylase (94.93%) and α-glucosidase (84.90%) inhibitory activities at a concentration of 1000 μg/mL in rats.[91] *Pleurotus tuberregium* is traditionally used as a decoction for the management of diabetes in Southern Nigeria. Onuekwuzu et al.[92] studied the antidiabetic potential of *P. tuberregium* Sclerotia aqueous extract against alloxan-induced diabetic rabbits. The authors found that extractant dose of 100, 200, and 300 mg/kg reduced BGL and improved serum lipid profile of diabetic rabbits (lowered triglycierides, LDL, VLDL, cholesterol, and increased HDL levels) and thus claimed the beneficial effects of mushroom in diabetes and related hyperlipidaemia.[92]

4.4 ANTIDIABETIC EFFECTS OF MUSHROOM DERIVED CONSTITUENTS

Mushrooms form an abundant source of various nutritional constituents due to which they have been a center for various medicinal researches. Structural characterization has shown that the majority of bioactive myco-constituents belong to the classes of polysaccharides, proteins, phenolic compounds, terpenoids, alkaloids, and sterols.[93] Due to diversity in high-quality medicinal and nutritive components, mushrooms have gain significant attention to be developed as functional food.

4.4.1 POLYSACCHARIDES

Polysaccharides are one of the most abundant components of mushrooms. These are combinations of multiple monosaccharides bound by glycosidic linkages and are generally considered as biodegradable, biocompatible, and nontoxic macromolecules.[94] These macromolecules contribute to various pharmacological properties,[95] including antihyperglycemic, antihypercholestrolemic, anticarcinogenic, immunomodulatory, and anti-inflammatory activities of mushrooms.[38] The polysaccharides derived from mushrooms form the basis of nutraceutical application and dietary supplements usage of mushrooms. Some of the prominent polysaccharides of mushrooms that have been explored as functional food include pleuran derived from the *Pleurotus* species, lentinan from the *Lentinus edodes*, calocyban derived from the *Calocybe indica*, and ganoderan derived from the *Ganoderma lucidium*.[93] Although mannose, glucose, fructose, arabinose, mannitol, rhamnose, and xylose are the most common mushroom ingredients. A multitude of investigations has revealed the association of polysaccharides with antidiabetic effects of mushroom (Table 4.2). Majority of the mushroom polysaccharides have been reported to modulate insulin levels and protect pancreatic beta-cells. In addition, mushroom-derived polysaccharides inhibit gut α-amylase and α-glucosidase enzymes that is beneficial in lowering postprandial BGL. The extracellular polysaccharides isolated from *Coriolus versicolor* (ePS-F2-1, ePS-F3-1, ePS-F4-1) showed potent antidiabetic effect by inhibiting the α-glucosidase enzyme with ePS-F4-1 (IC_{50} 1 mg/mL).[96] The intracellular polysaccharides of the same species also exhibited α-glucosidase inhibition. These effects were due to the presence of α-(1,4)-glycosidic linkages in the polysaccharides.[97] Bioactive polysaccharides with β-glycosidic linkage evolved from *Russula emetica* by ultrasonication assisted extraction had 56.3% antidiabetic activity.[98] Two polysaccharides with molecular weight of 4.062×10^6 and 4.189×10^6 Da from *P. eryngii* had concentration dependent in-vitro α-glucosidase inhibitory effects with 56.13% and 57.57% (maximum) inhibition of enzyme at 6mg/mL.[99] Two new polysaccharides named as TZP1-1 and TZP2-1 isolated from *Thelephora ganbajun* (a wild edible mushroom) showed moderate in-vitro α-amylase inhibitory activities (23% and 48.6% inhibition, respectively, at 400 μg/mL). The analysis of composition of these compounds showed the presence of mannose, rhamnose, galactose, and xylose.[100] The antidiabetic effects of polysaccharides obtained from some mushrooms was reviewed and is reported in Table 4.2.

4.4.2 PROTEINS

Proteins and peptides form another nutritive element of the mushroom responsible for their multiple health improving effects. The protein content ranges from 228 to 249 g/kg dry matter have been reported in some of the mushrooms, which is significantly higher than other protein sources. Some of the prominent bioactive proteins present in mushrooms are lectins, fungal immunomodulatory proteins, ribosome-inactivating proteins, ribonucleases, and laccases. These form the basis of antidiabetic, antitumor, antiviral, immunomodulatory, and antioxidant activities of the mushrooms.[134] Some of the proteins exhibiting antihyperglycemic effects are enlisted in Table 4.3.

TABLE 4.2 Antidiabetic Effects of Some Mushroom Derived Polysaccharides.

Polysaccharides	Mushroom species	In-vitro experimental model	Dose	Result	Reference
Exo-polysaccharides	*Cerrena unicolor*	STZ-induced diabetes in rats	100 mg/kg, p.o. for 7 days	Decreased BGL; preserved pancreatic Langerhans islet areas	[101]
Exo-polysaccharides	*C. comatus*	STZ-induced diabetes in rats	100 mg/kg	Decreased BGL; preserved pancreatic Langerhans islet areas	[101]
Intracellular and extracellular polysaccharides	*C. comatus*	In-vitro α-amylase inhibition	2–10 mg/mL	Dose dependent enzyme inhibition	[102]
Polysaccharides	*Cordyceps cicadae*	Alloxan-induced diabetes in mice	100, 200 and 400 mg/kg, p.o.	Reduced BGL	[103]
Exopolysaccharide (EPS-III)	*C. militaris*	STZ-induced diabetes in rats	0.1–3 mg/mL	Dose-dependant inhibition of α-glucosidase enzyme in-vitro and reduced BGL	[104]
Cultured mycelium polysaccharide composed of mannose, galactose and glucose	*C. sinesis*	STZ-induced diabetes in rats	50 mg/kg, i.p.	Enhanced glucokinase activity, reduced hepatic glucose output and GLUT-2	[104]
Polysaccharide fraction	*C. sinesis*, *C. militaris*, *Omphalia lapidescens*, and *Tricholomamongolicum*	STZ-induced diabetes in rats	10 and 100 mg/kg	Decreased BGL	[47]
Polysaccharides	*Cordyceps taii*	STZ-induced diabetes in mice	100, 200 and 400 mg/kg, p.o.	Reduce fasting BGL and increased serum insulin levels	[106]
Polysaccharide (PSG-1)	*Ganoderma atrum*	High-fat diet and STZ-induced diabetes in rats	200 and 400 mg/kg, p.o. for 4 weeks	Reduced fasting serum glucose levels	[107]

TABLE 4.2 *(Continued)*

Polysaccharides	Mushroom species	In-vitro experimental model	Dose	Result	Reference
PSG-1 (composed of glucose, mannose, galactose and galacturonic acid)	*G. atrum*	High-fat diet and STZ-induced diabetes in rats	200 and 400 mg/kg	Reduced fasting BGL, insulin resistance, LDL-C, triglycerides; decreased expression of Bax and increased expression of Bcl-2 in pancreatic cells	[108]
Ganoderan B	*G. lucidum*	Normal mice and alloxan-induced diabetes in mice	30 mg/kg, i.p.	Reduced BGL, increased plasma insulin levels in normal mice and in glucose tolerance test; increased glucokinase and phosphofructokinase activity; decreased glucose-6-phosphatase, glycogen synthetase activity	[109]
Ganoderan B and C	*G. lucidum*	Normal mice	10, 30 and 100 mg/kg	Reduced BGL	[110]
Polysaccharides	*G. lucidum*	STZ-induced diabetes in mice	50 and 100 mg/kg/day for 7 days	Reduced fasting serum glucose levels, hepatic glucose-6-phosphatase, fructose-1,6-bisphosphatase and glycogen Phosphorylase mRNA expression	[111]
Polysaccharides	*G. lucidum*	High fat diet and STZ-induced diabetes in rats	0.4 g/kg, p.o.	Enhanced glucose and lipid metabolism, insulin sensitivity, glycogen synthesis, glucose transportation, increased expressions of p85, GS and GLUT4 in skeletal muscles	[112]
Polysaccharide	*G. lucidum*	STZ-induced diabetes in rats	200 mg/kg/daily, p.o. for 8 weeks	Reduced BGL by increasing antioxidant status of pancreas, stimulated β-cell regeneration, upregulated Bcl-2 and PDX-1 expression and downregulated caspase-3 Bax expression	[113]

TABLE 4.2 *(Continued)*

Polysaccharides	Mushroom species	In-vitro experimental model	Dose	Result	Reference
Polysaccharide	*G. lucidum*	Alloxan-induced toxicity in pancreatic cell lines	50, 100 and 200 mg/kg/daily, p.o. for 10 days	Reduced BGL and increase serum insulin, prevented necrosis of β-cells, inhibited NF-kB activation	[114]
Polysaccharide	*G. lucidum*	High fat diet and STZ-induced diabetes in rats	50 and 100 mg/kg/daily, p.o. for 7 days	Reduced BGL by inhibiting hepatic glucose regulatory enzymes (reduced expression of glycogen phosphorylase and hosphoenolpyruvate carboxykinase)	[111]
MT-α-glucan	*G. frondosa*	KK-Ay mice (diabetes rat model)	150 and 450 mg/kg twice day, p.o. for 2 weeks	Reduced fasting BGL, glycosylated serum protein, serum insulin and lipid peroxidation; Increased levels of hepatic glycogen, reduced glutathione, insulin binding capacity to liver plasma membrane	[115]
Polysaccharides (F2, F3)	*G. frondosa*	Diabetes rat model	50 and 100 mg/kg/day	Reduced fasting BGL, serum insulin, insulin resistance; increased hepatic insulin receptors	[116]
Polysaccharides (GFPS1, GFPS2, GFPS3, GFPS4)	*G. frondosa*	High-fat diet and STZ-induced diabetes in rats	200 mg/kg/day, p.o., for 4 weeks	Improved animal body weight; lowered BGL, serum IL-2, IL-6 and TNF-α; increased serum metalloproteinase 9	[117]
α-glucan	*G. frondosa*	STZ-induced diabetes in mice	100 and 300 mg/kg	Lowered fasting BGL, triglycerides, cholesterol, IL-1 and nitric oxide production; increased insulin concentration and IL-2 production; preserve β-cells	[118]
Polysaccharides	*I. obliquus*	High-fat diet and STZ-induced diabetes in rats	300, 600 and 900 mg/kg for 4 weeks	Upregulated glycogen levels and suppressed BGL	[119]

TABLE 4.2 *(Continued)*

Polysaccharides	Mushroom species	In-vitro experimental model	Dose	Result	Reference
Polysaccharides	*I. obliquus*	STZ-induced diabetes in rats	10, 20, and 30 mg/kg/day, p.o. for 6 weeks	Reduced BGL, lipid peroxidation, LDL, IL-1β levels, TNF-α levels, increased HDL and protected pancreatic β-cells	[120]
Polysaccharides	*I. obliquus*	STZ-induced diabetes in rats	50 mg/kg/day, p.o. for 4 weeks	Reduced BGL; increased serum insulin, pyruvate kinase levels, glycogen synthesis, interleukin-2 levels; upregulated interleukin-2 receptor and matrix metalloproteinase-9	[121]
Polysaccharides	*I. obliquus*	STZ-induced diabetes in rats	900 mg/kg, p.o.	Reduced fasting BGL; improved glucose tolerance, insulin sensitivity; upregulated hepatic GLUT4, PI3K-p85, p-Akt; protected pancreatic cells	[119]
Exopolysaccharides	*Lenzites betulina*	STZ-induced diabetes in rats	100 mg/kg	Decreased BGL; preserved pancreatic Langerhans islet areas	[101]
Polysaccharide	*Paecilomyces hepiali*	db/db genetic mice	10, 20, and 40 mg/kg/day for 8 weeks	Lowered BGL in OGTT; reduced serum oxidative stress and inflammatory markers; enhanced endogenous antioxidants in serum	[122]
Exo-polysaccharides	*P. baumii*	STZ-induced diabetes in rats	200 mg/kg/day, p.o., for 14 days	Reduced BGL	[68]
Extracellular polysaccharides	*P. baumii*	STZ-induced diabetes in rats	200 mg/kg	Decreased BGL	[68]
Polysaccharides	*P. linteus*	High-fat high-fructose diet-induced diabetes in mice	50 mg/kg twice daily, p.o. for 4 weeks	Reduced BGL and glucose intolerance	[123]
Polysaccharide powder	*P. lintius*	Alloxan-induced diabetes in rats	300 and 600 mg/kg, p.o. for 8 weeks	Decreased the fasting BGL	[124]

TABLE 4.2 *(Continued)*

Polysaccharides	Mushroom species	In-vitro experimental model	Dose	Result	Reference
Water-soluble polysaccharides	*Pleurotus citrinopileatus*	STZ-induced diabetes in rats	0.4–0.12 g/kg	Decreased fasting BGL	[125]
Acidic, alkaline, enzymatically extractable mycelium zinc polysaccharides	*Pleurotus djamor*	STZ-induced diabetes in mice	200, 400, and 800 mg/kg, p.o. for 2 weeks	Reduced BGL	[126]
Extracellular polysaccharides (EPS1 and EPS2)	*P. eryngii*	STZ-induced diabetes in rats	5 mg/mL	Inhibited α-amylase and α-glucosidase activities and decreased BGL	[127]
Polysaccharide	*P. florida*	STZ-induced diabetes in mice	200 and 400 mg/kg, p.o.	Reduced BGL, serum triglycerides, urine glucose and ketones levels	[128]
Polysaccharides	*P. ostreatus*	STZ-induced diabetes in rats	100, 200, and 400 mg/kg, p.o. for 2 weeks	Dose-dependent lowering of fasting blood glucose, increase in fasting serum insulin levels and insulin sensitivity	[129]
Glucan rich polysaccharide (β-glucans)	*Pleurotus sajor caju*	C57BL/6J mice fed on a high diet.	60, 120, and 240 mg/kg	Dose-dependent elevation of serum insulin levels; improved glucose tolerance	[130]
Extracellular polysaccharides	*Pleurotus tuber-regium*	High-fat diet and STZ-induced diabetes in rats	20 mg/kg/day, po., for 8 weeks	Lowered BGL; increased serum insulin concentration; upregulated liver PPAR-α mRNA expression	[131]
Exopolysaccharides	*Tremella fuciformi*	C57BL/6J *ob/ob* mice	200 mg/kg/day, p.o., for 52 days	Reduced BGL; increased PPAR-γ expression	[132]
Acidic polysaccharide	*Tremella aurantia*	KK-Ay mice (Genetic mouse model)	0.5 g/l/day, p.o. for 10 weeks	Reduced BGL, insulin, triglycerides and cholesterol	[133]

TABLE 4.3 Mushroom Derived Antidiabetic Proteins.

Proteins	Mushroom species	Animal model in-vitro	Dose	Result	Reference
Ternatin	*Coriolus versicolor*	KK-Ay mice	Ternatin (8.5 or 17 nmol/day) or [D-Leu^7] ternatine (68 nmol/day) administered	Both of them suppressed the hyperglycemia. The levels of SREBP-1c mRNA were notably decreased in liver	[135]
SX-fraction of glycoprotein	*G. frondosa*	Spontaneously hypertensive rats	0.87, 1.75, 3.5 g/kg	Improved insulin sensitivity, improved glucose tolerance	[136]

4.4.3 POLYMERS

The mycelium being a complex, natural, polymeric fibrous material comprises of a combination of natural polymers such as chitin, cellulose, proteins, etc.[137] These polymers majorly formed from the combination of galactose with minute quantities of arabinose and glucose. The various bioactive polymers derived from the medicinal mushrooms have been found to exert antihyperglycemic activities having notable effects on glucose metabolism and pancreatic beta cells (Table 4.4).

4.4.4 TERPENOIDS

Terpenoids are volatile unsaturated complex organic compounds that significantly contribute to the antidiabetic effects of mushrooms. Among terpenoids, researchers have found sesquiterpenoids (aristolane, bisabolene, cuparene, fommanosane), diterpenoids (cyathane type), and triterpenoids (lanostane type) predominantly present in mushrooms.[142] Despite of the presence of diverse forms of terpenoids, few studies exploring the antidiabetic potential of these terpenoids could be found in literature. Lanostane triterpenes, namely Resinacein C (IC_{50} 1.049 mM), ganoderic acid Y (IC_{50} 0.17 mM), lucialdehyde C (IC_{50} 0.635 mM), 7-oxo-ganoderic acid Z3 (IC_{50} 0.106 mM), 7-oxo-ganoderic acid Z (IC_{50} 0.114 mM), and lucidadiol (IC_{50} 1.735 mM), isolated from *Ganoderma resinaceum* are reported to inhibit α-glucosidase activity in-vitro.[143] Few other mushroom-derived terpenes that showed in-vitro and/or in-vivo antidiabetic effects are enumerated in Table 4.5.

4.4.5 PHENOLS

A wide array of phenolic compounds having one or more aromatic rings is reported from mushroom. Phenolic acid, flavonoids, stilbenes, lignans, and tannins comprise the phenolic component of mushrooms. These compounds are known for their antioxidant-mediated biological effects specifically antidiabetic activities. Hispidin, a prominent phenolic compound from *P. linteus*, exhibited DDPH neutralising properties and protected RINm5F rat islet cell line from H_2O_2-induced apoptotic insult. Also, hispidin stimulated insulin release from RINm5F cells.[147] Lee et

TABLE 4.4 Mushroom-Derived Antidiabetic Polymers.

Polymers	Mushroom species	Animal model in-vitro	Dose	Result	Reference
Exopolymers	*Agrocybe cylindracea*	STZ-induced diabetes in rats	50 mg/kg, for 7 days	Reduced BGL	[138]
Exo-biopolymers	*Armillariella mellea*	STZ-induced diabetes in rats	100 mg/kg/day for 2 weeks	Reduced BGL, serum cholesterol and triglyceride	[139]
Exopolymers	*Auricularia polytricha*	STZ-induced diabetes in rats	50 mg/kg for 7 days	Reduced BGL	[138]
Exo-biopolymers	*Collybia confluens*	STZ-induced diabetes in rats	100 mg/kg/day, p.o. for 3 weeks	Reduced BGL, serum cholesterol and triglyceride	[140]
Exopolymers	*C. militaris*	STZ-induced diabetes in rats	50 mg/kg for 7 days	Reduced BGL and plasma triglyerides	[138]
Exo-biopolymers	*C. sinesis*	STZ-induced diabetes in rats	100 mg/kg/day for 2 weeks	Reduced BGL, serum cholesterol and triglyceride	[139]
Exo-biopolymers	*Coriolus versicolor*	STZ-induced diabetes in rats	100 mg/kg/day for 2 weeks	Reduced BGL, serum cholesterol and triglyceride	[139]
Exo-biopolymers	*Fomes fomentarius*	STZ-induced diabetes in rats	100 mg/kg/day for 2 weeks	Reduced BGL, serum cholesterol and triglyceride	[139]
Exo-biopolymers	*Ganoderma applanatum*	STZ-induced diabetes in rats	100 mg/kg/day, p.o. for 3 weeks	Reduced BGL, serum cholesterol and triglyceride	[140]
Exopolymers	*L. edodes*	STZ-induced diabetes in rats	50 mg/kg for 7 days	Reduced BGL and plasma triglyerides	[138]
Exopolymer (composed of glycoprotein, carbohydrate and protein)	*L. edodes*	STZ-induced diabetes in rats	50–200 mg/kg/day, p.o. for 7 days	Lowered BGL; increased serum insulin concentration; Reduced serum triglycerides and cholesterol	[141]

TABLE 4.4 *(Continued)*

Polymers	Mushroom species	Animal model in-vitro	Dose	Result	Reference
Exo-biopolymers	*Paecilomyces japonica*	STZ-induced diabetes in rats	100 mg/kg/day for 2 weeks	Reduced BGL, serum cholesterol and triglyceride	[139]
Exopolymers	*P. linteus*	STZ-induced diabetes in rats	50 mg/kg for 7 days	Reduced BGL	[138]

TABLE 4.5 Mushroom-Derived Antidiabetic Terpenoids.

Compound	Mushroom species	In-vitro/In-vivo assay	Dose	Result	Reference
25R-antcin K, dehydrosulphurenic acid, 25S-antcin B, dehydroeburicoic acid, eburicoic acid	*Antrodia cinnamomea*	In-vitro α-glycosidase inhibition	EC_{50} 0.054, 0.025, 0.21, 0.018 and 0.012 mg/mL, respectively	Inhibited enzyme activity	[144]
Ganoleuconin M, ganoleuconin N, Ganoleuconin P	*Ganoderma leucocontextum*	In-vitro α-glycosidase inhibition	IC_{50} 13.6, 2.5, and 5.9 μM	Inhibited enzyme activity	[57]
Caputmedusin A	*Hericium caput-medusae*	In-vitro α-glycosidase inhibition	IC_{50} 39.2 μM	Inhibited enzyme activity	[145]
Caputmedusin B	*Hericium caput-medusae*	In-vitro α-glycosidase inhibition	IC_{50} 36.2 μM	Inhibited enzyme activity	[145]
Caputmedusin C	*Hericium caput-medusae*	In-vitro α-glycosidase inhibition	IC_{50} 40.8 μM	Inhibited enzyme activity	[145]
Poricoic acid M, polyporenic acid C, eburicoic acid acetate, pinicolic acid E, poricoic acid D	*Wolfiporia cocos*	In-vitro glucose uptake stimulating effects in 3T3-L1 adipocytes cells	2.5 μM	Increased the insulin-stimulated glucose uptake	[79]
Alkaline-insoluble fraction comprised of dehydroeburiconic acid, dehydrotrametenolic acid, eburicoic acid, and trematenolic acid	*Mushroom Wolfiporia cocos*	High-fat-diet-induced obese mice	50 and 100 mg/kg, p.o. for 8 weeks	Reduced BGL and glycosylated hemoglobin A1c; improved glucose tolerance and insulin resistance; decreased serum triglyceride and total cholesterol	[79]
Dehydrotumulosic acid, dehydrotrametenolic acid, and pachymic acid	*Poria cocos*	STZ-induced diabetes in mice	1, 5 and 10 mg/kg	Insulin mediated reduction in BGL	[146]

al.[148] demonstrated the aldose reductase inhibitory effects of hispidin and thereby, suggesting the possible use of hispidin in diabetic and related complications.[148] Advanced glycation end products (hemoglobin A1C formation) are one of the hallmark pathological features of diabetes. Higher levels of advanced glycation end products activated nuclear factor-kappa B and initiate inflammatory and oxidative stress pathways leading to diabetic and associated complications. In search of protein glycation inhibitors, Lee et al.[149] isolated nine phenolic acids protocatechuic acid, protocatechualdehyde, caffeic acid, ellagic acid, hispidin, davallialactone, hypholomine B, interfungins A, and inoscavin A, with IC_{50} ranging from 144.28 to 1089 μM, isolated from *P. linteus* as protein glycation inhibitors.[149] Huang et al.[150] identified hispidin (IC_{50} 297.06 μg/mL), hispolon (IC_{50} 12.38 μg/mL) and inotilone (IC_{50} 18.62 μg/mL) as α-glucosidase inhibitors from *Phellinus merrillii* fruiting bodies.[150] Erinacenols D (IC_{50} 19.6 μM), 4-[3′,7′-dimethyl-2′,6′-octadienyl]-2-formyl-3-hydroxy-5-methyoxybenzylalcohol (IC_{50} 7.5 μM), hericene A (IC_{50} 6.7 μM), hericene D (IC_{50} 3.9 μM) and hericene D(IC_{50} 15.5 μM) from *H. erinaceus* exhibited strong α-glucosidase inhibitory effects.[151] Figure 4.3 summarizes the effects displayed by mushrooms species in experimental models.

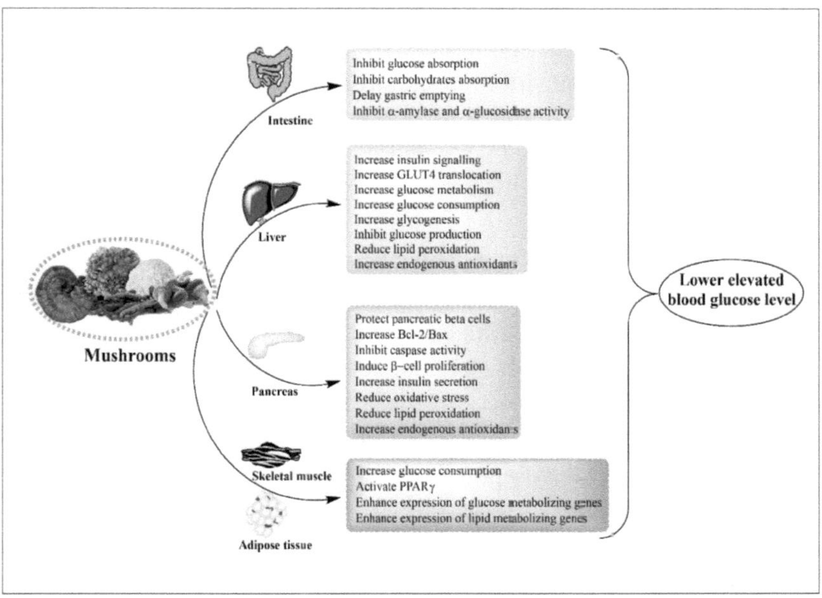

FIGURE 4.3 How mushrooms help to lower BGLs.

4.5 FUTURE DIRECTIONS

It is evident from the above review that many mushrooms and mushroom-derived products have strong antidiabetic potential in experimental models and preclinical studies. Hence their use for managing elevated blood sugar in traditional medicine is getting scientific support. Some known compounds (e.g., ellagic acid, hispidin, α-glucan, etc.), some novel constituents (ganoderans, ganoleuconins, caputmedusins, poricoic acid, etc.) and extracts/fractions have displayed marked antidiabetic activity. Some mechanisms have been elucidated, some need to be explored and in some fractions, synergistic effects are evident.

There is a multitude of investigations on mushrooms but why are not drugs derived from mushrooms available clinically? To make this possible and develop nutraceutical and/or pharmaceutical antidiabetic formulations from mushrooms, according to the authors the following need to be done:

- Since only about 10% of mushrooms species have been scientifically examined thus other genera/ species should be explored. This might yield novel and potent compounds.
- In order to ensure uniformity of content and a sustainable supply of the raw material, cultivation of bioactive mushrooms should be taken up.
- Biotechnology may be used to enhance biomass yield and secondary metabolite production in mushroom cultures.
- Processing of mushrooms should follow a standardized protocol to assure reproducibility thus making the extraction/isolation procedures commercially viable and dependable.
- Environment friendly—"Green" or solvent free extraction techniques maybe used.
- Quality control and standardization of bioactive mushroom extracts/ fractions/compounds shall ensure quality and stability of the products.
- Comprehensive pharmacological studies to confirm efficacy, mechanisms of action, targets, dosage, and toxicity.
- Systematic, placebo-controlled randomized clinical trials should further substantiate basic research and preclinical outcomes.
- Formulation development—including targeting and sustained delivery systems.
- Increased interface of academia, mushroom farmers, and pharmaceutical industry for technology transfer and development of commercially viable antidiabetic products.

The journey from raw state to commercial product is summarized in Figure 4.4.

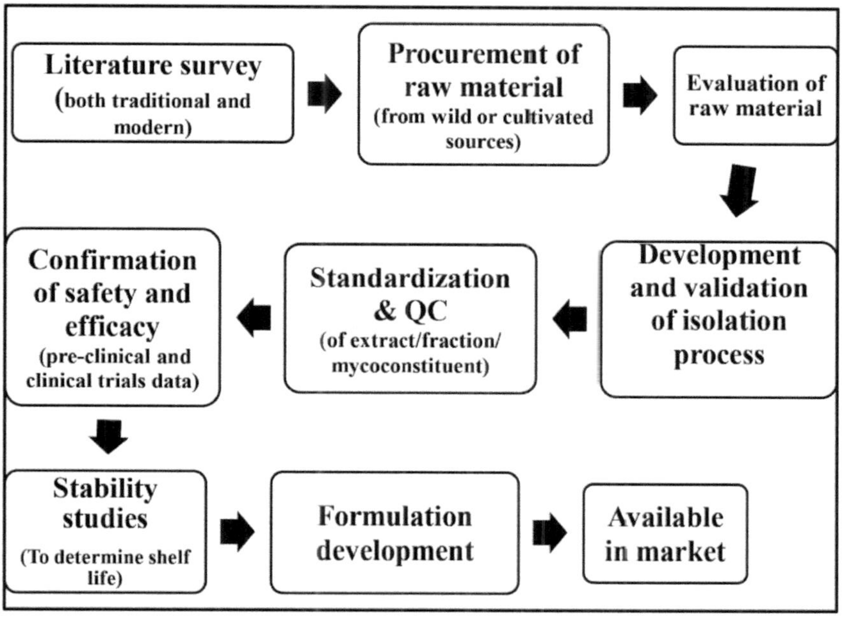

FIGURE 4.4 Drug development from mushrooms.

The aim is to understand nature, explore it judiciously, and develop mushroom derived drugs to bring relief to the millions afflicted with diabetes mellitus.

KEYWORDS

- **antidiabetic agents**
- **mushrooms**
- **mycoconstituents**
- **toxicity**
- **pharmacology**

REFERENCES

1. Rahi, D. K.; Malik, D. Diversity of Mushrooms and Their Metabolites of Nutraceutical and Therapeutic Significance. *J. Mycol.* **2016**. https://doi.org/10.1155/2016/7654123
2. Valverde, M. E.; Hernández-Pérez, T; Paredes-López, O. Edible Mushrooms: Improving Human Health and Promoting Quality Life. *Int. J. Microbiol.* **2015,** 1–14. https://doi.org/10.1155/2015/376387
3. Rizzo, G.; Goggi, S.; Giampieri, F.; Baroni, L. A Review of Mushrooms in Human Nutrition and Health. *Trends Food Sci. Technol.* **2021**. doi: 10.1016/j.tifs.2020.12.025.
4. Chowdhury, P.; Paul, S. The Potential Role of Mushrooms in the Prevention and Treatment of Diabetes: A Review. *J. Biol. Act. Prod. Nat.* **2020,** *10* (5), 429–454.
5. Antunes, F; Marçal, S; Taofiq, O; Morais, A; Freitas, A. C; Ferreira, I; Pintado, M. Valorization of Mushroom By-products as a Source of Value-added Compounds and Potential Applications. *Molecules* **2020,** *25* (11), 2672.
6. Mahari, W. A. W.; Peng, W.; Nam, W. L.; Yang, H.; Lee, X. Y.; Lee, Y. K.; Liew, R. K.; Ma, N. L.; Mohammad, A.; Sonne, C; Van Le, Q. A Review on Valorization of Oyster Mushroom and Waste Generated in the Mushroom Cultivation Industry. *J. Hazard. Mater.* **2020,** *400*, 123156.
7. Kalač, P. A Review of Chemical Composition and Nutritional Value of Wild-growing and Cultivated Mushrooms. *J. Sci. Food Agric.* **2013,** *93* (2), 209–218.
8. Islam, T.; Ganesan, K.; Xu, B. B. New Insight into Mycochemical Profiles and Antioxidant Potential of Edible and Medicinal Mushrooms: A Review. *Int. J. Med. Mushrooms* **2019,** *21* (3), 237–251.
9. Lu, H.; Lou, H.; Hu, J.; Liu, Z.; Chen, Q. Macrofungi: A Review of Cultivation Strategies, Bioactivity, and Application of Mushrooms. *Compr. Rev. Food Sci. Food Saf.* **2020,** *19* (5), 2333–2356.
10. Chaturvedi, V. K.; Agarwal, S.; Gupta, K. K.; Ramteke, P. W.; Singh, M. P. Medicinal Mushroom: Boon for Therapeutic Applications. *3 Biotech* **2018,** *8* (8), 1–20.
11. Chowdhury, P.; Paul, S. The Potential Role of Mushrooms in the Prevention and Treatment of Diabetes: A Review. *J. Biol. Act. Prod. Nat.* **2020,** *10* (5), 429–454.
12. Yadav, S. K.; Ir, R.; Jeewon, R.; Doble, M.; Hyde, K. D.; Kaliappan, I.; Jeyaraman, R.; Reddi, R. N.; Krishnan, J.; Li, M.; Durairajan, S. S. A Mechanistic Review on Medicinal Mushrooms-derived Bioactive Compounds: Potential Mycotherapy Candidates for Alleviating Neurological Disorders. *Planta Med.* **2020,** *86*, 1161–1175.
13. Martel, J.; Ojcius, D. M.; Chang, C. J.; Lin, C. S.; Lu, C. C.; Ko, Y. F.; Tseng, S. F.; Lai, H. C.; Young, J. D. Anti-obesogenic and Antidiabetic Effects of Plants and Mushrooms. *Nat. Rev. Endocrinol.* **2017,** *13* (3), 149–160.
14. Khursheed, R.; Singh, S. K.; Wadhwa, S.; Gulati, M.; Awasthi, A. Therapeutic Potential of Mushrooms in Diabetes Mellitus: Role of Polysaccharides. *Int. J. Biol. Macromol.* **2020,** *164*, 1194–1205.
15. Stojkovic, D.; Smiljkovic, M.; Ciric, A.; Glamoclija, J.; Van Griensven, L.; Ferreira, I. C.; Sokovic, M. An Insight into Antidiabetic Properties of Six Medicinal and Edible Mushrooms: Inhibition of α-Amylase and α-Glucosidase Linked to Type-2 Diabetes. *S. Afr. J. Bot.* **2019,** *120*, 100–103.

16. Wu, T.; Xu, B. Antidiabetic and Antioxidant Activities of Eight Medicinal Mushroom Species from China. *Int. J. Med. Mushrooms* **2015,** *17*, 129–140.
17. Ogbole, O. O.; Nkumah, A. O.; Linus, A. U.; Falade, M. O Molecular Identification, in Vivo and *in Vitro* Activities of *Calvatia gigantea* (Macro-fungus) as an Antidiabetic Agent. *Mycology* **2019,** *10* (3), 166–173.
18. Choi, S. B.; Park, C. H.; Choi, M. K.; Jun, D. W.; Park, S. Improvement of Insulin Resistance and Insulin Secretion by Water Extracts of *Cordyceps militaris*, *Phellinus linteus*, and *Paecilomyces tenuipes* in 90% Pancreatectomized Rats. *Biosci. Biotechnol. Biochem.* **2004,** *68* (11), 2257–2264.
19. Liu C, Song J, Teng M, Zheng X, Li X, Tian Y, et al. Antidiabetic and Antinephritic Activities of Aqueous Extract of *Cordyceps militaris* Fruit Body in Diet-streptozotocin-induced Diabetic Sprague Dawley Rats. *Oxid. Med. Cell Longev.* **2016,** *2016*, 9685257.
20. Chen, S. D.; Yong, T. Q.; Zhang, Y. F.; Hu, H. P.; Xie, Y. Z. Inhibitory Effect of Five *Ganoderma* Species (Agaricomycetes) against Key Digestive Enzymes Related to Type 2 Diabetes Mellitus. *Int. J. Med. Mushrooms* **2019,** *21* (7), 703–711.
21. Sarker, M. M. R. Antihyperglycemic, Insulin-sensitivity and Anti-hyperlipidemic Potential of *Ganoderma lucidum*, a Dietary Mushroom, on Alloxan- and Glucocorticoid-induced Diabetic Long-Evans Rats. *Funct. Foods Heal. Dis.* **2015,** *5* (12), 450–466.
22. Seto, S. W.; Lam, T. Y.; Tam, H. L.; Au, A. L. S.; Chan, S. W.; Wu, J. H.; Yu, P. H. F.; Leung, G. P. H.; Ngai, S. M.; Yeung, J. H.; Leung, P. S. Novel Hypoglycemic Effects of *Ganoderma lucidum* Water-extract in Obese/Diabetic (+db/+db) Mice. *Phytomedicine* **2009,** *16* (5), 426–436.
23. Ratnaningtyas, N. I.; Hernayanti, H.; Andarwanti, S.; Ekowati, N.; Purwanti, E. S.; Sukmawati, D. Effects of *Ganoderma lucidum* Extract on Diabetic Rats. *Biosaintif. J. Biol. Biol. Educ.* **2018,** *10* (3), 642–647.
24. Bach, E. E.; Hi, E. M. B.; Martins, A. M. C.; Nascimento, P. A. M.; Wadt, N. S. Y. Hypoglicemic and Hypolipedimic Effects of *Ganoderma lucidum* in Streptozotocin-induced Diabetic Rats. *Medicines* **2018,** *5* (3), 78.
25. Nyam, K. L.; Chow, C. F.; Tan, C. S.; Ng, S. T. Antidiabetic Properties of the Tiger's Milk Medicinal Mushroom, *Lignosus rhinocerotis* (Agaricomycetes), in Streptozotocin-induced Diabetic Rats. *Int. J. Med. Mushrooms* **2017,** *19* (7), 607–617.
26. Zheng, S.; Deng, S.; Huang, Y.; Huang, M.; Zhao, P.; Ma, X.; Wen, Y.; Wang, Q.; Yang, X. Anti-diabetic Activity of a Polyphenol-rich Extract from *Phellinus igniarius* in KK-Ay Mice with Spontaneous Type 2 Diabetes Mellitus. *Food Funct.* **2018,** *9* (1), 614–623.
27. Liu, Y.; Wang, C.; Li, J.; Mei., Y.; Liang, Y. Hypoglycemic and Hypolipidemic Effects of *Phellinus Linteus* Mycelial Extract from Solid-state Culture in a Rat Model of Type 2 Diabetes. *Nutrients* **2019,** *11* (2), 296.
28. Dubey, S.; Yadav, C.; Bajpeyee, A.; Singh, M. P. Effect of *Pleurotus fossulatus* Aqueous Extract on Biochemical Properties of Liver and Kidney in Streptozotocin-induced Diabetic Rat. *Diabetes, Metab. Syndr. Obes. Targets Ther.* **2020,** *13*, 3035.
29. Singh, V.; Bedi, G. K; Shri, R. *In vitro* and in Vivo Antidiabetic Evaluation of Selected Culinary-medicinal Mushrooms (Agaricomycetes). *Int. J. Med. Mushrooms* **2017,** *19* (1), 17–25.

30. Kaur, A.; Dhingra, G. S.; Shri, R. Evaluation of Carbohydrate Metabolism Inhibition by Some Species of Medicinal Mushrooms from India. *Int. J. Med. Mushrooms* **2005,** *17* (4), 351–360.
31. Karunarathna, S. C.; Chen, J.; Mortimer, P. E.; Xu, J. C.; Zhao, R. L.; Callac, P.; Hyde, K. D. Mycosphere Essay 8: A Review of Genus *Agaricus* in Tropical and Humid Subtropical Regions of Asia. *Mycosphere* **2016,** *7* (4), 417–439.
32. Mao, Y.; Mao, J.; Meng, X. Extraction Optimization and Bioactivity of Exopolysaccharides from *Agaricus bisporus*. *Carbohydr. Polym.* **2013,** *92* (2), 1602–1607.
33. Bhushan, A.; Kulshreshtha, M. The Medicinal Mushroom *Agaricus bisporus*: Review of Phytopharmacology and Potential Role in the Treatment of Various Diseases. *J. Nat. Sci. Med.* **2018,** *1* (1), 4–9.
34. Jeong, S. C.; Jeong, Y. T.; Yang, B. K.; Islam, R.; Koyyalamudi, S. R.; Pang, G.; Cho, K. Y.; Song, C. H. White Button Mushroom (*Agaricus bisporus*) Lowers Blood Glucose and Cholesterol Levels in Diabetic and Hypercholesterolemic Rats. *Nutr. Res.* **2010,** *30* (1), 49–56.
35. Zaid, O. A. R. A.; Sonbaty, S. E. L.; Hamam, M. A. Anti-diabetic Activity of *Agaricus bisporus*: A Biochemical and Pathological Study. *Int. J. Pharm. Sci.* **2017,** *7*, 1740–1745.
36. Ekowati, N.; Yuniati, N. I.; Hernayant, H.; Ratnaningtyas, N. I. Antidiabetic Potentials of Button Mushroom (*Agaricus bisporus*) on Alloxan-induced Diabetic Rats. *J. Biol. Biol. Educ.* **2018,** *10* (3), 655–662.
37. Cristine da Silva de Souza, A.; Gesser, C. V.; de Almeida, G. G.; Assuncao, S. A.; Bracht, A.; Marina, P. R. *Agaricus blazei* Bioactive Compounds and Their Effects on Human Health: Benefits and Controversies. *Curr. Pharm. Des.* **2017,** *23* (19), 2807–2834.
38. Firenzuoli, F.; Gori, L.; Lombardo, G. The Medicinal Mushroom *Agaricus blazei* Murrill: Review of Literature and Pharmaco-toxicological Problems. *Evid.-Based Complement. Altern. Med.* **2008,** *5* (1), 3–15.
39. Kim, Y. W.; Kim, K. H.; Choi, H. J.; Lee, D. S. Anti-diabetic Activity of β-Glucans and Their Enzymatically Hydrolyzed Oligosaccharides from *Agaricus blazei*. *Biotechnol. Lett.* **2005,** *27* (7), 483–487.
40. Oh, T. W.; Kim, Y. A.; Jang, W. J.; Byeon, J. I.; Ryu, C. H.; Kim, J. O.; Ha, Y. L. Semipurified Fractions from the Submerged-culture Broth of *Agaricus blazei* Murill Reduce Blood Glucose Levels in Streptozotocin-induced Diabetic Rats. *J. Agric. Food Chem.* **2010,** *58* (7), 4113–4119.
41. Wei, Q.; Zhan, Y.; Chen, B.; Xie, B.; Fang, T.; Ravishankar, S.; Jiang, Y. Assessment of Antioxidant and Antidiabetic Properties of *Agaricus blazei* Murill Extracts. *Food Sci. Nutr.* **2020,** *8* (1), 332–339.
42. Gray, A. M.; Flatt, P. R. Insulin-releasing and Insulin-like Activity of *Agaricus campestris* (Mushroom). *J. Endocrinol.* **1998,** *157* (2), 259–266.
43. Chen, P. X.; Wang, S.; Nie, S.; Marcone, M. Properties of *Cordyceps sinensis*: A Review. *J. Funct. Foods* **2013,** *5* (2), 550–569.
44. Shashidhar, M. G.; Giridhar, P.; Sankar, K. U.; Manohar, B. Bioactive Principles from *Cordyceps sinensis*: A Potent Food Supplement—A Review. *J. Funct. Foods* **2013,** *5* (3), 1013–1030.

45. Lo, H. C.; Tu, S. T.; Lin, K. C.; Lin, S. C. The Anti-hyperglycemic Activity of the Fruiting Body of *Cordyceps* in Diabetic Rats Induced by Nicotinamide and Streptozotocin. *Life Sci.* **2004,** *74* (23), 2897–2908.
46. Lo, H. C.; Hsu, T. H.; Tu, S. T.; Lin, K. C. Anti-hyperglycemic Activity of Natural and Fermented *Cordyceps sinensis* in Rats with Diabetes Induced by Nicotinamide and Streptozotocin. *Am. J. Chin. Med.* **2006,** *34* (5), 819–832.
47. Zhang, G.; Huang, Y.; Bian, Y.; Wong, J. H.; Ng, T. B.; Wang, H. Hypoglycemic Activity of the Fungi *Cordyceps militaris*, *Cordyceps sinensis*, *Tricholoma mongolicum*, and *Omphalia lapidescens* in Streptozotocin-induced Diabetic Rats. *Appl. Microbiol. Biotechnol.* **2006,** *72* (6), 1152–1156.
48. Kan, W. C.; Wang, H. Y.; Chien, C. C.; Li, S. L.; Chen, Y. C.; Chang, L. H.; Cheng, C. H.; Tsai, W. C.; Hwang, J. C.; Su, S. B.; Huang, L. H. Effects of Extract from Solid-state Fermented *Cordyceps sinensis* on Type 2 Diabetes Mellitus. *Evid.-Based Complement. Altern. Med.* **2012,** *2012*, 743107.
49. Kiho, T.; Hui, J. I.; Yamane, A.; Ukai, S. Polysaccharides in Fungi. XXXII. Hypoglycemic Activity and Chemical Properties of a Polysaccharide from the Cultural Mycelium of *Cordyceps sinensis*. *Biol. Pharm. Bull.* **1993,** *16* (12), 1291–1293.
50. Balon, T. W.; Jasman, A. P.; Zhu, J. S. A Fermentation Product of *Cordyceps sinensis* Increases Whole-body Insulin Sensitivity in Rats. *J. Altern. Complement. Med.* **2002,** *8* (3), 315–323.
51. Chiu, C. P.; Hwang, T. L.; Chan, Y.; El-Shazly, M.; Wu, T. Y.; Lo, I. W.; Hsu, Y. M.; Lai, K. H.; Hou, M. F.; Yuan, S. S.; Chang, F. Research and Development of *Cordyceps* in Taiwan. *Food Sci. Hum. Wellness* **2016,** *5* (4), 177–185.
52. Chu, H. L.; Chien, J. C.; Duh, P. D. Protective Effect of *Cordyceps militaris* against High Glucose-induced Oxidative Stress in Human Umbilical Vein Endothelial Cells. *Food Chem.* **2011,** *129* (3), 871–876.
53. Cheng, Y. W.; Chen, Y. I.; Tzeng, C. Y.; Chen, H. C.; Tsai, C. C.; Lee, Y. C.; Lin, J. G.; Lai, Y. K.; Chang, S. L. Extracts of *Cordyceps militaris* Lower Blood Glucose Via the Stimulation of Cholinergic Activation and Insulin Secretion in Normal Rats. *Phyther. Res.* **2012,** *26* (8), 1173–1177.
54. Yu, S. H.; Chen, S. Y. T.; Li, W. S.; Dubey, N. K.; Chen, W. H.; Chuu, J. J.; Leu, S. J.; Deng, W. P. Hypoglycemic Activity through a Novel Combination of Fruiting Body and Mycelia of *Cordyceps militaris* in High-fat Diet-induced Type 2 Diabetes Mellitus Mice. *J. Diabetes Res.* **2015,** *2015*, 723190.
55. Dong, Y.; Jing, T.; Meng, Q.; Liu, C.; Hu, S.; Ma, Y.; Liu, Y.; Lu, J.; Cheng, Y.; Wang, D.; Teng, L. Studies on the Antidiabetic Activities of *Cordyceps militaris* Extract in Diet-streptozotocin-induced Diabetic Sprague-Dawley Rats. *Biomed. Res. Int.* **2014,** *2014*, 160980.
56. Kim, D. J.; Kang, Y. H.; Kim, K. K.; Kim, T. W.; Park, J. B.; Choe, M. Increased Glucose Metabolism and Alpha-glucosidase Inhibition in *Cordyceps militaris* Water Extract-treated HepG2 Cells. *Nutr. Res. Pract.* **2017,** *11* (3), 180–189.
57. Wang, K.; Bao, L.; Xiong, W.; Ma, K.; Han, J.; Wang, W.; Yin, W.; Liu, H. Lanostane Triterpenes from the Tibetan Medicinal Mushroom *Ganoderma leucocontextum* and Their Inhibitory Effects on HMG-CoA Reductase and α-Glucosidase. *J. Nat. Prod.* **2015,** *78* (8), 1977–1989.

58. Okazaki, M.; Tanaka, A.; Hatta, Y.; Kawahara, Y.; Kamiuchi, S.; Iwata, N.; Asano, S.; Suzuki, F.; Iizuka, H.; Hibino, Y. Antioxidant Properties of a Water-soluble Extract from Culture Medium of *Ganoderma lucidum* (Rei-shi) Mycelia and Antidiabetic Effects in Streptozotocin-treated Mice. *Jpn. J. Complement. Altern. Med.* **2008,** *5* (3), 209–218.
59. Li, F.; Zhang, Y.; Zhong, Z. Antihyperglycemic Effect of *Ganoderma lucidum* Polysaccharides on Streptozotocin-induced Diabetic Mice. *Int. J. Mol. Sci.* **2011,** *12* (9), 6135–6145.
60. Teng, B. S.; Wang, C. D.; Zhang, D.; Wu, J. S.; Pan, D.; Pan, L. F.; Yang, H. J.; Zhou, P. Hypoglycemic Effect and Mechanism of a Proteoglycan from *Ganoderma lucidum* on Streptozotocin-induced Type 2 Diabetic Rats. *Eur. Rev. Med. Pharmacol. Sci.* **2012,** *16*, 166–175.
61. Cho, J. Y.; Sadiq, N. B.; Kim, J. C.; Lee, B.; Hamayun, M.; Lee, T. S.; Kim, H. S.; Park, S. H.; Nho, C. W.; Kim, H. Y. Optimization of Antioxidant, Anti-diabetic, and Anti-inflammatory Activities and Ganoderic Acid Content of Differentially Dried *Ganoderma lucidum* Using Response Surface Methodology. *Food Chem.* **2021,** *335*, 127645.
62. Jiang, Y.; Wu, N.; Fu, Y. J.; Wang, W.; Luo, M.; Zhao, C. J.; Zu, Y. G.; Liu, X. L. Chemical Composition and Antimicrobial Activity of the Essential Oil of Rosemary. *Environ. Toxicol. Pharmacol.* **2011,** *32* (1), 63–68.
63. Lee, W. Y.; Park, Y.; Ahn, J. K.; Ka, K. H.; Park, S. Y. Factors Influencing the Production of Endopolysaccharide and Exopolysaccharide from *Ganoderma applanatum*. *Enzyme Microb. Technol.* **2007,** *40* (2), 249–254.
64. Jung, S. H.; Lee, Y. S.; Shim, S. H.; Lee, S.; Shin, K. H.; Kim, J. S.; Kim, Y. S.; Kang, S. S. Inhibitory Effects of *Ganoderma applanatum* on Rat Lens Aldose Reductase and Sorbitol Accumulation in Streptozotocin-induced Diabetic Rat Tissues. *Phyther. Res.* **2005,** *19* (6), 477–480.
65. Costa, T. M.; Mayer, D. A.; Siebert, D. A.; Micke, G. A.; Alberton, M. D.; Tavares, L. B. B.; de Oliveira, D. Kinetics Analysis of the Inhibitory Effects of Alpha-glucosidase and Identification of Compounds from *Ganoderma lipsiense* Mycelium. *Appl. Biochem. Biotechnol.* **2020,** *191*, 1–14.
66. Rašeta, M.; Popović, M.; Čapo, I.; Stilinović, N.; Vukmirović, S.; Milošević, B.; Karaman, M. Antidiabetic Effect of Two Different *Ganoderma* Species Tested in Alloxan Diabetic Rats. *RSC Adv.* **2020,** *10* (17), 10382–10393.
67. Lu, X.; Chen, H.; Dong, P.; Fu, L.; Zhang, X. Phytochemical Characteristics and Hypoglycaemic Activity of Fraction from Mushroom *Inonotus obliquus*. *J. Sci. Food Agric.* **2010,** *90* (2), 276–280.
68. Hwang, H. J.; Kim, S. W.; Lim, J. M.; Joo, J. H.; Kim, H. O.; Kim, H. M.; Yun, J. W. Hypoglycemic Effect of Crude Exopolysaccharides Produced by a Medicinal Mushroom *Phellinus baumii* in Streptozotocin-induced Diabetic Rats. *Life Sci.* **2005,** *76* (26), 3069–3080.
69. Kim, Y. O.; Park, H. W.; Kim, J. H.; Lee, J. Y.; Moon, S. H.; Shin, C. S. Anti-cancer Effect and Structural Characterization of Endo-polysaccharide from Cultivated Mycelia of *Inonotus obliquus*. *Life Sci.* **2006,** *79* (1), 72–80.
70. Kim, H. G.; Yoon, D. H.; Kim, C. H.; Shrestha, B.; Chang, W. C.; Lim, S. Y.; Lee, W. H.; Han, S. G.; Lee, J. O.; Lim, M. H.; Kim, G. Y. Ethanol Extract of *Inonotus obliquus*

Inhibits Lipopolysaccharide-induced Inflammation in RAW 264.7 Macrophage Cells. *J. Med. Food* **2007,** *10* (1), 80–89.
71. Ko, S. K.; Jin, M.; Pyo, M. Y. *Inonotus obliquus* Extracts Suppress Antigen-specific IgE Production through the Modulation of Th1/Th2 Cytokines in Ovalbumin-sensitized Mice. *J. Ethnopharmacol.* **2011,** *137* (3), 1077–1082.
72. Saar, M. Fungi in Khanty Folk Medicine. *J. Ethnopharmacol.* **1991,** *31* (2), 175–179.
73. Cui, Y.; Kim, D. S.; Park, K. C. Antioxidant Effect of *Inonotus obliquus*. *J. Ethnopharmacol.* **2005,** *96* (1–2), 79–85.
74. Rhee, S. J.; Cho, S. Y.; Kim, K. M.; Cha, D. S.; Park, H. J. A Comparative Study of Analytical Methods for Alkali-soluble β-Glucan in Medicinal Mushroom, Chaga (*Inonotus obliquus*). *LWT—Food Sci. Technol.* **2008,** *41* (3), 545–549.
75. Duru, K. C.; Kovaleva, E. G.; Danilova, I. G.; van der Bijl, P. The Pharmacological Potential and Possible Molecular Mechanisms of Action of *Inonotus obliquus* from Preclinical Studies. *Phyther. Res.* **2019,** *33* (8), 1966–1980.
76. Cha, J. Y.; Jun, B. S.; Yoo, K. S.; Hahm, J. R.; Cho, Y. S. Fermented Chaga Mushroom (*Inonotus obliquus*) Effects on Hypolipidemia and Hepatoprotection in Otsuka Long-Evans Tokushima Fatty (OLETF) Rats. *Food Sci. Biotechnol.* **2006,** *15* (1), 122–127.
77. Sun, J. E.; Ao, Z. H.; Lu, Z. M.; Xu, H. Y.; Zhang, X. M.; Dou, W. F.; Xu, Z. H. Antihyperglycemic and Antilipidperoxidative Effects of Dry Matter of Culture Broth of *Inonotus obliquus* in Submerged Culture on Normal and Alloxan-diabetes Mice. *J. Ethnopharmacol.* **2008,** *118* (1), 7–13.
78. Chen, H.; Tian, T.; Miao, H.; Zhao, Y. Y. Traditional Uses, Fermentation, Phytochemistry and Pharmacology of *Phellinus linteus*: A Review. *Fitoterapia* **2016,** *113*, 6–26.
79. Chen, B.; Zhang, J.; Han, J.; Zhao, R.; Bao, L.; Huang, Y.; Liu, H. Lanostane Triterpenoids with Glucose-uptake-stimulatory Activity from Peels of the Cultivated Edible Mushroom *Wolfiporia cocos*. *J. Agric. Food Chem.* **2019,** *67* (26), 7348–7364.
80. Kim, H. M.; Kang, J. S.; Kim, J. Y.; Park, S. K.; Kim, H. S.; Lee, Y. J.; Yun, J.; Hong, J. T.; Kim, Y.; Han, S. B. Evaluation of Antidiabetic Activity of Polysaccharide Isolated from *Phellinus linteus* in Non-obese Diabetic Mouse. *Int. Immunopharmacol.* **2010,** *10* (1), 72–78.
81. Patel, Y.; Naraian, R.; Singh, V. K. Medicinal Properties of *Pleurotus* Species (Oyster Mushroom): A Review. *World J. Fung. Plant Biol.* **2012,** *3* (1), 1–12.
82. Kapahi, M.; Sachdeva, S. Mycoremediation Potential of *Pleurotus* Species for Heavy Metals: A Review. *Bioresour. Bioprocess.* **2017,** *4* (1), 1–9.
83. Corrêa, R. C. G.; Brugnari, T.; Bracht, A.; Peralta, R. M.; Ferreira, I. C. Biotechnological, Nutritional and Therapeutic Uses of *Pleurotus* spp. (Oyster Mushroom) Related with Its Chemical Composition: A Review on the Past Decade Findings. *Trends Food Sci. Technol.* **2017,** *50*, 103–117.
84. Barh, A.; Sharma, V. P.; Annepu, S. K.; Kamal, S.; Sharma, S.; Bhatt, P. Genetic Improvement in *Pleurotus* (Oyster Mushroom): A Review. *3 Biotech* **2019,** *9* (9), 1–14.
85. Ravi, B.; Renitta, R. E.; Prabha, M. L.; Issac, R.; Naidu, S. Evaluation of Antidiabetic Potential of Oyster Mushroom (*Pleurotus ostreatus*) in Alloxan-induced Diabetic Mice. *Immunopharmacol. Immunotoxicol.* **2013,** *35* (1), 101–109.

86. Johnny, I.; Okon, J. Antidiabetic Effect of *Pleurotus ostreatus* (Jacq. ex Fr) Kumm. Mushroom on Alloxan-induced Diabetic Rats. *Indian J. Pharm. Biol. Res.* **2013,** *1* (02), 31–36.
87. Sangi, S. M. A.; Bawadekji, A.; Al Ali, M. Comparative Effects of Metformin, *Pleurotus ostreatus*, *Nigella sativa*, and *Zingiber officinale* on the Streptozotocin-Induced Diabetes Mellitus in Rats. *Pharmacogn. Mag.* **2018,** *14* (55), 268.
88. Ghaly, I. S.; Ahmed, E. S.; Booles, H. F.; Farag, I. M.; Nada, S. A. Evaluation of Antihyperglycemic Action of Oyster Mushroom (*Pleurotus ostreatus*) and Its Effect on DNA Damage, Chromosome Aberrations and Sperm Abnormalities in Streptozotocin-induced Diabetic Rats. *Glob. Vet.* **2011,** *7* (6), 532–544.
89. Balaji, P.; Madhanraj, R. Rameshkumar, K.; Veeramanikandan, V.; Eyini, M.; Arun, A.; Thulasinathan, B.; Al Farraj, D. A.; Elshikh, M. S.; Alokda, A. M.; Mahmoud, A. H.; Evaluation of Antidiabetic Activity of *Pleurotus pulmonarius* against Streptozotocin-nicotinamide Induced Diabetic Wistar Albino Rats. *Saudi J. Biol. Sci.* **2020,** *27* (3), 913–924.
90. Ng, S. H.; Mohd Zain, M. S.; Zakaria, F.; Wan Ishak, W. R.; Wan Ahmad, W. A. N. Hypoglycemic and Antidiabetic Effect of *Pleurotus sajor-caju* Aqueous Extract in Normal and Streptozotocin-induced Diabetic Rats. *Biomed. Res. Int.* **2015,** 214918. https://doi.org/10.1155/2015/214918
91. Prabu, M.; Kumuthakalavalli, R. Antidiabetic Potential of the Oyster Mushroom *Pleurotus florida* (Mont.) Singer. *Int. J. Curr. Pharm. Res.* **2017,** *9* (4), 51–54.
92. Onuekwuzu, I. M.; Chidinma, I. C.; Chigozie, I. J. Anti-diabetic Effect of a Flavonoid and Sitosterol-rich Aqueous Extract of *Pleurotus tuberregium* Sclerotia in Alloxan-induced Diabetic Rabbits. *Endocrine, Metab. Immune Disord. Targets* **2019,** *19* (8), 1148–1156.
93. Ma, G.; Yang, W.; Zhao, L.; Pei, F.; Fang, D.; Hu, Q. A Critical Review on the Health Promoting Effects of Mushrooms Nutraceuticals. *Food Sci. Hum. Wellness* **2018,** *7* (2), 125–133.
94. Cassano, R.; Mellace, S.; Trombino, S. Responsive Polymer-biomacromolecule Conjugates for Drug Delivery. In *Stimuli Responsive Polymeric Nanocarriers for Drug Delivery Applications*; Makhlouf, A. S. H., Ed.; Woodhead Publishing: Sawston, United Kingdom, 2018; pp 433–452.
95. Sari, M.; Prange, A.; Lelley, J. I.; Hambitzer, R. Screening of Beta-glucan Contents in Commercially Cultivated and Wild Growing Mushrooms. *Food Chem.* **2017,** *216*, 45–51.
96. Yang, J. P.; Hsu, T.; Lin, F.; Hsu, W.; Chen, Y. Potential Antidiabetic Activity of Extracellular Polysaccharides in Submerged Fermentation Culture of *Coriolus versicolor* LH1. *Carbohydr. Polym.* **2012,** *90* (1), 174–180.
97. Hsu, W. K.; Hsu, T. H.; Lin, F. Y.; Cheng, Y. K.; Yang, J. P. W. Separation, Purification, and α-Glucosidase Inhibition of Polysaccharides from *Coriolus versicolor* LH1 Mycelia. *Carbohydr. Polym.* **2013,** *92* (1), 297–306.
98. Kaewnarin, K.; Suwannarach, N.; Kumla, J.; Choonpicharn, S.; Tanreuan, K.; Lumyong, S. Characterization of Polysaccharides from Wild Edible Mushrooms from Thailand and Their Antioxidant, Antidiabetic, and Antihypertensive Activities. *Int. J. Med. Mushrooms* **2020,** *22* (3), 221–233.

99. Zheng, X.; Sun, H.; Wu, L.; Kong, X.; Song, Q.; Zhu, Z. Structural Characterization and Inhibition on α-Glucosidase of the Polysaccharides from Fruiting Bodies and Mycelia of *Pleurotus eryngii*. *Int. J. Biol. Macromol.* **2020,** *156*, 1512–1519.
100. Gong, L. L.; Meng, F. J. Hou, Y. C.; Liu, Y.; Xu, J. J.; Zhang, W. N.; Chen, Y. Purification, Characterization, and Bioactivity of Two New Polysaccharide Fractions from *Thelephora ganbajun* Mushroom. *J. Food Biochem.* **2020,** *44* (1), e13092.
101. Yamac, M.; Zeytinoglu, M.; Kanbak, G.; Bayramoglu, G.; Senturk, H. Hypoglycemic Effect of Crude Exopolysaccharides Produced by *Cerrena unicolor*, *Coprinus comatus*, and *Lenzites betulina* Isolates in Streptozotocin-induced Diabetic Rats. *Pharm. Biol.* **2009,** *47* (2), 168–174.
102. Cao, H.; Ma, S.; Guo, H.; Cui, X.; Wang, S.; Zhong, X.; Wu, Y.; Zheng, W.; Wang, H.; Yu, J.; Ma, L. Comparative Study on the Monosaccharide Compositions, Antioxidant and Hypoglycemic Activities *in Vitro* of Intracellular and Extracellular Polysaccharides of Liquid Fermented *Coprinus comatus*. *Int. J. Biol. Macromol.* **2019,** *139*, 543–549.
103. Zhang, Q.; Olatunji, O. J.; Chen, H.; Tola, A. J.; Oluwaniyi, O. O. Evaluation of the Anti-diabetic Activity of Polysaccharide from *Cordyceps cicadae* in Experimental Diabetic Rats. *Chem. Biodivers.* **2018,** *15* (8), e1800219.
104. Sun, H.; Yu, X.; Li, T.; Zhu, Z. Structure and Hypoglycemic Activity of a Novel Exopolysaccharide of *Cordyceps militaris*. *Int. J. Biol. Macromol.* **2021,** *166*, 496–508.
105. Kiho, T.; Ookubo, K.; Usui, S.; Ukai, S.; Hirano, K. Structural Features and Hypoglycemic Activity of a Polysaccharide (CS-F10) from the Cultured Mycelium of *Cordyceps sinensis*. *Biol. Pharm. Bull.* **1999,** *22* (9), 966–970.
106. Liu, R. M.; Dai, R.; Luo, Y.; Xiao, J. H. Glucose-lowering and Hypolipidemic Activities of Polysaccharides from *Cordyceps taii* in Streptozotocin-induced Diabetic Mice. *BMC Complement. Altern. Med.* **2019,** *19* (1), 230.
107. Zhu, K. X.; Nie, S. P.; Li, C.; Gong, D.; Xie, M. Y. *Ganoderma atrum* Polysaccharide Improves Aortic Relaxation in Diabetic Rats Via PI3K/Akt Pathway. *Carbohydr. Polym.* **2014,** *103*, 520–527.
108. Zhu, K.; Nie, S.; Li, C.; Lin, S.; Xing, M.; Li, W.; Gong, D.; Xie, M. A Newly Identified Polysaccharide from *Ganoderma atrum* Attenuates Hyperglycemia and Hyperlipidemia. *Int. J. Biol. Macromol.* **2013,** *57*, 142–150.
109. Hikino, H.; Ishiyama, M.; Suzuki, Y.; Konno, C. Mechanisms of Hypoglycemic Activity of Ganoderan B: A Glycan of *Ganoderma lucidum* Fruit Bodies. *Planta Med.* **1989,** *55* (5), 423–428.
110. Tomoda, M.; Gonda, R.; Kasahara, Y.; Hikino, H. Glycan Structures of Ganoderans B and C, Hypoglycemic Glycans of *Ganoderma lucidum* Fruit Bodies. *Phytochemistry* **1986,** *25* (12), 2817–2820.
111. Xiao, C.; Wu, Q. P.; Cai, W.; Tan, J. B.; Yang, X. B.; Zhang, J. M. Hypoglycemic Effects of *Ganoderma lucidum* Polysaccharides in Type 2 Diabetic Mice. *Arch. Pharm. Res.* **2012,** *35* (10), 1793–1801.
112. Liu, Y.; Li, Y.; Zhang, W.; Sun, M.; Zhang, Z. Hypoglycemic Effect of Inulin Combined with *Ganoderma lucidum* Polysaccharides in T2DM Rats. *J. Funct. Foods* **2019,** *55*, 381–390.

113. Zheng, J.; Yang, B.; Yu, Y.; Chen, Q.; Huang, T.; Li, D. *Ganoderma lucidum* Polysaccharides Exert Anti-hyperglycemic Effect on Streptozotocin-induced Diabetic Rats through Affecting β-Cells. *Comb. Chem. High Throughput Screen.* **2012,** *15* (7), 542–550.
114. Zhang, H. N.; He, J. H.; Yuan, L; Lin, Z. B. In Vitro and in Vivo Protective Effect of *Ganoderma lucidum* Polysaccharides on Alloxan-induced Pancreatic Islets Damage. *Life Sci.* **2003,** *73* (18), 2307–2319.
115. Hong, L.; Xun, M.; Wutong, W. Anti-diabetic Effect of an α-Glucan from Fruit Body of Maitake (*Grifola frondosa*) on KK-Ay Mice. *J. Pharm. Pharmacol.* **2007,** *59* (4), 575–582.
116. Xiao, C.; Wu, Q.; Xie, Y.; Zhang, J.; Tan, J. Hypoglycemic Effects of *Grifola frondosa* (Maitake) Polysaccharides F2 and F3 through Improvement of Insulin Resistance in Diabetic Rats. *Food Funct.* **2015,** *6* (11), 3567–3575.
117. Kou, L.; Du, M.; Liu, P.; Zhang, B.; Zhang, Y.; Yang, P.; Shang, M.; Wang, X. Anti-diabetic and Anti-nephritic Activities of *Grifola frondosa* Mycelium Polysaccharides in Diet-streptozotocin-induced Diabetic Rats Via Modulation on Oxidative Stress. *Appl. Biochem. Biotechnol.* **2019,** *187* (1), 310–322.
118. Lei, H.; Guo, S.; Han, J.; Wang, Q.; Zhang, X.; Wu, W. Hypoglycemic and Hypolipidemic Activities of MT-α-glucan and Its Effect on Immune Function of Diabetic Mice. *Carbohydr. Polym.* **2012,** *89* (1), 245–250.
119. Wang, J.; Wang, C.; Li, S.; Li, W.; Yuan, G.; Pan, Y.; Chen, H. Anti-diabetic Effects of *Inonotus obliquus* Polysaccharides in Streptozotocin-induced Type 2 Diabetic Mice and Potential Mechanism Via PI3K-Akt Signal Pathway. *Biomed. Pharmacother.* **2017,** *95*, 1669–1677.
120. Diao, B. Z.; Jin, W. R.; Yu, X. J. Protective Effect of Polysaccharides from *Inonotus obliquus* on Streptozotocin-induced Diabetic Symptoms and Their Potential Mechanisms in Rats. *Evid.-Based Complement. Altern. Med.* **2014,** *2014*, 841496. https://doi.org/10.1155/2014/841496
121. Wang, J.; Hu, W.; Li, L.; Huang, X.; Liu, Y.; Wang, D.; Teng, L. Antidiabetic Activities of Polysaccharides Separated from *Inonotus obliquus* Via the Modulation of Oxidative Stress in Mice with Streptozotocin-induced Diabetes. *PLoS One* **2017,** *12* (6), e0180476.
122. Hu, W.; Wang, J.; Guo, W.; Liu, Y.; Guo, Z.; Miao, Y.; Wang, D. Studies on Characteristics and Anti-diabetic and -nephritic Effects of Polysaccharides Isolated from *Paecilomyces hepiali* Fermentation Mycelium in db/db Mice. *Carbohydr. Polym.* **2020,** *232*, 115766.
123. Feng, H.; Zhang, S.; Wan, J. M. F.; Gui, L.; Ruan, M.; Li, N.; Zhang, H.; Liu, Z.; Wang, H. Polysaccharides Extracted from *Phellinus linteus* Ameliorate High-fat High-fructose Diet Induced Insulin Resistance in Mice. *Carbohydr. Polym.* **2018,** *200*, 144–153.
124. Zhao, C.; Liao, Z.; Wu, X.; Liu, Y.; Liu, X.; Lin, Z.; Huang, Y.; Liu, B. Isolation, Purification, and Structural Features of a Polysaccharide from *Phellinus linteus* and Its Hypoglycemic Effect in Alloxan-induced Diabetic Mice. *J. Food Sci.* **2014,** *79* (5), H1002–H1010.

125. Hu, S. H.; Wang, J. C.; Lien, J. L.; Liaw, E. T.; Lee, M. Y. Antihyperglycemic Effect of Polysaccharide from Fermented Broth of *Pleurotus citrinopileatus*. *Appl. Microbiol. Biotechnol.* **2006,** *70* (1), 107–113.
126. Zhang, J.; Meng, G.; Zhang, C.; Lin, L.; Xu, N.; Liu, M.; Cui, F.; Jia, L. The Antioxidative Effects of Acidic-, Alkalic-, and Enzymatic-extractable Mycelium Zinc Polysaccharides by *Pleurotus djamor* on Liver and Kidney of Streptozocin-induced Diabetic Mice. *BMC Complement. Altern. Med.* **2015,** *15* (1), 440.
127. Zhang, C.; Zhang, L.; Liu, H.; Zhang, J.; Hu, C.; Jia, L. Antioxidation, Anti-hyperglycaemia and Renoprotective Effects of Extracellular Polysaccharides from *Pleurotus eryngii* SI-04. *Int. J. Biol. Macromol.* **2018,** *111*, 219–228.
128. Ganeshpurkar, A.; Kohli, S.; Rai, G. Antidiabetic Potential of Polysaccharides from the White Oyster Culinary-medicinal Mushroom *Pleurotus florida* (Higher Basidiomycetes). *Int. J. Med. Mushrooms* **2014,** *16* (3), 207–217.
129. Zhang, Y.; Hu, T.; Zhou, H.; Zhang, Y.; Jin, G.; Yang, Y. Antidiabetic Effect of Polysaccharides from *Pleurotus ostreatus* in Streptozotocin-induced Diabetic Rats. *Int. J. Biol. Macromol.* **2016,** *83*, 126–132.
130. Kanagasabapathy, G.; Kuppusamy, U. R.; Abd Malek, S. N.; Abdulla, M. A.; Chua, K. H.; Sabaratnam, V. Glucan-rich Polysaccharides from *Pleurotus sajor-caju* (Fr.) Singer Prevents Glucose Intolerance, Insulin Resistance and Inflammation in C57BL/6J Mice Fed a High-fat Diet. *BMC Complement. Altern. Med.* **2012,** *12* (1), 261–269.
131. Huang, H. Y.; Korivi, M.; Yang, H. T.; Huang, C. C.; Chaing, Y. Y.; Tsai, Y. C. Effect of *Pleurotus tuber-regium* Polysaccharides Supplementation on the Progression of Diabetes Complications in Obese-diabetic Rats. *Chin. J. Physiol.* **2014,** *57* (4), 198–208.
132. Cho, E. J.; Hwang, H. J.; Kim, S. W.; Oh, J. Y.; Baek, Y. M.; Choi, J. W.; Bae, S. H.; Yun, J. W. Hypoglycemic Effects of Exopolysaccharides Produced by Mycelial Cultures of Two Different Mushrooms *Tremella fuciformis* and *Phellinus baumii* in ob/ob mice. *Appl. Microbiol. Biotechnol.* **2007,** *75* (6), 1257–1265.
133. Kiho, T.; Kochi, M.; Usui, S.; Hirano, K.; Aizawa, K.; Inakuma, T. Antidiabetic Effect of an Acidic Polysaccharide (TAP) from *Tremella aurantia* and Its Degradation Product (TAP-H). *Biol. Pharm. Bull.* **2001,** *24* (12), 1400–1403.
134. Xu, X.; Yan, H.; Chen, J.; Zhang, X. Bioactive Proteins from Mushrooms. *Biotechnol. Adv.* **2011,** *29* (6), 667–674.
135. Kobayashi, M.; Kawashima, H.; Takemori, K.; Ito, H.; Murai, A.; Masuda, S.; Yamada, K.; Uemura, D.; Horio, F. Ternatin, a Cyclic Peptide Isolated from Mushroom, and Its Derivative Suppress Hyperglycemia and Hepatic Fatty Acid Synthesis in Spontaneously Diabetic KK-Ay Mice. *Biochem. Biophys. Res. Commun.* **2012,** *427* (2), 299–304.
136. Preuss, H. G.; Echard, B.; Bagchi, D.; Perricone, N. V.; Zhuang, C. Enhanced Insulin-Hypoglycemic Activity in Rats Consuming a Specific Glycoprotein Extracted from Maitake Mushroom. *Mol. Cell Biochem.* **2007,** *306* (1), 105–113.
137. Haneef, M.; Ceseracciu, L.; Canale, C.; Bayer, I. S.; Heredia-Guerrero, J. A.; Athanassiou, A. Advanced Materials from Fungal Mycelium: Fabrication and Tuning of Physical Properties. *Sci. Rep.* **2017,** *7* (1), 41292.

138. Jeong, S. C. A Preliminary Study on the Hypoglycemic Effect of the Exo-polymers Produced by Five Different Medicinal Mushrooms. *J. Microbiol. Biotechnol.* **2000,** *11*, 167.
139. Yang, B. K.; Kim, G. N.; Jeong, Y. T.; Jeong, H.; Mehta, P.; Song, C. H. Hypoglycemic Effects of Exo-biopolymers Produced by Five Different Medicinal Mushrooms in STZ-induced Diabetic Rats. *Mycobiology* **2008,** *36* (1), 45–49.
140. Yang, B. K.; Jung, Y. S.; Song, C. H. Hypoglycemic Effects of *Ganoderma applanatum* and *Collybia confluens* Exo-polymers in Streptozotocin-induced Diabetic Rats. *Phyther. Res.* **2007,** *21* (11), 1066–1069.
141. Yang, B. K.; Kim, D. H.; Jeong, S. C.; Das, S.; Choi, Y. S.; Shin, J. S.; Lee, S. C.; Song, C. H. Hypoglycemic Effect of a Lentinus Edodes Exo-polymer Produced from a Submerged Mycelial Culture. *Biosci. Biotechnol. Biochem.* **2002,** *66* (5), 937–942.
142. Duru, M. E.; Çayan, G. T. Biologically Active Terpenoids from Mushroom Origin: A Review. *Rec. Nat. Prod.* **2015,** *4*, 456.
143. Chen, X. Q.; Zhao, J.; Chen, L. X.; Wang, S. F.; Wang, Y.; Li, S. P. Lanostane Triterpenes from the Mushroom *Ganoderma resinaceum* and Their Inhibitory Activities against α-Glucosidase. *Phytochemistry* **2018,** *149*, 103–115.
144. Huang, H. T.; Wang, S. L.; Nguyen, V. B.; Kuo, Y. H. Isolation and Identification of Potent Antidiabetic Compounds from *Antrodia cinnamomea*—An Edible Taiwanese Mushroom. *Molecules* **2018,** *23* (11), 1–12.
145. Chen, L.; Li, Z. H.; Yao, J. N.; Peng, Y. L.; Huang, R.; Feng, T.; Liu, J. K. Isoindolinone-containing Meroterpenoids with α-Glucosidase Inhibitory Activity from Mushroom *Hericium caput-medusae*. *Fitoterapia* **2017,** *122*, 107–114.
146. Li, T. H.; Hou, C. C.; Chang, C. L. T.; Yang, W. C. Anti-hyperglycemic Properties of Crude Extract and Triterpenes from *Poria cocos*. *Evid.-Based Complement. Altern. Med.* **2011,** 128402. https://doi.org/10.1155/2011/128402.
147. Jang, J. S.; Lee, J. S.; Lee, J. H.; Kwon, D. S.; Lee, K. E.; Lee, S. Y.; Hong, E. K. Hispidin Produced from *Phellinus linteus* Protects Pancreatic β-Cells from Damage by Hydrogen Peroxide. *Arch. Pharm. Res.* **2010,** *33* (6), 853–861.
148. Lee, Y. S.; Kang, Y. H.; Jung, J. Y.; Lee, S.; Ohuchi, K.; Shin, K. H.; Kang, I. J.; Park, J. H. Y.; Shin, H. K.; Lim, S. S. Protein Glycation Inhibitors from the Fruiting Body of *Phellinus linteus*. *Biol. Pharm. Bull.* **2008,** *31* (10), 1968–1972.
149. Lee, Y. S.; Kang, Y. H.; Jung, J. Y.; Kang, I. J.; Han, S. N.; Chung, J. S.; Shin, H. K.; Lim, S. S. Inhibitory Constituents of Aldose Reductase in the Fruiting Body of *Phellinus linteus*. *Biol. Pharm. Bull.* **2008,** *31* (4), 765–768.
150. Huang, G. J.; Hsieh, W. T.; Chang, H. Y.; Huang, S. S.; Lin, Y. C.; Kuo, Y. H. α-Glucosidase and Aldose Reductase Inhibitory Activities from the Fruiting Body of *Phellinus merrillii*. *J. Agric. Food Chem.* **2011,** *59* (10), 5702–5706.
151. Ho, L. H.; Zulkifli, N. A.; Tan, T. C. Edible Mushroom: Nutritional Properties, Potential Nutraceutical Values, and Its Utilisation in Food Product Development. In *An Introduction to mushroom*; Passari, A. K., and Sánchez, S., Eds.; IntechOpen, 2020; pp 19–38.

CHAPTER 5

Mechanism of Actions of Antidiabetic Mushrooms

WASIM SAJAD MALIK, MOHD YAQUB BHAT*, ABDUL HAMID WANI, ANEES UN NISA, and LATIF A. PEER

Plant Pathology, Mycology and Microbiology Laboratory, Department of Botany, University of Kashmir, Srinagar 19006, Jammu and Kashmir, India

**Corresponding author. E-mail: myaqub35@gmail.com*

ABSTRACT

Mushrooms are commonly used as a health-promoting food. These health-promoting properties of mushrooms have been attributed to various valuable components like carbohydrates, proteins, minerals, and dietary fibers present in the mushrooms. These bioactive molecules seem to be a promising and possibly more efficient alternate for the production of antidiabetic drugs. The most potent antidiabetic molecule present in mushrooms is β-glucan, a homopolysaccharide present in the fungal cell wall. It controls diabetes in both insulin-dependent and insulin-independent manner. The bioactive compounds of mushrooms with antidiabetic potential act on pancreatic cells and regulate the insulin concentration by various mechanisms. β-Glucan protects the pancreatic cells against oxidative damage and by regeneration of the pancreatic islets of Langerhans thereby increasing the production of insulin. It also upregulates the expression of insulin-response protein GLUT-4 and PPAR-α expression in the liver cells, which in turn control hyperglycemia via regulation of

Therapeutic Mushrooms for Diabetes Mellitus: Current Evidences and Future Scope. Uzma Azeem, Khalid Rehman Hakeem, (Eds.)

lipid metabolism. It also binds to β-glucan receptors presents in the mucus lining of the intestine and prevents the absorption of cholesterol in the gut. It inhibits α-glucosidase enzyme aldose reductase, tyrosine kinase (TK) and aldosereductase (AR) which are associated with the induction of postprandial hyperglycemia. Mushroom also contains certain compounds like ergosterol peroxide (EPO), glucagon-like peptide 1 (GLP-1), galacto-glucan, lovastatin, hispidin which inhibits the carbohydrate metabolizing enzymes (α-glucosidase and α-amylase) thereby reducing the postrandial elevation of blood glucose level. Besides these direct effects on the cycle of diabetics, mushroom polysaccharides also enhance the formation of probiotics which improve glucose metabolism and insulin resistance associated with type 2 diabetes and reduce the symptoms associated with diabetes.

5.1 INTRODUCTION

Diabetes, a chronic metabolic disorder that results from the deficit or resistance to insulin is one among the top 10 causes of death globally. Along with cancer, cardiovascular and respiratory ailments, diabetes accounts for nearly 80% of all the premature noncommunicable disease deaths.[1] The International Diabetes Federation (IDF) have projected that there were 451 million people suffering from diabetes worldwide in 2017 if it goes unchecked the number may rise to 693 million by 2045.[2] Up to now, three types of diabetes have been characterized: type 1, type 2 and gestational diabetes. Type 1 diabetes is associated with the impaired postprandial insulin secretion due to destructive lesions of pancreatic β-cells.[3] Type 2 diabetes is related to the increased resistance of cellular receptors to insulin. Gestational diabetes occurs during pregnancy and is related with the elevation of glucose in blood above the level of normal but below the diagnosis of diabetics.[4] All of these defects result in the abnormal elevation of blood glucose known as hyperglycemia, which causes several life-threatening complications like nephropathy and retinopathy.[5] From time-to-time, various drugs have been designed for the control of diabetes yet its management remains highly unsatisfactory. Therefore, it is important to design biomolecules, which help to prevent diabetes and have fewer side effects. Wild edible mushrooms are enriched with abundant bioactive compounds some of which are having antidiabetic properties.[6] Some of the most potent antidiabetic bioactive compounds characterized from mushrooms are β-glucan, ergosterol peroxide (EPO), GLP-1, galactoglucan, lovastatin, hispidin. Some of the common mechanisms through which antidiabetic mushroom acts are as under.

5.2 MECHANISM OF ACTION OF ERGOSTEROL PEROXIDE IN PALMITATE (PA) INDUCED C2C12 CELLS

EPO (Fig. 5.1) is an important constituent of fungal cell wall and its content in *Grifola frondosa* was found about 75 µg/g dry weight.[7] It is a sterol derivative with a chemical formulae $C_{28}H_{44}C_3$ (5α,8α-epidioxy-22E-ergosta-6,22-dien-3-β-ol). EPO is a major bioactive compound found in many edible mushrooms and was isolated from *Cordyceps sinensis*,[8] *Ganoderma lucidum*,[9] *Hericium erinaceum*,[10] *G. frondosa*,[11] *Cordyceps cicadae*,[12] *Inonotus obliquus*,[13] and *Xylaria nigripes*,[14] etc.

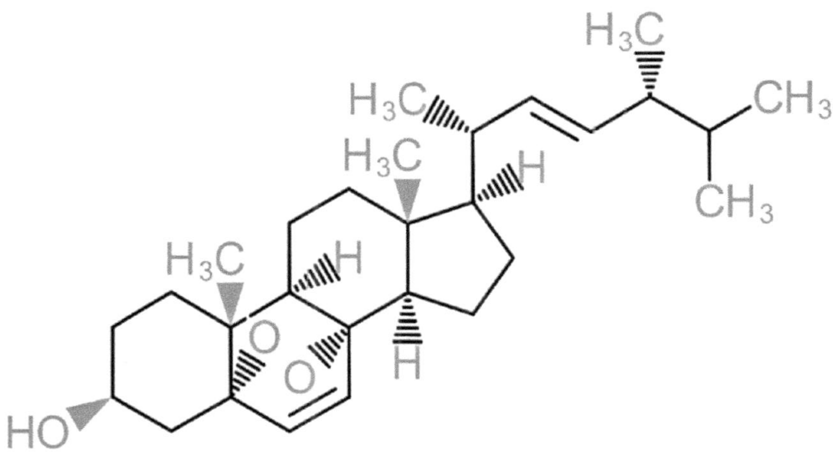

FIGURE 5.1 Chemical structure of ergosterol peroxide.

The antidiabetic effects of EPO from *G. frondosa* and its related molecular signaling pathways in palmitate-induced C2C12 cells was studied in detail by Wu et al.[7]

5.2.1 EFFECT OF EPO ON GLUCOSE UPTAKE IN C2C12 CELLS

They observed that EPO increased the glucose absorption at 5–10 μM but at 20 μM cytotoxicity was observed and cell viability was only 88.75%. The cell viability decreases further to 81.43% when the cells were treated with PA. The pretreated C2C12 with 0.5–5 μM EPO showed 100% protection against PA-induced cytotoxicity. The increase in glucose uptake by C2C12 cells when treated with 5 μM EPO was similar to that of insulin treated cells as shown in Table 5.1.

TABLE 5.1 Effect of EPO on Cell Viability and Glucose Uptake.

Treatments		Cell viability %	Glucose uptake ratio
Control		100.00 ± 5.6	1.00 ± 0.08
Insulin (150 nM)		ND	1.95 ± 0.18
EPO (μM)	0.5	100.00 ± 2.45	0.83 ± 0.25
	1	100.00 ± 4.30	1.05 ± 0.38
	5	100.00 ± 6.32	1.86 ± 0.08
	10	100.00 ± 3.38	1.90 ± 0.08
	20	88.75 ± 5.41	1.28 ± 0.03

5.2.2 EFFECTS OF EPO ON REACTIVE OXYGEN SPECIES FORMATION

There was an increase in reactive oxygen species (ROS) production in C2C12 cells when induced with PA, but when co-treated with EPO there was a significant decrease in ROS production[7] as shown in Table 5.2.

TABLE 5.2 Effect of EPO on PA-Induced ROS Formation.[7]

Treatment	Fluorescence intensity %
Control	55
PA	70
EPO (1 μM)	60
PA + EPO (1 μM)	65
EPO (5 μM)	45
PA + EPO (5 μM)	50

The results indicate that the ROS production was significantly reduced when the C2C12 cells were treated with 5 μM EPO.

5.2.3 EFFECT OF EPO ON IRS-1, PI3K, PKB, AND GLUT-4 SIGNALING PATHWAYS

The cells treated with 5 μM EPO upregulate the expression of IRS-1, phosphatidylinositol 3-kinase (PI3K) and protein kinase B (PKB) genes by phosphorylation. It also downregulates the expression of p-JNK and P38 genes. In addition, the EPO treated cells shows an increase in the translocation GLUT-4 gene to the plasma membrane in dose dependent manner.

The complete mechanism of action of EPO as an antidiabetic molecule was studied on *G. frondosa*.[7] It was found that 5 μM EPO significantly upregulated glucose absorption and was as good for glucose absorption as that of insulin. Hence is used to treat type 2 diabetics.

5.2.3.1 MECHANISM

Step 1: Binding of signaling molecule (EPO) at cell membrane receptor tyrosine kinase (TK) and its activation by phosphorylation.

Step 2: Phosphorylation of insulin receptor substrate 1 (IRS-1) by receptor TK.

Step 3: Activation of phosphatidylinositol 3-kinase (PI3K) by IRS-1.

Step 4: Activation of protein kinase B (PKB) also known as AKT by PI3K promotes the translation of glucose transporter 4 (GLUT4). Beside this Akt molecule has also been found to supress the gluconeogenesis in the liver and hence used to control type 2 diabetes.[15]

Step 5: GLUT4 facilitates the diffusion of circulating glucose into muscle cells.

The EPO with the combination of palmitate (PA) effectively reduces the ROS production. ROS are linked with the disruption of insulin signaling by phosphorylating IRS serine/threonine kinases. Besides ROS also plays a great role in deactivating transcription of GLUT 4 genes and hinders mitochondrial activities.[16,17] Hence EPO with the combination of PA attenuate the disruption of insulin signaling. The same phenomenon of upregulation of GLUT4 by treating the cells with polysaccharides of *Inonotus obliquus* has also been reported[18] as shown in Figure 5.2.

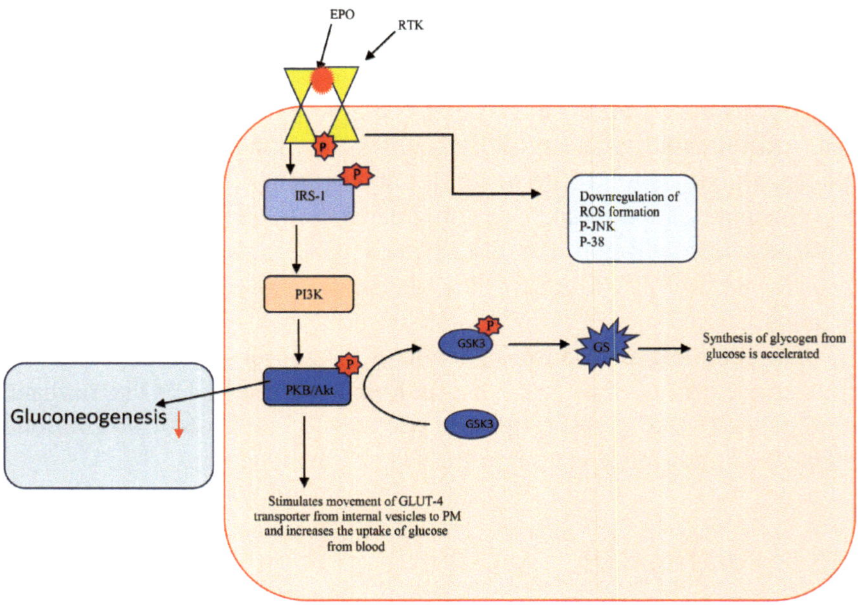

FIGURE 5.2 Molecular signaling pathway of ergosterol peroxide in palmitate-induced C2C12 cells (modified from Wu et al.[7]).

5.3 INHIBITION OF LIPID DEPOSITION VIA AUTOPHAGY ENHANCEMENT BY MUSHROOM POLYSACCHARIDES

Autophagy is a body's way of transporting cytoplasmic contents of a cell to lysosomes for degradation. It is an important mechanism for nutrient recycling and cellular homeostasis.[19] The disruption in the mechanism of autophagy is a major cause of type 2 diabetes.[20] The autophagy level decreases with the increase in plasma insulin level in mice.[21] In addition, autophagy also helps to maintain structure and function of β-cells and also protects them from damage caused due to high fat diet.[22]

5.3.1 MUSHROOM POLYSACCHARIDES ACTIVATE AUTOPHAGY

Many polysaccharide compounds have been shown to induce autophagy.[23] Yang et al.[24] examined the autophagic capacity of *Amillariella mellea* by using HeLa cells stably expressing GFP-tagged LC3 (an autophagosome marker). When these cells were treated with mushroom polysaccharides the number of GFP-LC3 puncta increased indicating the increase in the formation of autophagosomes. Many biochemical markers such as decrease in p62 and elevation in the conversion of LC3-I to LC3-II established the elevation in the concentration of formation of autophagosomes (Table 5.3).[24]

5.3.2 MUSHROOM POLYSACCHARIDES REGULATES LIPID ACCUMULATION

Free fatty acid deposition by hepatocytes results in the suppression of autophagic function and insulin resistance.[25] Yang et al.[24] studied the effect of *A. mellea* polysaccharides on lipid accumulation in Hepa1-6 cells. They found that the addition of mushroom polysaccharides reduces ALT and AST level in db/db mice (Table 5.3).

TABLE 5.3 Effect of Mushroom Polysaccharides on Autophagy and Lipid Accumulation.[24]

Treatments	p62/Actin	LC3-I TO LC3-II	ALT (IU/l)	AST (IU/l)
C_{57}BL/6J	0.70	1.25	14	17
Db	1.80	0.90	85	62
Db + MET	0.80	1.45	50	30
Db + polysaccharides	1.00	1.65	60	35

The extract of oyster mushroom shows hypocholesterolemic effect on liver and kidney. The intake of 5% powder of *Pleurotus ostreatus* and *P. sajor-caju* reduces the total cholesterol level by 37% and 21%, respectively. After certain experiments, it was found that the bioactive compound showing hypocholesterolemic effect is lovastatin.[26] The chemical formula of lovastatin is $C_{24}H_{36}O_5$ and its chemical structure is given in Figure 5.3.

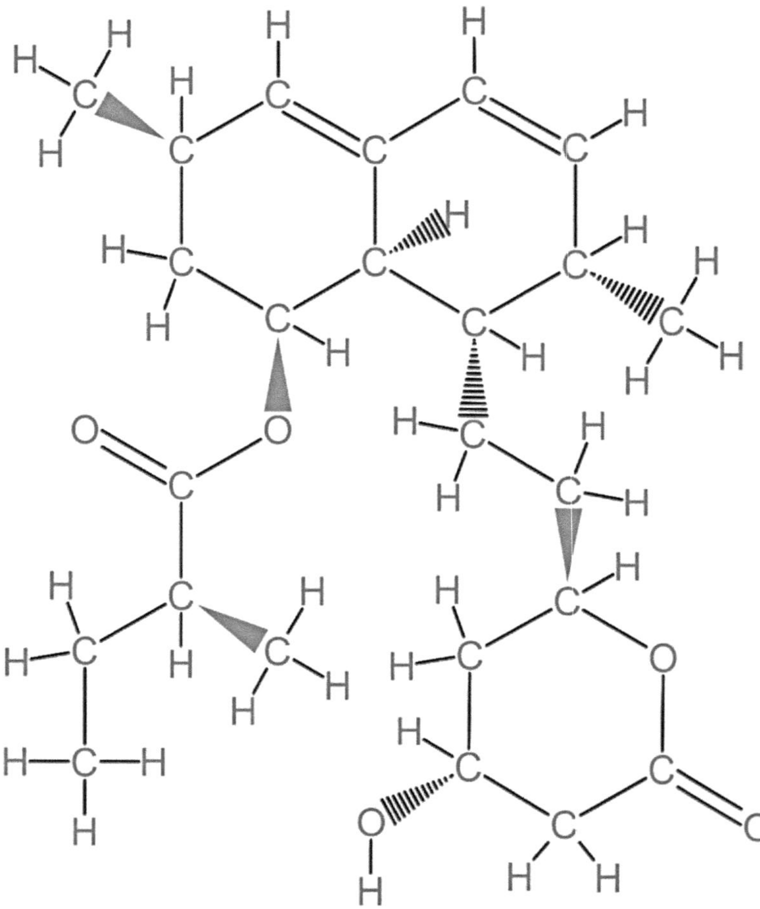

FIGURE 5.3 Chemical structure of lovastatin.

5.3.3 EFFECT OF MUSHROOM POLYSACCHARIDES ON INSULIN-STIMULATED GLUCOSE UPTAKE

Yang et al.[24] studied the effect of *A. mellea* polysaccharides on insulin-stimulated glucose uptake in Hepa1-6 cells and found that the treatment of FG significantly reduces the glucose uptake in Hepa1-6 cells. Metformin an antidiabetic drug significantly reduced FG-induced insulin resistance by 60%. When the cells were treated with alkali soluble polysaccharides even at a low concentration (0.01 mg/mL) from the fruiting bodies of *A. mellea* (AAMP), *Gomphidius rutilus* (AGRP), *Agrocybe cylindracea*, *Hypsizygus marmoreus*, *Pleurotus eryngii* (APEP) and *P. ostreatus* (APOP), they enhanced the glucose uptake. They also perform monosaccharide composition analysis and found glucose and mannose as the main alkali soluble polysaccharides. The potent antidiabetic molecule was found to be galactoglucan. Galactoglucan activates autophagy by inhibiting the lysosomal inhibitor bafilomycin A1 (BafA1) and by degrading p62 protein an autophagy substrate. Treatment of cells with FG (high glucose and fatty acid) resulted in the elevation of number and size of intracellular lipid droplets. The co-treatment of BafA1 (a lysosomal inhibitor) along with galactoglucan suppresses the insulin sensitization effect of galactoglucan (Fig. 5.4).[24]

5.3.4 AAMP ENLARGED PANCREATIC ISLETS

The pancreatic islets of db/db diabetic mice were significantly enlarged as compared to normal mice due to insulin resistance. But when db/db diabetic mice were treated by the mushroom polysaccharides from *A. mellea* (AAMP) the pancreatic islets cells become significantly smaller and denser. This suggests that AAMP restored the size of pancreatic islets and protects them from compensatory expansion. Besides it enlarges pancreatic islets and enhances insulin signaling by phosphorylating IR, Akt/PKB, and AMPK.[24]

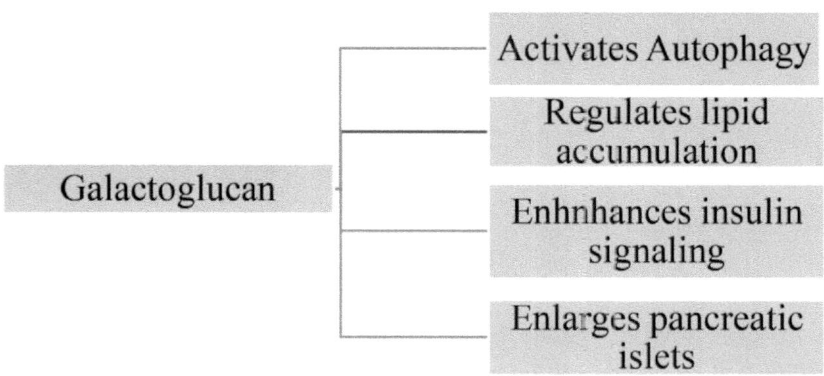

FIGURE 5.4 Effects of galactoglucan.

5.4 INHIBITION OF α-GLUCOSIDASES AND α-AMYLASEENZYMES

α-Glucosidases are the enzymes that catalysis the hydrolysis of terminal nonreducing (α-1,4) linked α-glucose into a single α-glucose molecule for intestinal absorption. Whereas, α-amylases are the enzymes that catalysis the hydrolysis of the internal (α-1,4) linked starch molecules into two or three glucose units such as maltose.[27] Both of these enzymes lead to the elevation of blood glucose levels and hence are a major cause of diabetes. Koike et al.[28] suggested that the inhibition of α-glucosidases and α-amylases in type 2 patients may reduce hyperglycaemia. The α-glucosidase inhibition activity was demonstrated with maximum inhibition and EC_{50} values. Some of the potent α-glucosidase inhibitor mushrooms and their EC_{50} value are shown in Table 5.4. Huang et al.[29] found eight biologically potent molecules in *Antrodia cinnamomea* which acts as the inhibitors of α-glucosidases. These molecules are 25R-antcin B, 25R-antcin K, 25S-anticin B, 25S-antcin I, 25S-antcin K, dehydrosulphurenic acid, dehydroeburicoic acid, and euburicoic acid.[29]

TABLE 5.4 α-Glucosidase Inhibition by Various Mushrooms.

Sr. no.	Mushroom	EC_{50} value	Reference
1.	Acarbose (+ve control)	0.27	[29]
2.	*A. cinnamomea*	0.21	[29]
3.	*G. lucidum*	0.08	[30]
4.	*Trametes versicolor*	0.12	[30]
5.	*T. pubescence*	≥1.0	[31]
6.	*Pleurotus eous*	0.28	[32]
7.	*P. cornucopiae*	23.20	[33]
8.	*Phellinus linteus*	0.16	[30]
9.	*Agaricus blazei*	0.05	[30]
10.	*G. frondosa*	0.04	[30]
11.	*Hericium erinaceum*	0.04	[30]

Stojkovic et al.[34] studied the inhibitory effect of *A. blazei*, *Coprinus comatus*, *Cordyceps militaris*, *Inonotus obliquus*, *Morchella conica* and *P. linteus* on α-glycosidases and α-amylasesandfound *Inonotus obliquus* to be most effective in inhibiting α-glucosidases and α-amylases in type-2 patients. The polysaccharides isolated from *Pleurotus ostreatus*, *Astragalus* sp. and *Yacon* sp. shows the inhibitory effect on α-glucosidase over 40% at the conc. of 0.4 mg/mL. The IC_{50} value of *Pleurotus ostreatus* and *Astragalus* sp. was 0.424 and 0.28 mg/mL, respectively.[35] In a similar experiment Azeem et al.[36] compared the half-maximal inhibitory concentration (IC_{50}) of hydroalcoholic extracts of *Inonotus pachyphloeus*, *P. gilyus*, *P. sanfordii*, *P. tortulosus*, *P. fastuosus* and *Phellinus allardii*. They concluded that these hydroalcoholic mushroom extracts cause a concentration dependent inhibition of α-glucosidases and α-amylases. The *P. fastuosus*showed the highest cumulative inhibitory effect on α-glucosidases and α-amylases with an IC_{50} value of 27.33 ± 1.45 mg/mL followed by *P. sanfordii* and *I. pachyphloeus* with their respective IC_{50} values of 30.33 ± 0.88 mg/mL and 52.00 ± 1.15 mg/mL. *P. allardii* with a considerably higher IC_{50} value of 98.00 ± 0.57 mg/mL as depicted in Figure 5.5.[36]

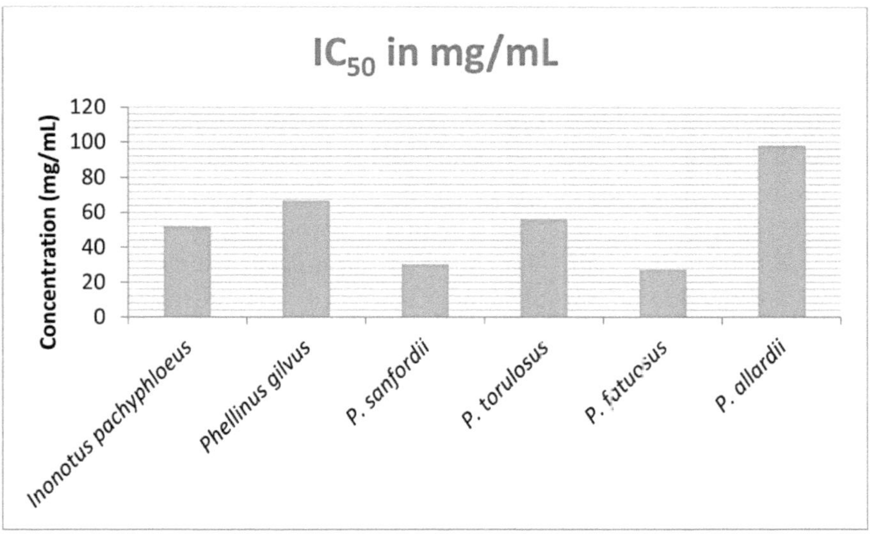

FIGURE 5.5 Hydroalcoholic extracts of different mushroom species with their cumulative IC_{50} values against α-amylase and α-glucosidase.[36]

In a similar experiment it was found that the polysaccharides ICPs (intracellular crude polysaccharides), ECPs (extracellular crude polysaccharides), IDPs (intracellular deproteinized polysaccharides) and EDPs (extracellular deproteinized polysaccharides) from *Coprinus comatus* possess significant ($P < 0.05$) α-amylase inhibitory effect at a concentration of 2–10 mg/mL.[37] The highest inhibitory effect was that of ICPs at the inhibition rate of 87.15 ± 0.99% at 10 mg/mL, whereas EDPs possess the lowest inhibitory effect at the inhibition rate of 36.04 ± 0.22% at 10 mg/mL. The mechanism by which these polysaccharides inhibit the activity of α-amylase remains unclear.

5.5 PROTECTION OF PANCREATIC B-CELLS FROM DAMAGE BY HYDROGEN PEROXIDE

Hydrogen peroxide (H_2O_2) is the main reactive oxygen species (ROS) formed in all the biological systems.[38] It is experimentally proved that the enhancement in the level of H_2O_2 is closely related to diabetes and its related complications.[39,40] Rolo and Palmeira[41] proved that the inhibition of H_2O_2 production or enhancement of its scavengers could be beneficial in the treatments of metabolic disorders like diabetes. Even though certain synthetic antioxidants like butylated hydroxyanisole (BHA) and butylated hydroxytoluene (BHT) are commercially available, but due to their toxicological effects they are least preferred as compared to natural antioxidants. Thus, there is a gradual surge in the demand for natural antioxidants.[42] The first report of mushroom compound with antioxidant properties was hispidin isolated from *Inonotus xeranticus*.[43] Jang et al.[44] isolated the similar antioxidant compound hispidin from *Phellinus linetus* and studied its mechanism in detail. The chemical formula of hispidin is $C_{13}H_{10}O_5$ [6-(3,4-dihydroxystyryl)-4-hydroxy-2-pyrone]. Its chemical structure is similar to that of several strong antioxidants like resveratrol, which is present in many plant species.[45] The antioxidant property of hispidin is attributed to its catechol moiety.[46]

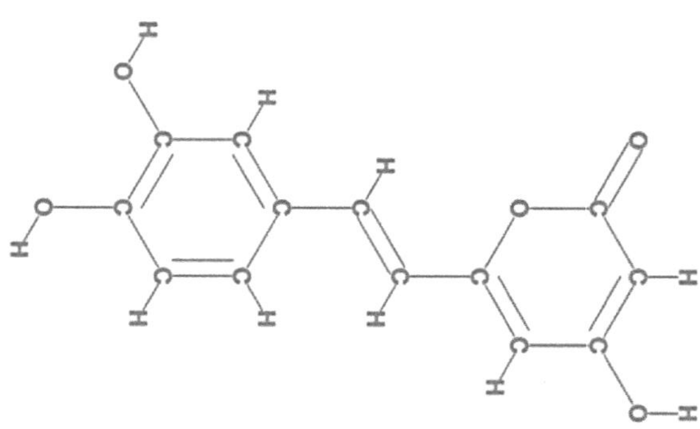

FIGURE 5.6 Chemical structure of hispidin.

5.5.1 RADICAL SCAVENGING ACTIVITY OF HISPIDIN

The radical scavenging ability of Hispidin was determined by according to standard methods.[47] They found that hispidin exhibit its effect in a dose dependent manner. Hispidin shows scavenging effects against super oxide radicals (SOD), DPPH radicals, and 2,2′-azino-bis-3-ethylbenzothiazoline-6-sulfonjic acid (ABTS) radical with IC_{50} values of 3.84 mM, 0.65 Mm and 0.83 μg/mL respectively. The radical scavenging activity of Hispidin was 55% at 30 μM which is higher than certain strong antioxidants like vitamin C and *N*-acetyl cysteine (NAC). When the RinM5F cell line treated with hispidin was observed under fluorescent microscope image it shows that there is a reduction in green fluorescence intensity. It indicates that due to the treatment of hispidin there is a reduction in the generation of ROS. Both of these experiments indicate that Hispidin has a strong antioxidant capacity.[48]

5.5.2 EFFECT OF HISPIDIN ON PANCREATIC Β-CELLS AND INSULIN SECRETION

Evans et al. verified that the elevation of reactive oxygen species (ROS) in mitochondria triggers the apoptosis of pancreatic β-cells.[49] Jang et al.[44] conducted an experiment on mushroom polysaccharides and found that the Hispidin possess strong antioxidant properties and protects the Pancreatic β-cells from oxidative damage. In addition, they also found that hispidin acts as a potent antioxidant molecule. They found that when the cells were exposed only to H_2O_2 certain apoptotic features like membrane blebbing and elevation in the concentration of annexin V were clearly visible. But when the cells were pre-treated with hispidin there was a decrease in the apoptotic features and in the concentration of annexin V. The cell survival rate was also increased by 14% which is higher as compared to Vitamin C (6%) and NAC (9%). H_2O_2 inhibited the secretion of insulin in RINm5F cells from 9.29 to 4.81 ng/mL. But when the cells were pre-treated with Hispidin the secretion of insulin was enhanced to 8.26 ng/mL. These results suggests that hispidin has shown antidiabetic properties through the inhibition of H_2O_2.[44]

5.6 ROLE OF MUSHROOM AS PREBIOTIC IN DIABETIC CONTROL

A well responsible factor for diabetic is gut dysbiosis. Gut dysbiosis leads to the suppression of useful lactic acid producing bacteria like *Lactobacillus* spp. *Streptococcus* spp. *Streptomyces* spp. etc. and the enhancement of gram-negative bacteria like *Actinobacillus* spp. *Escherichia* spp. *Brucella* spp. etc. These gram-negative bacteria lead to the production of lipopolysaccharides in the human gut which leads to insulin resistance.[50] The effect of mushroom polysaccharides on gut microflora is given in Table 5.5. Mushrooms are rich in polysaccharides like β-(1→3)-D-glucans, Xylans, mannans and Galactans which acts as prebiotics to stimulate the growth of gut microflora. They are nondigestible post-ingestional fermentable polysaccharides which confers health benefits to the host.[51] β-Glucans are an important component of the fungal cell wall which remains undigested in the human gut and thus acts as an important source of prebiotics.[52] The mushroom β-glucan protects the pancreatic cells against oxidative damage and by regeneration of the pancreatic islets of Langerhans thereby increasing the production of insulin. It also upregulates the expression of insulin-response protein GLUT-4 and PPAR-α expression in the liver cells, which in turn control hyperglycaemia via regulation of lipid metabolism. It also binds to β-glucan receptors presents in the mucus lining of the intestine and prevents the absorption of cholesterol in the gut. In small intestine these mushroom polysaccharides remain undigested and get converted into short chain fatty acids (SCFAs) in the large intestine. SCFAs elevate glucagon-like peptide-1 (GLP-1) protein secretion into the blood by large intestine.[53] The GLP-1 acts as a signaling molecule and binds to glucagon-like peptide-1 receptor (GLP-1R) in pancreatic (Islet alpha and beta) cells. GLP-1R is a G-protein coupled receptor (GPCR) which enhances the secretion of insulin by passing the signal downward as shown in the following steps and in Figure 5.6.[54,55]

Step 1: Conversion of polysaccharides into SCFA in the large intestine.

Step 2: Increase in the secretion of GLP-1 protein into the blood by large intestine.

Step 3: Binding of signaling molecule (GLP-1) to the receptor molecule (GLP-1R) in the pancreatic cells.

Step 4: Activation of PDX-1 (pancreatic duodenal homeobox-1) transcription factor (TF) by GLP-1R.

Step 5: Translocation of PDX-1 TF to nucleus and transcription of the preproinsulin, GLUT-2 and glucokinase genes which are involved

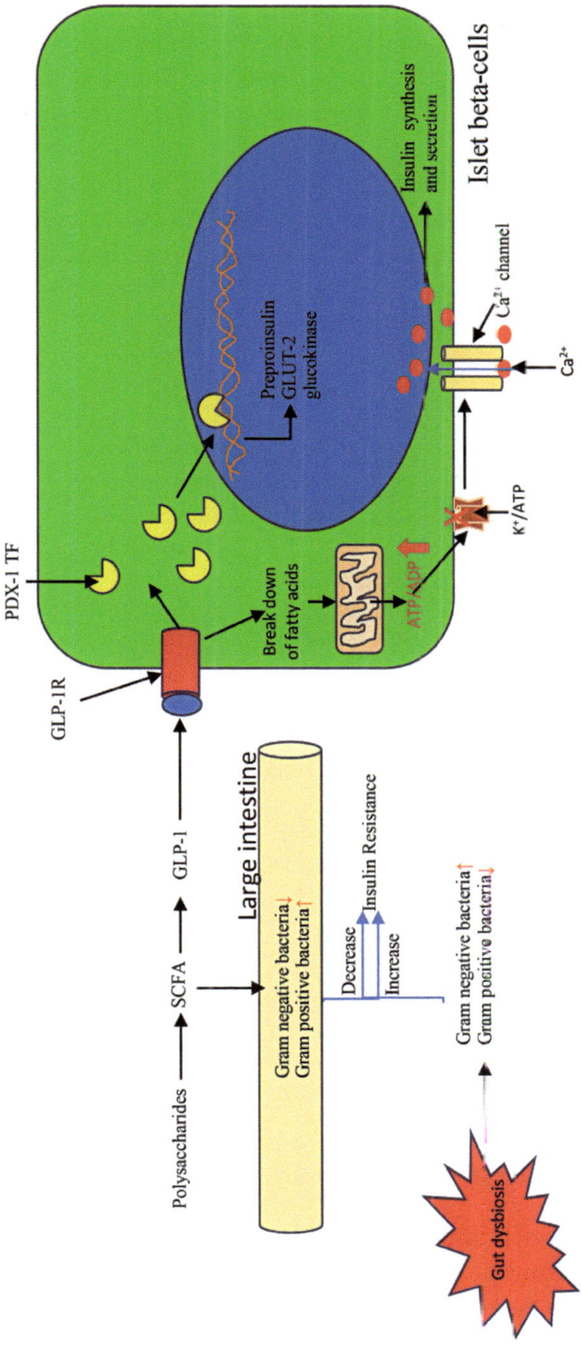

FIGURE 5.7 Mechanism of action of Polysaccharides on gut dysbiosis (modified from Khursheed et al.[54] and Reed and Kanamarlapudi[53]).

in insulin production, besides it also induces the transcription of genes involved in neogenesis, apoptotic and cell proliferation.

Step 6: Glut-2 removes excess of glucose from blood in kidney and liver whereas in pancreas along with glucokinase it enhances the insulin production.

Besides the activation of insulin genes GLP-1R also provides more metabolic fuel to mitochondria and raises the ATP/ADP ratio which closes the K^+ ATP channel. Closure of ATP channel opens the Ca^{2+} channel and the influx of Ca^{2+} occurs. High level of CA^{2+} is required for both the processes of insulin synthesis and secretion.

TABLE 5.5 Mushroom Polysaccharides as Prebiotics.

S. no.	Mushroom species	Extracted prebiotics	Effect on gut microflora		Reference
			Enhancement of	Suppression of	
1.	*A. blazei murill*	ABMP	Bacteroides	Firmicutes and proteobacteria	[55]
2.	*Agaricus bisporus*	GLP	*Lactobacillus*, Bacilli and *Helicobacter*	*Clostridium* and peptostreptococcaceae	[56]
3.	*Grifola frondose*	GFP	*Clostridum* and *Turicibacter*	*Helicobacter*, *Barnesiella* and *Flavonifracter*	[57]
4.	*Pleurotus eryngii*	PEP	*Anaerostipes* and *Clostridum*		[58]
5.	*P. linteus*	PLP	*Roseburia*, *Blautia* and *Eubacterium*		[59]
6.	*Ganoderma lucidum*	GLP	Parabacteroides and bacteroides	*Corynebacterium* and *Ruminococcus*	[60]
7.	*Hirsutella sinensis*	HSP	*Parabacteroides goldsteinii*		[61]

ABMP—Agaricus blazei polysaccharide; GLP—Glucagon like peptide; GFP—G. frondosa polysaccharide; PEP—Pleurotus eryngii polysaccharide; PLP—Phellinus linteus polysaccharide; HSP—Hirsutella sinensis polysaccharide.

5.7 ANTIDIABETIC ACTIVITY OF β-GLUCANS

Mushrooms are rich in polysaccharides like β-glucans, which consists of glucopyronase molecules comprised of linear chains with β-(1→3) and side chains with β-(1→6) linkages.[62]

5.7.1 EFFECT OF β-GLUCAN ON BODY WEIGHT OF DIABETIC RATS

While studying the effect of β-glucans from *A. blazei* on the diabetic rats Kim et al.[63] found that the final body weight of the control group decreased by 228.8 ± 12.2 g and that of β-glucan treated group decreased by 252.6 ± 6.9 g. Feeding the diabetic rats with β-glucans results in 6% reduction in the body weight suggesting that β-glucans helps to loose body weight and move towards normalcy. The food efficiency ratio for the β-glucan was −0.46 ± 0.2 while that of control was -1.2 ± 0.4 suggesting that β-glucans facilitated food utilization of diabetic rats.[63]

5.7.2 ANTI-HYPERGLYCEMIC AND ANTI-HYPERLIPEMIC EFFECTS OF β-GLUCANS IN DIABETIC RATS

The antihyperglycemic and antihyperlipemic effects of β-glucans from *Agaricus blazei* on the diabetic rats were studied by Kim et al.[63] They studied the effect of consumption of β-glucans for 6 weeks on the level of serum glucose, insulin, triglycerides and on cholesterol in diabetics rats and the observations are given in Table 5.6.

TABLE 5.6 Effect of β-Glucans on Glucose, Insulin, Triglycerides and Total Cholesterol.[63]

Serum component	Treatments					
	Normal control		Diabetic control		β-Glucans	
	Initial	Final	Initial	Final	Initial	Final
Glucose (mg/dl)	99.8 ± 6.4	108.7 ± 7	331.7 ± 37.6	787.3 ± 32.1	334.0 ± 38.4	643.0 ± 43.5
Insulin (ng/dl)	0.76 ± 0.06	0.62 ± 0.10	0.44 ± 0.08	0.43 ± 0.10	0.44 ± 0.10	0.76 ± 0.23
Triglycerides (mg/dl)	29.6 ± 1.3	51.3 ± 6.6	102.7 ± 18.0	406.4 ± 89.9	102.5 ± 17.1	214.1 ± 34.8
Total cholesterol (mg/dl)	88.1 ± 2.1	94.2 ± 4.3	98.9 ± 6.8	131.9 ± 12.4	100.3 ± 7.5	99.9 ± 6.8

The level of serum glucose, insulin, triglycerides, and total cholesterol in β-glucans treated diabetic rats was significantly reduced as compared to the control group. This lower level of serum glucose and insulin indicates that the β-glucans promotes the viability and proliferation of islets of pancreatic cells and hence upregulate the glucose metabolism in diabetics rats. The decrease in the level of triglycerides and total cholesterol in β-glucans treated diabetic rats suggests that it leads to the suppression of triglyceride synthesis in the liver. This would help to reduce hyperlipemia and arteriosclerosis.[64]

5.8 INHIBITION OF ADVANCED GLYCATION END PRODUCTS BY ANTIDIABETIC MUSHROOMS

Advanced glycation end products (AGEs) are chemically diverse group of molecules produced in cells or in long-lived extracellular proteins by a complex series of sequential reactions collectively known as classical Maillard reaction. The common AGEs include carboxymethyl-hydroxylysine, 2-(2-furoyl)-4(5)-(2-furanyl)-1*H*-imaidazole, Nε-(carbonylmethyl) lysine, 1*H*-imidazole, crossline and pyrroline. It was for the first time discovered by Maillard in 1912.[65] Later on it was Monnier et al.[66] and Sell and Monnier[67] who proposed that these molecules alter the structure and function of many proteins and established a strong link between AGEs and diabetics. Since the cytotoxicity of AGEs is associated with the increase in free-radical production.[68] It was reported that ROS scavengers can decrease the generation of free-radical production.[69] So, there was a search for molecules that possess antiglycation potential.

5.8.1 ANTIOXIDANT ACTIVITY OF L. RHINOCERUS EXTRACT SEPHADEX® FRACTIONS

The antioxidant potential of different Sephadex® fractions was calculated as their free radical-scavenging and ferric reducing abilities. Different Saphadex® fractions showed a constant but much slower increase in the reaction to reduce ferric to ferrous complexes as shown in Table 5.7. It indicates the weak reducing capacity of the Saphadex® fractions of *L. rhinocerus.* However, Pulido et al.[70] have proposed that dietary polyphenols require more time (≥30 min) to complete reaction. The free-radical scavenging ability of antioxidants highly depends on their capacity in inhibiting lipid peroxidation.[71] Yap et al.[72] found a strong positive correlation between the phenolic content and the free-radical scavenging activity of the Saphadex® fractions of *L. rhinocerus.* Such a correlation between secondary metabolites and their antioxidant capacities has also been reported earlier by several workers.[73,74] The medium molecular weight (MMW) Saphadex® fraction exhibited the strongest $O_2^{\cdot -}$ scavenging activity comparable to that of rutin and quercetin which suggests the presence of superoxide dismutase (SOD) like compounds in the extract.[75] Such SOD (manganese SOD) have been previously identified in the Sephadex® fraction of *L. rhinocerus* by 2D gel electrophoresis and MALDI and LCMS analysis.[76]

TABLE 5.7 Antioxidant Activities of Sephadex® Fractions from *L. rhinocerus*.[72]

Sephadex® fractions	Antioxidant activities by different methods			
	FRAP	**DPPH·**	**ABTS·+**	**O2·−**
HMW	0.25 ± 0.0	Nil	0.31 ± 0.2	7.36 ± 0.1
MMW	1.25 ± 0.0	Nil	0.49 ± 0.1	10.12 ± 0.1
LMW	2.00 ± 0.0	0.11 ± 0.1	0.56 ± 0.0	8.28 ± 0.1
Quercetin	3380 ± 150	4.10 ± 0.1	2.34 ± 0.2	11.73 ± 0.3
Rutin	570 ± 40	4.08 ± 0.2	1.51 ± 0.5	10.99 ± 0.24

HMW—high molecular weight fraction; MMV—medium molecular weight fraction; LMW—low molecular weight fraction.

The antioxidant capacity is expressed as Trolox equivalent antioxidant capacity.

5.8.2 GLYCATION INHIBITORY ACTIVITIES OF THE SEPHADEX® FRACTION

The Sephadex® fraction of *L. rhinocerus* for glycation inhibition was investigated by Yap et al.[72,77] They quantified the fluorescent AGEs at an excitation wavelength of 370 nm and at an emission wavelength of 445 nm. The quantification of CML, Pent, and other AGEs was done by ELISA kit as shown in Table 5.8.

TABLE 5.8 Quantification of Fluorescent AGEs, CML., Pent, etc.[72]

Sephadex® fraction	Glucose-induced AGEs	
	Fluorescent AGEs	**CML, Pent. etc.**
AGs	0.12	0.52
TM-CW	5.30	0.02
HMW	10.0	0.02
MMW	7.70	0.01
LMW	5.20	4.00

From Table 5.8 it is clear that the Sephadex® fraction reduces glucose-induced AGEs in the order LMMW > MMW > HMW, which corresponds to their secondary metabolite content. Methylglyoxal, a vital precursor of AGEs reacts with lysine and arginine residues of proteins to produce fluorescent products.[77,78] Yap et al.[76] have identified the gene from *L. rhinocerus* (GM3225_g) that encodes glyoxalase I. It plays a critical role in the detoxification of methylglyoxal by inhibiting protein modifications that causes the formation of AGEs and by blocking the conversions of dicarbonyl and methylglyoxal into AGEs.[79] Certain other studies have also shown that the antioxidant protects the cell against glycation derived free radicals.[80,81]

5.9 CONCLUSION

Wild mushrooms are enriched with numerous secondary metabolites some of which are having antidiabetic properties. Some of the most potent antidiabetic bioactive compounds characterized from wild mushrooms are ergosterol peroxide (EPO), β-glucan, glucagon-like peptide 1 (GLP-1), galactoglucan, lovastatin, hispidin, glyoxalase I enzyme, etc. EPO significantly upregulated glucose absorption and was as good for glucose absorption as that of insulin. Polysaccharides from certain mushroom enlarges pancreatic islets and enhances insulin signaling by phosphorylating IR, Akt/PKB and AMPK and are found to be effective in inhibiting α-glucosidases and α-amylases in type-2 patients. In addition to these mushroom polysaccharides are used to treat gut dysbiosis and serves a potent antioxidant molecule. Yet the precise standards for the utilization of mushroom as an alternative drug to insulin is lacking, because of lack of a proper molecular mechanism. Hence, the need of hour is to further unravel the exact mechanism of action of antidiabetic mushrooms.

KEYWORDS

- **diabetes mellitus**
- **antidiabetic roles of mushrooms**
- **mechanisms**

REFERENCES

1. Forouzanfar, M. H.; Afshin, A.; Alexander, L. T.; Anderson, H. R.; Bhutta, Z. A.; Biryukov, S.; Carrero, J. J. Global, Regional, and National Comparative Risk Assessment of 79 Behavioural, Environmental and Occupational, and Metabolic Risks or Clusters of Risks, 1990–2015: A Systematic Analysis for the Global Burden of Disease Study. *Lancet* **2015,** *388* (10053), 1659–1724.
2. Cho, N.; Shaw, J. E.; Karuranga, S.; Huang, Y. D.; da Rocha Fernandes, J. D.; Ohlrogge, A. W.; Malanda, B. IDF Diabetes Atlas: Global Estimates of Diabetes Prevalence for 2017 and Projections for 2045. *Diabetes Res. Clin. Pract.* **2018,** *138*, 271–281.
3. Kuzuya, T.; Nakagawa, S.; Satoh, J.; Kanazawa, Y.; Iwamoto, Y.; Kobayashi, M.; Nanjo, K.; Sasaki, A.; Seino, Y.; Ito, C.; Shima, K.; Committee of the Japan Diabetes Society on the Diagnostic Criteria of Diabetes Mellitus. Report of the Committee on the Classification and Diagnostic Criteria of Diabetes Mellitus. *Diabetes Res. Clin. Pract.* **2002,** *55* (1), 65–85.
4. Lende, M.; Rijhsinghani, A. Gestational Diabetes: Overview with Emphasis on Medical Management. *Int. J. Environ. Res. Publ. Health* **2020,** *17* (24), 9573.
5. Puri, S.; Hebrok, M. Diabetic β Cells: To Be or Not to Be? *Cell* **2012,** *150* (6), 1103–1104.
6. Altaf, U.; Lalotra, P.; Sharma, Y. P. Nutritional and Mineral Composition of Four Wild Edible Mushrooms from Jammu and Kashmir, India. *Indian Phytopathol.* **2020,** *73* (2), 313–320.
7. Wu, S. J.; Tung, Y. J.; Ng, L. T. Anti-diabetic Effects of *Grifola frondosa* Bioactive Compound and Its Related Molecular Signaling Pathways in Palmitate-induced C2C12 Cells. *J. Ethnopharmacol.* **2020,** *260*, 112962.
8. Nam, K. S.; Jo, Y. S.; Kim, Y. H.; Hyun, J. W.; Kim, H. W. Cytotoxic Activities of Acetoxyscirpenediol and Ergosterol Peroxide from *Paecilomyces tenuipes*. *Life Sci.* **2001,** *69* (2), 229–237.
9. Ziegenbein, F. C.; Hanssen, H. P.; König, W. A. Secondary Metabolites from *Ganoderma lucidum* and *Spongiporus leucomallellus*. *Phytochemistry* **2006,** *67* (2), 202–211.
10. Krzyczkowski, W.; Malinowska, E.; Suchocki, P.; Kleps, J.; Olejnik, M.; Herold, F. Isolation and Quantitative Determination of Ergosterol Peroxide in Various Edible Mushroom Species. *Food Chem.* **2009,** *113* (1), 351–355.
11. Wu, S. J.; Lu, T. M.; Lai, M. N.; Ng, L. T. Immunomodulatory Activities of Medicinal Mushroom *Grifola frondosa* Extract and Its Bioactive Constituent. *Am. J. Chin. Med.* **2013,** *41* (01), 131–144.
12. Zhu, R.; Zheng, R.; Deng, Y.; Chen, Y.; Zhang, S. Ergosterol Peroxide from *Cordyceps cicadae* Ameliorates TGF-β1-Induced Activation of Kidney Fibroblasts. *Phytomedicine* **2014,** *21* (3), 372–378.
13. Kang, J. H.; Jang, J. E.; Mishra, S. K.; Lee, H. J.; Nho, C. W.; Shin, D.; Jin, M.; Kim, M. K.; Choi, C.; Oh, S. H. Ergosterol Peroxide from Chaga Mushroom (*Inonotus obliquus*) Exhibits Anti-cancer Activity by Down-regulation of the β-Catenin Pathway in Colorectal Cancer. *J. Ethnopharmacol.* **2015,** *173*, 303–312.

14. Liaw, C. C.; Wu, S. J.; Chen, C. F.; Lai, M. N.; Ng, L. T. Anti-inflammatory Activity and Bioactive Constituents of Cultivated Fruiting Bodies of *Xylaria nigripes* (Ascomycetes), a Chinese Medicinal Fungus. *Int. J. Med. Mushrooms* **2017,** *19* (10), 915–924.
15. Khorami, S. A. H.; Movahedi, A. R. I. Y. O.; Huzwah, K.; Sokhini, A. M. M. PI3K/AKT Pathway in Modulating Glucose Homeostasis and Its Alteration in Diabetes. *J. Med. Biomed. Sci.* **2015,** *1* (2), 46–55.
16. Higaki, Y.; Mikami, T.; Fujii, N.; Hirshman, M. F.; Koyama, K.; Seino, T.; Tanaka, K.; Goodyear, L. J. Oxidative Stress Stimulates Skeletal Muscle Glucose Uptake through a Phosphatidylinositol 3-Kinase-Dependent Pathway. *Am. J. Physiol.—Endocrinol. Metab.* **2008,** *294* (5), 889–897.
17. Rains, J. L.; Jain, S. K. Oxidative Stress, Insulin Signaling, and Diabetes. *Free Radic. BioMed.* **2011,** *50* (5), 567–575.
18. Gulati, V.; Singh, M. D.; Gulati, P. Role of Mushrooms in Gestational Diabetes Mellitus. *AIMS Med. Sci.* **2019,** *6* (*1*), 49–66.
19. Mizushima, N.; Komatsu, M. Autophagy: Renovation of Cells and Tissues. *Cell* **2011,** *147* (4), 728–741.
20. Levine, B.; Kroemer, G. Autophagy in the Pathogenesis of Disease. *Cell* **2008,** *132* (1), 27–42.
21. Yang, L.; Li, P.; Fu, S.; Calay, E. S.; Hotamisligil, G. S. Defective Hepatic Autophagy in Obesity Promotes ER Stress and Causes Insulin Resistance. *Cell Metab.* **2010,** *11* (6), 467–478.
22. Singh, R.; Kaushik, S.; Wang, Y.; Xiang, Y.; Novak, I.; Komatsu, M.; Tanaka, K.; Cuervo, A. M. Czaja, M. J. Autophagy Regulates Lipid Metabolism. *Nature* **2009,** *458* (7242), 1131–1135.
23. Zheng, Y.; Ren, W.; Zhang, L.; Zhang, Y.; Liu, D.; Liu, Y. A Review of the Pharmacological Action of *Astragalus* Polysaccharide. *Front. Pharmacol.* **2020,** *11*, 349.
24. Yang, S.; Yan, J.; Yang, L.; Meng, Y.; Wang, N.; He, C.; Fan, Y.; Zhou, Y. Polysaccharides from Mushroom Fruiting Bodies Improve Insulin Resistance by Inhibiting Lipid Deposition Via Autophagy Enhancement. **2018**. Available at SSRN 3248625. http://dx.doi.org/10.2139/ssrn.3248625
25. Dong, H.; Czaja, M. J. Regulation of Lipid Droplets by Autophagy. *Trends Endocrinol. Metab.* **2011,** *22* (6), 234–240.
26. Alam, N.; Amin, R.; Khan, A.; Ara, I.; Shim, M. J.; Lee, M. W.; Lee, U. Y.; Lee1, T. S. Comparative Effects of Oyster Mushrooms on Lipid Profile, Liver and Kidney Function in Hypercholesterolemic Rats. *Mycobiology* **2009,** *37* (1), 37–42.
27. Rajagopalan, G.; Krishnan, C. α-Amylase Production from Catabolite Derepressed *Bacillus subtilis* KCC103 Utilizing Sugarcane Bagasse Hydrolysate. *Bioresour. Technol.* **2008,** *99* (8), 3044–3050.
28. Koike, D.; Yamadera, K.; Dimagno, E. P. Effect of a Wheat Amylase Inhibitor on Canine Carbohydrate Digestion, Gastrointestinal Function, and Pancreatic Growth. *Gastroenterology* **1995,** *108* (4), 1221–1229.
29. Huang, H. T.; Wang, S. L.; Nguyen, V. B.; Kuo, Y. H. Isolation and Identification of Potent Antidiabetic Compounds from *Antrodia cinnamomea*—An Edible Taiwanese Mushroom. *Molecules* **2018,** *23* (11), 2864.

30. Wang, S. L. New Novel α-Glucosidase Inhibitors Produced by Microbial Conversion. *Process Biochem.* **2018,** *65*, 228–232.
31. Su, C. H.; Lai, M. N.; Ng, L. T. Inhibitory Effects of Medicinal Mushrooms on α-Amylase and α-Glucosidase–Enzymes Related to Hyperglycemia. *Food Funct.* **2013,** *4* (4), 644–649.
32. Shoba, K.; Krishnakumari, S. In Vitro Studies on Antioxidant and Antidiabetic Activity of *Pleurotus eous* Mushroom in Methanol and Aqueous Extract. *Asian J. Pharm. Clin. Res.* **2018,** *11*, 259–285.
33. Bae, S. M.; Han, S. M.; Lee, Y. H.; Jung, Y. K.; Ji, J. H.; Lee, J. S. Extraction and Characterization of an Anti-hyperglycemic α-Glucosidase Inhibitor from Edible Mushroom, *Pleurotus cornucopiae. Microbiol. Biotechnol. Lett.* **2016,** *44* (2), 124–129.
34. Stojkovic, D.; Smiljkovic, M.; Ciric, A.; Glamoclija, J.; Van Griensven, L.; Ferreira, I. C.; Sokovic, M. An Insight into Antidiabetic Properties of Six Medicinal and Edible Mushrooms: Inhibition of α-Amylase and α-Glucosidase Linked to Type-2 Diabetes. *S. Afr. J. Bot.* **2019,** *120*, 100–103.
35. Zhen-Yuan, Z.; Zhang, J. Y.; Li-Jing, C. H. E. N.; Xiao-Cui, L.; Yang, L. I. U.; Wan-Xiao, W.; Zhang, Y. M. Comparative Evaluation of Polysaccharides Isolated from *Astragalus*, Oyster Mushroom, and Yacon as Inhibitors of α-Glucosidase. *Chin. J. Nat. Med.* **2014,** *12* (4), 290–293.
36. Azeem, U.; Shri, R.; Dhingra, G. S. In Vitro and In Vivo Anti-hyperglycemia Activities of Medicinal Mushrooms (Hymenochaetaceae) from India. *Int. J. Med. Mushrooms* **2021,** *23* (2), 29–41.
37. Cao, H.; Ma, S.; Guo, H.; Cui, X.; Wang, S.; Zhong, X.; Wu, Y.; Zheng, W.; Yu, J.; Ma. L. Comparative Study on the Monosaccharide Compositions, Antioxidant and Hypoglycemic Activities in Vitro of Intracellular and Extracellular Polysaccharides of Liquid Fermented *Coprinus comatus. Int. J. Biol. Macromol.* **2019,** *139*, 543–549.
38. Rojkind, M.; Dominguez-Rosales, J. A.; Nieto, N.; Greenwel, P. Role of Hydrogen Peroxide and Oxidative Stress in Healing Responses. *Cell Mol. Life Sci.* **2002,** *59* (11), 1872–1891.
39. Pi, J.; Bai, Y.; Zhang, Q.; Wong, V.; Floering, L. M.; Daniel, K.; Reece, J. M.; Deeney, J. T.; Andersen, M. E.; Corkey, B. E.; Collins, S. Reactive Oxygen Species as a Signal in Glucose-Stimulated Insulin Secretion. *Diabetes* **2007,** *56* (7), 1783–1791.
40. Nishikawa, T.; Araki, E. Impact of Mitochondrial ROS Production in the Pathogenesis of Diabetes Mellitus and Its Complications. *Antioxid. Redox Signall.* **2007,** *9* (3), 343–353.
41. Rolo, A. P.; Palmeira, C. M. Diabetes and Mitochondrial Function: Role of Hyperglycemia and Oxidative Stress. *Toxicol. Appl. Pharm.* **2006,** *212* (2), 167–178.
42. Saito, M.; Sakagami, H.; Fujisawa, S. Cytotoxicity and Apoptosis Induction by Butylated Hydroxyanisole (BHA) and Butylated Hydroxytoluene (BHT). *Anticancer Res.* **2003,** *23* (6C), 4693–4701.
43. Lee, I. K.; Seok, S. J.; Kim, W. K.; Yun, B. S. Hispidin Derivatives from the Mushroom *Inonotus xeranticus* and Their Antioxidant Activity. *J. Nat. Prod.* **2006,** *69* (2), 299–301.

44. Jang, J. S.; Lee, J. S.; Lee, J. H.; Kwon, D. S.; Lee, K. E.; Lee, S. Y.; Hong, E. K. Hispidin Produced from *Phellinus linteus* Protects Pancreatic β-Cells from Damage by Hydrogen Peroxide. *Arch. Pharm. Res.* **2010,** *33* (6), 853–861.
45. Martín, A. R.; Villegas, I.; La Casa, C.; de la Lastra, C. A. Resveratrol, a Polyphenol Found in Grapes, Suppresses Oxidative Damage and Stimulates Apoptosis during Early Colonic Inflammation in Rats. *Biochem. Pharmacol.* **2004,** *67* (7), 1399–1410.
46. Park, I. H.; Chung, S. K.; Lee, K. B.; Yoo, Y. C.; Kim, S. K.; Kim, G. S.; Song, K. S. An Antioxidant Hispidin from the Mycelial Cultures of *Phellinus linteus*. *Arch. Pharm. Res.* **2004,** *27* (6), 615–618.
47. Blois, M. S. Antioxidant Determinations by the Use of a Stable Free Radical. *Nature* **1958,** *181* (4617), 1199–1200.
48. Marklund, S.; Marklund, G. Involvement of the Superoxide Anion Radical in the Autoxidation of Pyrogallol and a Convenient Assay for Superoxide Dismutase. *Eur. J. Biochem.* **1974,** *47* (3), 469–474.
49. Evans, J. L.; Goldfine, I. D.; Maddux, B. A.; Grodsky, G. M. Are Oxidative Stress-Activated Signaling Pathways Mediators of Insulin Resistance and β-Cell Dysfunction?. *Diabetes* **2003,** *52* (1), 1–8.
50. Bulam, S.; Üstün, N. Ş.; Pekşen, A. β-Glucans: An Important Bioactive Molecule of Edible and Medicinal Mushrooms. *Türkmen A* **2018,** *1*, 1242–1258.
51. Wang, X.; Liu, H.; Chen, J.; Li, Y.; Qu, S. Multiple Factors Related to the Secretion of Glucagon-Like Peptide-1. *Int J Endocrinol* **2015**. doi: 10.1155/2015/651757.
52. De Graaf, C.; Donnelly, D.; Wootten, D.; Lau, J.; Sexton, P. M.; Miller, L. J.; Ahn, J. M.; Liao, J.; Fletcher, M. M.; Yang, D.; Brown, A. J. Glucagon-Like Peptide-1 and Its Class BG Protein–Coupled Receptors: A Long March to Therapeutic Successes. *Pharmacol. Rev.* **2016,** *68* (4), 954–1013.
53. Reed, J.; Bain, S. C.; Kanamarlapudi, V. Recent Advances in Understanding the Role of Glucagon-Like Peptide 1. *F1000 Biol. Rep.* **2020,** *9*, F1000.
54. Khursheed, R.; Singh, S. K.; Wadhwa, S.; Gulati, M.; Awasthi, A. Therapeutic Potential of Mushrooms in Diabetes Mellitus: Role of Polysaccharides. *Int. J. Biol. Macromol.* **2020,** *164*, 1194–1205.
55. Vincent, M.; Philippe, E.; Everard, A.; Kassis, N.; Rouch, C.; Denom, J.; Taked, Y.; Uchiyama, S.; Delzenne, N. M.; Cani, P. D.; Migrenne, S. Dietary Supplementation with *Agaricus blazei* Murill Extract Prevents Diet-induced Obesity and Insulin Resistance in Rats. *Obesity* **2013,** *21* (3), 553–561.
56. Tian, Y.; Nichols, R. G.; Roy, P.; Gui, W.; Smith, P. B.; Zhang, J.; Lin, Y.; Weaver, V. J.; Patterson, A. D.; Cantorna, M. T. Prebiotic Effects of White Button Mushroom (*Agaricus bisporus*) Feeding on Succinate and Intestinal Gluconeogenesis in C57BL/6 Mice. *J. Funct. Food* **2018,** *45*, 223–232.
57. Chen, Y.; Liu, D.; Wang, D.; Lai, S.; Zhong, R.; Liu, Y.; Yang, C.; Liu, B.; Sarkar, M. R.; Zhao, C. Hypoglycemic Activity and Gut Microbiota Regulation of a Novel Polysaccharide from *Grifola frondosa* in Type 2 Diabetic Mice. *Food Chem. Toxicol.* **2019,** *126*, 295–302.
58. Nakahara, D.; Nan, C.; Mori, K.; Hanayama, M.; Kikuchi, H.; Hirai, S.; Egashira, Y. Effect of Mushroom Polysaccharides from *Pleurotus eryngii* on Obesity and Gut Microbiota in Mice Fed a High-Fat Diet. *Eur. J. Nutr.* **2020,** *59* (7), 3231–3244.

59. Liu, Y.; Wang, C.; Li, J.; Li, T.; Zhang, Y.; Liang, Y.; Mei, Y. *Phellinus linteus* Polysaccharide Extract Improves Insulin Resistance by Regulating Gut Microbiota Composition. *FASEB J.* **2020,** *34* (1), 1065–1078.
60. Zhu, F.; Du, B.; Bian, Z.; Xu, B. Beta-Glucans from Edible and Medicinal Mushrooms: Characteristics, Physicochemical and Biological Activities. *J. Food Compos. Anal.* **2015,** *41*, 165–173.
61. Wu, T. R.; Lin, C. S.; Chang, C. J.; Lin, T. L.; Martel, J.; Ko, Y. F.; Ojcius, D. M.; Lu, C. C.; Young, J. D.; Lai, H. C. Gut Commensal *Parabacteroides goldsteinii* Plays a Predominant Role in the Anti-obesity Effects of Polysaccharides Isolated from *Hirsutella sinensis*. *Gut* **2019,** *68* (2), 248–262.
62. Taylor, K. A. A Modification of the Phenol/Sulfuric Acid Assay for Total Carbohydrates Giving More Comparable Absorbances. *Appl. Biochem. Biotechnol.* **1995,** *53* (3), 207–214.
63. Kim, K. H.; Kim, Y. O.; Ko, B. S.; Youn, H. J.; Lee, D. S. Over-expression of the Gene (bglBC1) from *Bacillus circulans* Encoding an Endo-β-(1→3),(1→4)-Glucanase Useful for the Preparation of Oligosaccharides from Barley β-Glucan. *Biotechnol. Lett.* **2004,** *26* (22), 1749–1755.
64. Prince, P. S. M.; Menon, V. P.; Pari, L. Hypoglycaemic Activity of *Syzigium cumini* Seeds: Effect on Lipid Peroxidation in Alloxan Diabetic Rats. *J. Ethnopharmacol.* **1998,** *61* (1), 1–7.
65. Maillard, L. C. Action des acides amines sur les sucres; formation des melanoidines par voie methodique. *C. R. Acad. Sci.* **1912,** *154*, 66–68.
66. Monnier, V. M.; Sell, D. R.; Abdul-Karim, F. W.; Emancipator, S. N. Collagen Browning and Cross-linking Are Increased in Chronic Experimental Hyperglycemia: Relevance to Diabetes and Aging. *Diabetes* **1988,** *37* (7), 867–872.
67. Sell, D. R.; Monnier, V. M. Structure Elucidation of a Senescence Cross-link from Human Extracellular Matrix: Implication of Pentoses in the Aging Process. *J. Biol. Chem.* **1989,** *264* (36), 21597–21602.
68. Kazeem, M. I.; Akanji, M. A.; Hafizur, R. M.; Choudhary, M. I. Antiglycation, Antioxidant and Toxicological Potential of Polyphenol Extracts of Alligator Pepper, Ginger and Nutmeg from Nigeria. *Asian Pac. J. Trop. Med.* **2012,** *2* (9), 727–732.
69. Wu, C. H.; Huang, S. M.; Lin, J. A.; Yen, G. C. Inhibition of Advanced Glycation Endproduct Formation by Foodstuffs. *Food Funct* **2011,** *2* (5), 224–234.
70. Pulido, R.; Bravo, L.; Saura-Calixto, F. Antioxidant Activity of Dietary Polyphenols as Determined by a Modified Ferric Reducing/Antioxidant Power Assay. *J. Agric. Food Chem.* **2000,** *48* (8), 3396–3402.
71. Bagchi, D.; Swaroop, A.; Preuss, H. G.; Bagchi, M. Free Radical Scavenging, Antioxidant and Cancer Chemoprevention by Grape Seed Proanthocyanidin: An Overview. *Mutat. Res.—Fundam. Mol. Mech.* **2014,** *768*, 69–73.
72. Yap, H. Y. Y.; Tan, N. H.; Ng, S. T.; Tan, C. S.; Fung, S. Y. Inhibition of Protein Glycation by Tiger Milk Mushroom [*Lignosus rhinocerus* (cooke) Ryvarden] and Search for Potential Anti-diabetic Activity-related Metabolic Pathways by Genomic and Transcriptomic Data Mining. *Front. Pharmacol.* **2018,** *9*, 103.
73. Grassmann, J. Terpenoids as Plant Antioxidants. *Vitam. Horm.* **2005,** *72*, 505–535.

74. Surveswaran, S.; Cai, Y. Z.; Corke, H.; Sun, M. Systematic Evaluation of Natural Phenolic Antioxidants from 133 Indian Medicinal Plants. *Food Chem.* **2007,** *102* (3), 938–953.
75. Nishikimi, M.; Rao, N. A.; Yogi, K. Colorimetric Determination of Super Oxide Dismutase. *Biochem. Biophys. Commun.* **1972,** *46*, 849–854.
76. Yap, H. Y. Y.; Fung, S. Y.; Ng, S. T.; Tan, C. S.; Tan, N. H. Genome-based Proteomic Analysis of *Lignosus rhinocerotis* (Cooke) Ryvarden Sclerotium. *Int. J. Med. Sci.* **2015,** *12* (1), 23.
77. Thormalley, P.; Langborg, A.; Minhas, H. Formation of Glyoxal, Methylglyoxal, and 3-DG in the Glycation of Proteins. *Biochem. J.* **1999,** *344*, 109–116.
78. Tang, S. J.; Suen, T. C.; McInnes, R. R.; Buchwald, M. Association of the TLX-2 Homeodomain and 14-3-3η Signaling Proteins. *J. Biol. Chem.* **1998,** *273* (39), 25356–25363.
79. Wu, C. H.; Yen, G. C. Inhibitory Effect of Naturally Occurring Flavonoids on the Formation of Advanced Glycation Endproducts. *J. Agric. Food Chem.* **2005,** *53* (8), 3167–3173.
80. Elosta, A.; Ghous, T.; Ahmed, N. Produtos naturais como agentes anti-glicação: possível potencial terapêutico para complicações diabéticas. *Curr. Diabetes Rev.* **2012,** *8* (2), 92–108.
81. Bahmani, M.; Zargaran, A.; Rafieian-Kopaei, M.; Saki, K. Ethnobotanical Study of Medicinal Plants Used in the Management of Diabetes Mellitus in the Urmia, Northwest Iran. *Asian Pac. J. Trop. Med.* **2014,** *7*, 348–354.

CHAPTER 6

Effects of Mushrooms in Gestational Diabetes Mellitus

MOHD YAQUB BHAT*, ASIF HAMID DAR, ABDUL HAMID WANI, AADIL RASHID SHEIKH, WASIM SAJAD MALIK, and PALLAKI SHRIKHANDIA

Plant Pathology and Mycology Lab, Department of Botany, University of Kashmir, Srinagar 190006, Jammu and Kashmir, India

**Corresponding author. E-mail: myaqub35@gmail.com*

ABSTRACT

Gestational diabetes is a form of hyperglycemia, which is a common metabolic disorder during pregnancy. The synthetic hypoglycemic drugs used to cure gestational diabetes, due to their side effects after prolonged use fail significantly to change the course of diabetic complications. Mushrooms as a source of various bioactive metabolites, namely, terpenoids, polysaccharides, dietary fibers, proteins, lectins, sterols, alkaloids, phenolic compounds, and many other biomolecules of numerous health benefits act as nature's pharmacy store. Medicinal mushrooms have been used traditionally as antidiabetic agents for centuries especially by Korea, Japan, China, and India. The experimental validation to such uses has been established by various in vivo clinical studies on pregnant human and animal models. This chapter emphasizes on some promising medicinal mushrooms, which have been experimentally validated by scientific community for the prevention and treatment of gestational diabetes mellitus.

Therapeutic Mushrooms for Diabetes Mellitus: Current Evidences and Future Scope. Uzma Azeem, Khalid Rehman Hakeem, (Eds.)

6.1 INTRODUCTION

Diabetes mellitus, a chronic disorder marked by increased blood glucose, results due to abnormal insulin secretion or insulin dysfunction.[1] This disorder is of three types, namely, type 1 diabetes mellitus, type 2 diabetes mellitus, and gestational diabetes mellitus (GDM). GDM is the manifestation of hyperglycemia along the course of pregnancy and is mostly presumed to progress into the development of type 2 diabetes mellitus in the later life.[2–5] Evidence suggests that after every 2 min, a woman dies from pregnancy comorbidities and a principal illness among these; the gestational diabetes which is believed to affect one in six women is increasing at an alarming pace. As per the recent International Diabetes Federation (IDF) report, GDM affects approximately 14% of pregnancies worldwide, perturbing around 18,000,000 births annually.[6] Gestational diabetes further aggravates the problem by putting the lives of both the mother and neonate in danger of developing conditions like pre-eclampsia, gestational hypertension, fetal macrosomia, and obstructed labor.[7,8,9] A newborn from a female with GDM is likely to be macrosomic and thus prone to prenatal death; and if survived, is susceptible to birth injuries, neonatal hypoglycemia, metabolic syndrome and obesity in later life.[4,10–12] In the beginning of gestation insulin sensitivity increases due to an underlying increase in energy demand to meet the needs of mother and fetus,[13] however, with progress in gestation a surge of placental and local hormones such as progesterone, leptin, placental lactogen, estrogen, cortisol, and placental growth hormone lead to insulin resistance, thereby elevating the maternal blood glucose level.[14] Regular physiological adaptations to pregnancy like, hypertrophy of pancreatic β-cells and enhanced glucose-stimulated insulin secretion come into action which tend to maintain the maternal glycemic level.[15] However, due to various reasons like β-cell dysfunction; chronic insulin resistance; neurohormonal dysfunction; prolonged leptin resistance; decreased adiponectin; adipose tissue inflammation; increased gut permeability (facilitating the inflammatory mediator uptake from the gut into the circulation leading to systemic insulin resistance) associated with particular gut microbiome; oxidative stress, the normal metabolic adaptations to pregnancy do not occur sufficiently in all women, which leads to the development of gestational diabetes mellitus.[16] Currently, there is no standard treatment or prevention strategy for gestational diabetes other than lifestyle intervention. Though, certain chemical and biochemical agents like glyburide, metformin, humulin, phenformin, troglitazone are available in the market and are quite effective against GDM, but concerns arise regarding their harmful side-effects and long-term safety for the maternal and neonatal health.[17–19] Therefore, need of the hour is to find out new treatments which are safe, have high efficacy and do not impart their side effects on maternal and fetal health. Mushrooms being used as traditional antidiabetic remedies since ancient times represent an exquisite field for generating new types of therapeutics to combat diabetes. Moreover, several mushroom species due to the presence of vast array of important bioactive constituents have successfully regulated the blood glucose level, altered the course of diabetic complications, and attenuated the various mechanisms of carbohydrate metabolism under clinical and/or experimental trails without posing harmful side effects.[20,21] Therefore, mushrooms could ameliorate GDM and may bring potential benefits to the maternal-fetal health. Thus, use of mushrooms paves a new way in complementary therapy for alleviating gestational diabetes mellitus.[22,23]

6.2 IN VITRO STUDIES IN FAVOR OF ANTI-GDM EFFECTS OF MUSHROOMS

6.2.1 INHIBITION OF A-GLUCOSIDASE

α-Glucosidase, an enzyme in the small intestinal epithelium converts oligosaccharides and disaccharides into glucose. Inhibiting α-glucosidase notably masks the breakdown of oligosaccharides and disaccharides into glucose, which thus, serves as an effective strategy to combat the increase in postprandial blood glucose level in pregnant females.[24] Several studies have reported that terpenes and their structurally oxidized forms, that is, lanostane triterpenoids from various mushroom species including *Inonotus obliquus*, *Ganoderma lucidum*, *Ganoderma lingzhi*, *Ganoderma leucocontextum* exhibit remarkable inhibitory effect against α-glucosidase under in vitro conditions.[25–29] Moreover, methanol extract of *Ganoderma resinaceum* showed inhibitory activity against α-glucosidase.[30] Triterpenes like, Resinacein C, ganoderic acid Y, lucialdehyde C, 7-oxo-ganoderic acid Z3, 7-oxo-ganoderic acid Z, and lucidadiol isolated from ethanol extract of *G. resinaceum* have displayed very strong inhibitory effect against α-glucosidase in comparison to standard drug acarbose.[31,32]

In a study polysaccharides from the mushroom *Inonotus obliquus* have been reported to show remarkable inhibition on the said enzyme.[33] Likewise, many studies have reported that crude extracts of mushrooms such as *Ganodermaphilippii*, *Lenzites elegans*, *Rigidoporus ulmarius*, *Antrodia cinnamomea*, *Calvatiagigantea*, *Coprinus comatus*, *Cordyceps militaris*, *Morchella conica*, *Phellinus linteus*, *Inonotus obliquus*, *P. linteus*, *Clitocybe maxima*, *Agaricus blazei*, *Pleurotus florida*, *Grifola frondosa*, *Hericium erinaceus*, *A. blazei*, *Coriolus versicolor*, *Catathelasma ventricosum*, *G. lucidum*, *Strophariarugoso annulata*, *Craterellus cornucopioides* and *Laccaria amethystea* possess significant α-glucosidase enzyme inhibitory activity.[34–40]

6.2.2 INHIBITION OF ALDOSE REDUCTASE

Similarly an enzyme namely aldose reductase involved in polyol pathway known to intensify diabetic complications under hyperglycaemic condition, is also a potent target for inhibition by mushroom extracts and mushroom-derived constituents. Mushrooms namely *Agrocybe aegerita*, *Auricularia auricula-judae*, *G. lucidum*, *Lentinula edodes*, *Russula sanguinea*, *G. frondosa*, *H. erinaceus*, and *Tremella fuciformis* were evaluated for their in vitro aldose reductase inhibition and of these *G. lucidum* was found to be most effective.[41] Lanostane-type triterpenoids obtained from *G. lucidum* have shown considerable inhibitory effect on aldose reductase.[42,43] Similarly there are reports that polycyclic meroterpenoids of *Ganoderma leucocontextum* have shown significant inhibitory effect against bovine lens aldose red.[44] Lee et al.[45] in their study has reported considerable in vitro inhibition of dichloromethane extract of *Ganoderma applanatum* on rat aldose reductase. These in vitro study models exhibiting antidiabetic properties of the said mushroom species validate these mushrooms for their putative therapeutic use against gestational diabetes mellitus.

6.3 IN VIVO EFFECTS OF MUSHROOMS ON GDM DEMONSTRATED BY STUDIES ON ANIMAL MODELS

As there is paucity of data regarding the experimental protocols employed for studying in vivo effects of mushrooms in treating gestational diabetes, a suitable model methodology, adapted from the study of Laurino et al.[46] is presented here. GDM-STZ rats represent a well-established experimental model for the evaluation of insulin deficiency and hyperglycaemic effects on foetuses. Pregnant rats are induced for gestational diabetes by STZ/Streptozotocin treatment on 8th day of pregnancy. Rats with more than 120 mg/dl fasting blood glucose level are considered diabetic and are utilized as reliable experimental model for studying the effects of mushroom extracts\constituents on GDM.[47] These GDM-STZ rats are categorized as, positive control group, negative control group, preimplantation group, postimplantation group and treated differently. Positive control group rats are treated with prodiabetic substance and 0.9% saline solution from the beginning of gestation; negative control group is treated with saline solution only, from 1st to 19th day of gestational; preimplantation group is given mushroom treatment from day 1 to day 19, and postimplantation group is given mushroom treatment from day 9 to day 19. Different parameters including, hematologic, maternal biochemical-profile, embryo-fetal progression, oxidative stress biomarkers and ovary size are scrutinized from the beginning of gestation. Caesarean sections are done on 20th day of pregnancy and blood samples are collected from hepatic veins for analysis of biochemical parameters such as albumin, creatinine, urea, glucose, triglycerides, alanine aminotransferase, aspartate aminotransferase, total cholesterol and HDL-cholesterol. These are measured in an automated spectrophotometry system. Blood is further screened for haemoglobin, hematocrit, RBCs, WBCs and platelet counts. Amniotic fluid is collected from gestational sacs and the samples are stored immediately at −80°C. Females are then euthanized and their womb and ovaries are removed, weighed, and maintained at −80°C until further examination. Uterine canal is examined to find out the number of foetuses, implantation issues if any and visible resorptions. Oxidative stress biomarkers like catalase, glutathione peroxidase (GPx), reduced glutathione (GSH) and thiobarbituric acid reactive substances (TBARS) are analyzed by following the methodologies of Aebi,[48] Paglia and Valentine,[49] Ellman,[50] and Ohkawa; Ohishi; Yagi.[51] For measuring the abovementioned biomarkers of placenta, placental homogenate is taken in phosphate buffer followed by addition of hydrogen peroxide to start the reaction and catalase activity is evaluated by UV/VIS spectrophotometry. Whereas for blood, a constant of variation (k) related to hemoglobin (Hb) value is employed to obtain blood catalase activity in terms of k/g Hb. GPx level in blood plasma is correlated with the oxidation of the reduced form of NADPH. GSH and TBARS are quantified by making use of calibration curves with predefined concentrations of the respective standards. Lyophilized and reconstituted powder of *L. edodes* orally given to rats with streptozotocin-induced gestational diabetes mellitus during the first 19 days of gestation reduced the plasma levels of catalase, glucose, urea, and triglycerides. Though, it could not omit the deleterious effects caused by streptozotocin; however, *L. edodes* at this dosage alleviated the preimplantation issues significantly.[52]

In a similar study, rats with streptozotocin-induced gestational diabetes mellitus (GDM-STZ) were fed with *L. edodes* fruiting body powder either before or after fetus implantation and the effects were evaluated by performing hematologic, oxidative stress and metabolic assessments.[46] The oral glucose tolerance test (OGTT) showed significant differences among the glycemic profiles of rats treated prior and post-fetus implantation. Insulin level of the blood plasma and amniotic fluid of GDM-STZ rats was reduced by STZ treatment and was not reversed by the postimplantation treatment. Plasma and amniotic fluid glucose, triglycerides, and hematocrit levels were found to be increased by STZ treatment in pregnant mice; however, post-fetus implantation treatment with *L. edodes* showed a significant decrease in these parameters as shown in Figure 6.1. On the other hand, postimplantation treatment exhibited increase in total cholesterol level, whereas the prior implantation treatment decreased it. The decreased ovary size and increased placental mass in GDM-STZ rats was not reversed by postimplantation treatment; however, prior treatment had significant effect. GDM-STZ mice experienced high postimplantation losses which were found to be reduced by prior-implantation *L. edodes* diet; however, postimplantation treatment had no impact over this. Similarly, fetal weight was found to be decreased in GDM-STZ untreated and postimplantation treated mice, whereas fetal weight was found to be increased by preimplantation treatment. Both prior and postimplantation treatments had no effect on GPx (an oxidative stress inducible enzyme) in the blood, however TBARS (thiobarbituric acid reactive substance) in plasma was found to be decreased.

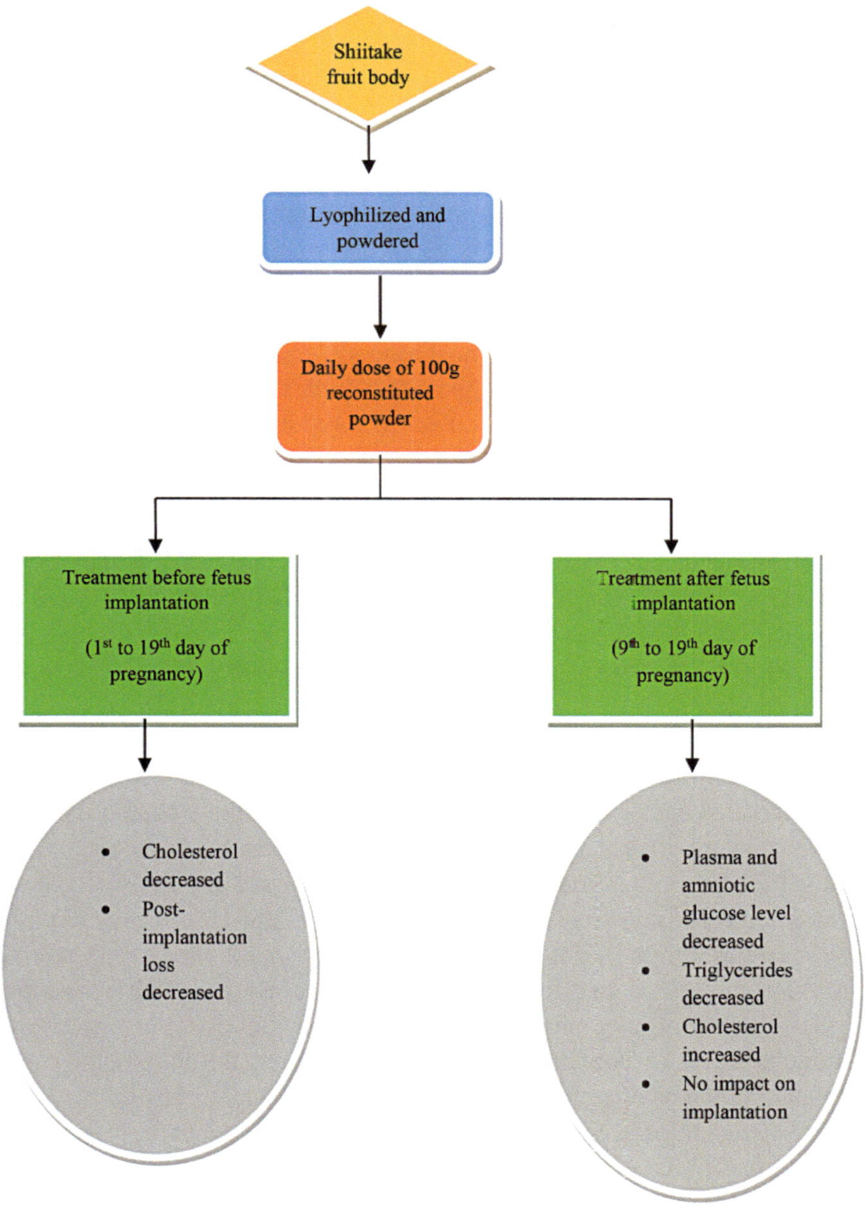

FIGURE 6.1 The effect of oral treatment of *L. edodes* powder on GDM-STZ rats, Laurino et al.[46]

Pregnant rats induced for gestational diabetes with streptozotocin treatment on day 8 of pregnancy were given reconstituted lyophilized powder of mushroom species namely *L. edodes*, *G. lucidum,* and *A. blazei* at the dosage of 100 mg/kg per day from day 1 to 19 (batch A) or from day 9 to 20 (batch B). OGTT assessment performed on day 17 of pregnancyrevealed that *G. lucidum* treatment in batch A exhibited considerable reduction in glycemic levels after 10, 20, 30, and 60 min after dextrose administration, whereas *G. lucidum*in batch B showed a decrease only after 20, 30, and 60 min. Likewise, *L. edodes* in batch A and batch B showed reduction at 30 and 120 min, respectively; whereas *A. blazei* had no significant impact in any of the batches. In briefthe mushrooms *G. lucidum* and *L. edodes* at a dosage of 100 mg/kg/day when given to pregnant rats before or after streptozotocin treatment have been observed toreduce the glucose levels and thus the peak of glycemic curve.[53] Caetano et al.[54] in while evaluating the effects of *Agaricus brasiliensis* diet on rats with streptozotocin-induced gestational diabetes mellitus, reported that it reduced the blood glucose level prior to STZ treatment, and successfully maintained the normal glycemic level even after STZ treatment. The authors in the aforementioned study also observed that *A. brasiliensis* diet successfully declined the levels of alanine aminotransferase, aspartate aminotransferase, triglycerides and LDL cholesterol, and elevated the HDL cholesterol level. Moreover, this mushroom demonstrated significant antioxidant activity neutralizing the oxidative stress and protecting the fetus from STZ induced damage. The principal mushroom bioactive compounds with well know antidiabetic activity employed for treatment of diabetes/GDM constitute terpenoids and mushroom polysaccharides especially β-glucans extracted from mushroom sporocarps, cultured mushroom mycelium, or their culture broth. Various in vivo and *in vitro* studies have reported that mushroom polysaccharides exhibit their antidiabetic effects by, inhibiting glucose absorption along gut; enhancing insulin-signalling pathways; modulating the carbohydrate metabolism; balancing the antioxidant status, enhancing the pancreatic β-cell mass thereby enhancing insulin secretion. *L. edodes*, *A. blazei*, *Schizophyllum commune*, *G. lucidum*, *A. brasiliensis*, *P. florida*, and *Lentinus squarrosulus* are the edible mushrooms abundant in β-glucans.[55] β-glucans a class of dietary fibres present in mushrooms act as prebiotics favoring the growth of good bacteria thereby causing the modulation of gut micro-flora which in turn results in the amelioration of diabetes.[56,57] β-glucan administration under diabetic conditions has

TABLE 6.1 Some Mushrooms with Anti-GDM Potential as Exhibited in Vivo on Diabetic Rats.

Mushroom species	Form used	Results	Mechanism involved	References
L. edodes	Reconstituted powder	Decreased blood glucose level, urea and triglycerides in GDM-STZ mice	Improved liver function and stabilized insulin response	[52]
P. florida	Polysaccharides	Reduced BGL and cholesterol level	Enhance SOD, catalase and glutathione peroxidase	[64]
G. frondosa	Mycelial broth	Antihyperglycemic and anti-inflammatory	Downregulates various inflammatory mediators	[65]
Pleurotus ostreatus	Whole polysaccharide extract	Lowered BGL and cholesterol level	Attenuates insulin resistance and oxidation stress, enhances GSK3 phosphorylation and GLUT4 translocation	[66]
Coprinus comatus	Polysaccharide fraction of ethanol extract	Hypoglyceamic effect	Immune modulation improving insulin secretion	[67]
Pleurotus tuberregium	Polysaccharides	Hypoglyceamic effect and oxidation stress attenuating effect	Attenuates gut microbiota	[68]
P. linteus	Polysaccharides	Significant antidiabetic effect	Changes composition of gastrointestinal microbiota	[69]
Armillaria mellea	Neural polysaccharide fraction	Hypoglyceamic and hypolipideamic effect	Enhances insulin sensitivity and reduces lipid accumulation by activating autophagy	[70]
Agaricus bisporus	Sporocarp extract	Hypoglyceamic and cholesterol lowering effect in STZ-treated diabetic rats	Protects pancreatic islets from STZ induced damage	[71]
Agaricus campestris	Fruiting body aqueous extract	Blood glucose lowering effect	Enhances insulin secretion and has insulin like activity	[72]

TABLE 6.1 *(Continued)*

Mushroom species	Form used	Results	Mechanism involved	References
A. auricula-judae	Mycelial powder	Reduction of BGL, triglycerides and cholesterol levels	Improves antioxidant status	[73]
C. comatus	Isolated compound Comatin	Lowering of BGL and improvement of glucose tolerance	Prevents the formation of Advanced glycated end-products (AGEs)	[74]
H. erinaceus	Methanolic extract of fruiting body	Hypoglycemic effects with significantly lower elevation rates of postprandial blood glucose level		[75]
Inonotus obliquus	Culture broth	Antihyperglycemic, antilipid peroxidative and antioxidant effects in alloxan-induced diabetic mice	Increase in insulin production, decrease in LDL-C, increase in hepatic glycogen	[76]
	Ethyl acetate fraction	Reduction of BGL	Increases antioxidant enzymes which thereby protect pancreatic β-cells	[77]
Laetiporus sulphureus var. *miniatus*	Extracellular polysaccharides (EPS)	Increased insulin level	Proliferation and regeneration of pancreatic β-cells	[78]
Lentinus strigosus	Exopolysaccharides (EPS) from mycelial culture	Decreased plasma glucose level up to 21.1% at the dose of 150 mg/kg bw	Regeneration of pancreatic islets	[79]

TABLE 6.1 *(Continued)*

Mushroom species	Form used	Results	Mechanism involved	References
Tremella fuciformis	Exopolysaccharides of submerged mycelial culture	Reduced fasting blood glucose level, improved glucose tolerance and glucose sensitivity	Acts through peroxisome proliferator-activated receptor (PPAR-γ)-mediated lipid metabolism	[80]
Tremella mesenterica	Fruiting body extract	Reduced fasting blood glucose level in diabetic and prediabetic impaired glucose tolerant rats		[81]
Wolfiporia extensa	Crude extract and triterpenes	Reduced postprandial blood glucose level in diabetic mice	Enhancing insulin sensitivity	[82, 83]

been shown to cause the systemic improvement of body which makes the organism to withstand the onset of diabetic complications.[58–60] Histopathological report of the diabetic rats administered with polysaccharides of *Ganoderma atrum*[61] demonstrated increase in β-cell mass, elongation of pancreatic islets, and pancreas restoration.[62] Similarly a protein linked polysaccharide obtained from *G. lucidum* sporocarps revealed the similar antidiabetic potential by inhibiting the β-cell apoptosis in streptozotocin (STZ)-induced diabetic rats.[63]

6.4 CLINICAL TRIALS DEMONSTRATING ANTI-GDM EFFECTS OF MUSHROOMS

Mushrooms being rich in minerals like potassium, phosphorus, calcium, phosphorus, and magnesium; vitamins like vitamin B complex, vitamin C, vitamin D, digestible proteins, carbohydrates, antioxidants and dietary fibre, could serve as an ideal food commodity.[84] Proper dietary pattern is linked with decreased gestational diabetes risk. The nutrient patterns consisting of vitamin A, vitamins B2 and B6, vitamin C, calcium, potassium, dietary fiber, and folate have been positively linked with gestational diabetes in several studies.[47] Various studies have confirmed the correlation between dietary fiber of the diets like those having mushrooms in the menu and the risk of GDM development.[85] The GDM ameliorating effects of such high-fiber diets can mainly be attributed to soluble dietary fiber which performs various pharmacological activities, like enhancement of insulin sensitivity, decrease in adiposity, modulation of inflammatory markers, and attenuation of various gut and adipocyte-derived hormones.[86,87] Calcium and vitamin D supplement have shown the beneficial effects on the metabolic profile of women suffering from GDM.[88] In close agreement to the aforementioned evidence, a prospective cohort study reported that women taking calcium rich low-fat foods like mushrooms, whole grains and skimmed dairy products during prepregnancy experienced relatively less incidence of GDM.[89] The biological mechanism anticipated to be attenuated by such kind of calcium rich-low fat foods could be the modulation of intracellular calcium level which in turn affects insulin sensitivity and insulin release.[90,91] The oxidation of excess glucose and subsequent nonenzymatic glycation of proteins increases ROS which thereby aggravates the diabetic complications in pregnant women.

Therefore, exogenous antioxidants rich functional food has the potential to prevent the GDM associated complications from worsening.[22,23] Various mushroom species including, *L. edodes*, *L. sulphureus*, *A. auricula-judae*, *G. frondosa*, *H. erinaceus*, *A. bisporus*, *P. ostreatus*, etc. having ample essential nutrients and being low in calorific value qualify as promising functional food in the prevention of diseases like GDM.[92] Sun and Niu[93] while performing studies on effects of button mushroom (*A. bisporus*) on gestational comorbidities reported that mushroom diet significantly lowered the risk of gestational diabetes ($P = 0.047$). The study was carried out on two groups of female subjects; 582 in MD group (MD stands for mushroom diet) and 580 in placebo group. Females of the MD group were fed 100 g of button mushroom daily from prepregnancy up to the 20th week of gestation. The study was further extended to evaluate the efficacy of mushroom diet with respect to BMI and chronological age of female subjects in both the study groups and it was observed that, within the placebo group the subjects with normal prepregnancy BMI were 2.7 times more prone to develop gestational diabetes (OR = 2.66, 95% CI = 1.38–3.62, $P = 0.024$). Likewise, subjects in the placebo group aged between 25 and 29 years experienced the incidence of gestational diabetes 2.4-folds (OR = 2.35, 95% CI = 1.77–4.62, $P = 0.018$) than that of females of same age within MD group; and placebo subjects of age >30 years developed gestational diabetes 3 times (OR = 3.04, 95% CI = 1.98–6.26, $P = 0.007$) more than that of females of same age group within the MD group.

6.5 CONCLUSION

Gestational diabetes is a form of hyperglycemia, which is common metabolic disorder during pregnancy. Synthetic hypoglycemic drugs used to cure GDM owing to their side effects, pose a threat on fetal health after their prolonged use, and could even lead to problems like fetal disgenesis and miscarriage. Mushrooms being rich in various bioactive metabolites and biomolecules with numerous pharmacological benefits behave like nature's pharmacy store which is to be explored for harnessing potential therapeutic agents to treat this ever expanding epidemic of gestational diabetes in women without posing harmful effects on developing fetus.

KEYWORDS

- **gestation**
- **diabetes mellitus**
- **GDM-STZ**
- **mushrooms**

REFERENCES

1. Kaur, A.; Dhingra, G. S.; Shri, R. Evaluation of Carbohydrate Metabolism Inhibition by Some Species of Medicinal Mushrooms from India. *Int. J. Med. Mushrooms* **2015,** *17* (4), 351–360.
2. Ratner, R. E.; Christophi, C. A.; Metzger, B. E.; Dabelea, D.; Bennett, P. H.; Pi-Sunyer, X.; Fowler, S.; Kahn, S. E. Diabetes Prevention Program Research Group. Prevention of Diabetes in Women with a History of Gestational Diabetes: Effects of Metformin and Lifestyle Interventions. *J. Clin. Endocrmetab.* **2008,** *93* (12), 4774–4779.
3. Bellamy L.; Casas J.; Hingorani A. D. Type 2 Diabetes Mellitus after Gestational Diabetes: A Systematic Review and Meta-analysis. *Lancet* **2009,** *373* (9677), 1773–1779.
4. Kampmann, U.; Madsen, L. R.; Skajaa, G. O.; Iversen, D. S.; Moeller, N.; Ovesen, P. Gestational Diabetes: A Clinical Update. *World J. Diabetes* **2015,** *6* (8), 1065.
5. Lauenborg, J.; Hansen, T.; Jensen, D. M.; Vestergaard, H.; Molsted-Pedersen, L.; Hornnes, P.; Damm, P. Increasing Incidence of Diabetes after Gestational Diabetes: A Long-term Follow-up in a Danish Population. *Diabetes Care* **2004,** *27* (5), 1194–1199.
6. Cho, N.; Shaw, J. E.; Karuranga, S.; Huang, Y. D.; DaRocha-Fernandes, J. D.; Ohlrogge, A. W.; Malanda, B. IDF Diabetes Atlas: Global Estimates of Diabetes Prevalence for 2017 and Projections for 2045. *Diabetes Res. Clin. Pract.* **2018,** *138*, 271–281.
7. Sheshiah, V.; Kapur, A.; Balaji, V.; Balaji, M. S. Hyperglycemia in Pregnancy—Consequences and Salvation. *Austin Diabetes Res.* **2016,** *1* (2), 1008.
8. Hod, M.; Kapur, A.; Sacks, D. A.; Hadar, E.; Agarwal, M.; Di-Renzo, G. C.; Divakar, H. The International Federation of Gynecology and Obstetrics (FIGO) Initiative on Gestational Diabetes Mellitus: A Pragmatic Guide for Diagnosis, Management, and Care. *Int. J. Gynaecol. Obstet.* **2015,** *131* (3), 173–211.
9. Carpenter, M. W.; Coustan, D. R. Criteria for Screening Tests for Gestational Diabetes. *Am. J. Obstetr. Gynecol.* **1982,** *144 (7)*, 768–773.
10. Hartling, L.; Dryden, D. M.; Guthrie, A.; Muise, M.; Vandermeer, B.; Donovan, L. Diagnostic Thresholds for Gestational Diabetes and Their Impact on Pregnancy Outcomes: A Systematic Review. *Diabetes Med.* **2014,** *31* (3), 319–331.

11. Metzger, B. E.; Contreras, M.; Sacks, D. A.; Watson, W.; Dooley, S. L.; Foderaro, M.; King, J. Hyperglycemia and Adverse Pregnancy Outcomes. *New Engl. J. Med.* **2008,** *358* (19), 1991–2002.
12. Hillier, T. A.; Pedula, K. L.; Schmidt, M. M.; Mullen, J. A.; Charles, M. A.; Pettitt, D. J. Childhood Obesity and Metabolic Imprinting: The Ongoing Effects of Maternal Hyperglycemia. *Diabetes Care* **2007,** *30* (9), 2287–2292.
13. Di-Cianni, G.; Miccoli, R.; Volpe, L.; Lencioni, C.; Del-Prato, S. Intermediate Metabolism in Normal Pregnancy and in Gestational Diabetes. *Diabetes Metab. Res. Rev.* **2003,** *19* (4), 259–270.
14. Catalano, P. M.; Tyzbir, E. D.; Roman, N. M.; Amini, S. B.; Sims, E. A. Longitudinal Changes in Insulin Release and Insulin Resistance in Nonobese Pregnant Women. *Am. J. Obstetgynecol.* **1991,** *165* (6), 1667–1672.
15. Parsons, J. A.; Brelje, T. C.; Sorenson, R. L. Adaptation of Islets of Langerhans to Pregnancy: Increased Islet Cell Proliferation and Insulin Secretion Correlates with the Onset of Placental Lactogen Secretion. *Endocrinology* **1992,** *130* (3), 1459–1466.
16. Plows, J. F.; Stanley, J. L.; Baker, P. N.; Reynolds, C. M.; Vickers, M. H. The Pathophysiology of Gestational Diabetes Mellitus. *Int. J. Mol. Sci.* **2018,** *19* (11), 3342.
17. Feig, D. S.; Moses, R. G. Metformin Therapy during Pregnancy: Good for the Goose and Good for the Gosling too? *Diabetes Care* **2011,** *34* (10), 2329–2330.
18. Castillo, W. C.; Boggess, K.; Stürmer, T.; Brookhart, M. A.; Benjamin, D. K.; Funk, M. J. Association of Adverse Pregnancy Outcomes with Glyburide Vs. Insulin in Women with Gestational Diabetes. *JAMA Pediatr.* **2015,** *169* (5), 452–458.
19. Li, W. L.; Zheng, H. C.; Bukuru, J.; De-Kimpe, N. Natural Medicines Used in the Traditional Chinese Medical System for Therapy of Diabetes Mellitus. *J. Ethnopharmacol.* **2004**, *92* (1), 1–21.
20. Lo, H. C.; Wasser, S. P. Medicinal Mushrooms for Glycemic Control in Diabetes Mellitus: History, Current Status, Future Perspectives, and Unsolved Problems. *Int. J. Med. Mushrooms* **2011,** *13* (5), 401–426.
21. Jovanovic, J. A.; Mihailovic, M.; Uskokovic, A. S.; Grdovic, N.; Dinic, S.; Poznanovic, G.; Vidakovic, M. Evaluation of the Antioxidant and Antiglycation Effects of *Lactarius deterrimus* and *Castanea sativa* Extracts on Hepatorenal Injury in Streptozotocin-Induced Diabetic Rats. *Front. Pharmacol.* **2017,** *8*, 793.
22. Maritim, A. C.; Sanders, A.; Watkins I. J. B. Diabetes, Oxidative Stress, and Antioxidants: A Review. *J. Biochem. Mol. Toxicol.* **2003,** *17* (1), 24–38.
23. Zhang, J. J.; Li, Y.; Zhou, T.; Xu, D. P.; Zhang, P.; Li, S.; Li, H. B. Bioactivities and Health Benefits of Mushrooms Mainly from China. *Molecules* **2016,** *21* (7), 938.
24. Sales, P. M.; Souza, P. M.; Simeoni, L. A.; Magalhaes, P. O.; Silveira, D. α-Amylase Inhibitors: A Review of Raw Material and Isolated Compounds from Plant Source. *J. Pharm. Sci.* **2012,** *15* (1), 141–183.
25. Ying, Y. M.; Zhang, L. Y.; Zhang, X.; Bai, H. B.; Liang, D. E.; Ma, L. F.; Shan, W. G.; Zhan, Z. J. Terpenoids with Alpha-glucosidase Inhibitory Activity from the Submerged Culture of *Inonotus obliquus*. *Phytochemistry* **2014,** *108*, 171–176.
26. Fatmawati, S.; Shimizu, K.; Kondo, R. Ganoderol B: A Potent α-Glucosidase Inhibitor Isolated from the Fruiting Body of *Ganoderma lucidum*. *Phytomedicine* **2011,** *18* (12), 1053–1055.

27. Fatmawati, S.; Shimizu, K.; Kondo, R. Ganoderic Acid Df, a New Triterpenoid with Aldose Reductase Inhibitory Activity from the Fruiting Body of *Ganoderma lucidum*. *Fitoterapia* **2010,** *81* (8), 1033–1036.
28. Fatmawati, S.; Kondo, R.; Shimizu, K. Structure–Activity Relationships of Lanostane-Type Triterpenoids from *Ganoderma lingzhi* as α-Glucosidase Inhibitors. *Bioorg. Med. Chem. Lett.* **2013,** *23* (21), 5900–5903.
29. Wang, K.; Bao, L.; Xiong, W.; Ma, K.; Han, J.; Wang, W.; Yin, W.; Liu, H. Lanostane triterpenes from the Tibetan Medicinal Mushroom *Ganoderma leucocontextum* and Their Inhibitory Effects on HMG-CoA Reductase and α-Glucosidase. *J. Nat. Prod.* **2015,** *78* (8), 1977–1989.
30. Zengin, G.; Sarikurkcu, C.; Gunes, E.; Uysal, A.; Ceylan, R.; Uysal, S.; Gungor, H.; Aktumsek, A. Two *Ganoderma* Species: Profiling of Phenolic Compounds by HPLC–DAD, Antioxidant, Antimicrobial and Inhibitory Activities on Key Enzymes Linked to Diabetes Mellitus, Alzheimer's Disease and Skin Disorders. *Food Funct* **2015,** *6* (8), 2794–2802.
31. Satria, D.; Tamrakar, S.; Suhara, H.; Kaneko, S.; Shimizu, K. Mass-Spectrometry-Based Untargeted Metabolomics and α-Glucosidase Inhibitory Activity of Lingzhi (*Ganoderma lingzhi*) during the Developmental Stages. *Molecules* **2019,** *24* (11), 2044.
32. Satria, D.; Amen, Y.; Niwa, Y.; Ashour, A.; Allam, A. E.; Shimizu, K. Lucidumol D, a New Lanostane-Type Triterpene from Fruiting Bodies of Reishi (*Ganoderma lingzhi*). *Nat. Prod. Res.* **2019,** *33* (2), 189–195.
33. Wang, C.; Gao, X.; Santhanam, R. K.; Chen, Z.; Chen, Y.; Xu, L.; Wang, C.; Ferri, N.; Chen, H. Effects of Polysaccharides from *Inonotus obliquus* and Its Chromium(III) Complex on Advanced Glycation End-products Formation, α-Amylase, α-Glucosidase Activity and H_2O_2-Induced Oxidative Damage in Hepatic L02 Cells. *Food Chem. Toxicol.* **2018,** *116* (12), 335–345.
34. Kaur, A.; Dhingra, G. S.; Shri, R. Evaluation of Carbohydrate Metabolism Inhibition by Some Species of Medicinal Mushrooms from India. *Int. J. Med. Mushrooms* **2015,** *17* (4), 351–360.
35. Huang, H. T.; Wang, S. L.; Nguyen, V. B.; Kuo, Y. H. Isolation and Identification of Potent Antidiabetic Compounds from *Antrodia cinnamomea*—An edible Taiwanese Mushroom. *Molecules* **2018,** *23* (11), 2864.
36. Ogbole, O. O.; Nkumah, A. O.; Linus, A. U.; Falade, M. O. Molecular Identification, in Vivo and in Vitro Activities of *Calvatia gigantea* (Macro-fungus) as an Antidiabetic Agent. *Mycyology* **2019,** *10* (3), 166–173.
37. Stojkovic, D.; Smiljkovic, M.; Ciric, A.; Glamoclija, J.; Van-Griensven, L.; Ferreira, I. C.; Sokovic, M. An Insight into Antidiabetic Properties of Six Medicinal and Edible Mushrooms: Inhibition of α-Amylase and α-Glucosidase Linked to Type-2 Diabetes. *S. Afr. J. Bot.* **2019**, *120* (1), 100–103.
38. Prabu, M.; Kumuthakalavalli, R. Antidiabetic Potential of the Oyster Mushroom *Pleurotus florida* (Mont.) Singer. *Int. J. Curr. Pharm. Res.* **2017**, *9* (4), 51–54.
39. Su, C. H.; Lai, M. N.; Ng, L. T. Inhibitory Effects of Medicinal Mushrooms on α-Amylase and α-Glucosidase–Enzymes Related to Hyperglycemia. *Food Funct.* **2013**, *4* (4), 644–649.

40. Liu, Y. T.; Sun, J.; Luo, Z. Y.; Rao, S. Q.; Su, Y. J.; Xu, R. R.; Yang, Y. Chemical Composition of Five Wild Edible Mushrooms Collected from Southwest China and Their Antihyperglycemic and Antioxidant Activity. *Food Chem. Toxicol.* **2012**, *50* (5), 1238–1244.
41. Wu, T.; Xu, B. B. Antidiabetic and Antioxidant Activities of Eight Medicinal Mushroom Species from China. *Int. J. Med. Mushrooms* **2015,** *17* (2), 129–140.
42. Fatmawati, S.; Shimizu, K.; Kondo, R. Ganoderic acid Df, a New Triterpenoid with Aldose Reductase Inhibitory Activity from the Fruiting Body of *Ganoderma lucidum*. *Fitoterapia* **2010,** *81* (8), 1033–1036.
43. Fatmawati, S.; Shimizu, K.; Kondo, R. Structure–Activity Relationships of Ganoderma Acids from *Ganoderma lucidum* as Aldose Reductase Inhibitors. *Bioorg. Med. Chem. Lett.* **2011,** *21* (24), 7295–7297.
44. Zhang, J.; Ma, K.; Chen, H.; Wang, K.; Xiong, W.; Bao, L.; Liu, H. A Novel Polycyclic Meroterpenoid with Aldose Reductase Inhibitory Activity from Medicinal Mushroom *Ganoderma leucocontextum*. *J. Antibiot.* **2017,** *70* (8), 915–917.
45. Lee, S. H.; Shim, S. H.; Kim, J. S.; Kang, S. S. Constituents from the Fruiting Bodies of *Ganoderma applanatum* and Their Aldose Reductase Inhibitory Activity. *Arch. Pharm. Res.* **2006,** *29* (6), 479–483.
46. Laurino, L. F.; Viroel, F. J.; Caetano, E.; Spim, S.; Pickler, T. B.; Rosa-Castro, R. M.; Gerenutti, M. *Lentinus edodes* Exposure Before and After Fetus Implantation: Materno-fetal Development in Rats with Gestational Diabetes Mellitus. *Nutrients* **2019,** *11* (11), 2720.
47. Chen, Q.; Feng, Y.; Yang, H.; Wu, W.; Zhang, P.; Wang, K.; Wang, Y.; Ko, J.; Shen, J.; Guo, L.; Zhao, F.; Du, W.; Ru, S.; Wang, S.; Zhang, Y. A Vitamin Pattern Diet Is Associated with Decreased Risk of Gestational Diabetes Mellitus in Chinese Women: Results from a Case Control Study in Taiyuan, China. *J. Diabetes Res.* **2019,** *2019*, 5232308.
48. Aebi, H. Catalase in Vitro Methods. *Enzymology* **1984,** *105*, 121–126.
49. Paglia, D. E.; Valentine, W. N. Studies on the Quantitative and Qualitative Characterization of Erythrocyte Glutathione Peroxidase. *J. Lab. Clin. Med.* **1967,** *70* (1), 158–169.
50. Ellman, G. L. Tissue sulfhydryl groups. *Arch. Biol. Phys.* **1959,** *82* (1), 70–77.
51. Ohkawa, H.; Ohishi, N.; Yagi, K. Assay for Lipid Peroxides in Animal Tissues by Thiobarbituric Acid Reaction. *Anal. Biochem.* **1979,** *95* (2), 351–358.
52. Maschio, B. H.; Gentil, B. C.; Caetano, E.; Rodrigues, L. S.; Laurino, L. F.; Spim, S.; Jozala, A. F.; Dos-Santos, C. A.; Grotto, D.; Gerenutti, M. Characterization of the Effects of the Shiitake Culinary-Medicinal Mushroom, *Lentinus edodes* (Agaricomycetes), on Severe Gestational Diabetes Mellitus in Rats. *Int. J. Med. Mushrooms* **2017,** *19* (11), 991–1000.
53. Laurino, L. F.; Viroel, F. J.; Pickler, T. B.; Gerenutti, M. Functional Foods in Gestational Diabetes: Evaluation of the Oral Glucose Tolerance Test (OGTT) in Pregnant Rats Treated with Mushrooms. *Reprod. Toxicol.* **2017,** *72*, 36.
54. Caetano, E. L. A.; Viroel, F. J. M.; Laurino, L. F.; Camargo, I. F.; Castro, R. D. M. R.; Pickler, T. B.; Gerenutti, M. Royal Sun Culinary-Medicinal Mushroom *Agaricus brasiliensis* (Agaricomycetes) as a Functional Food in Gestational Diabetes Mellitus before and after Fetus Implantation. *Int. J. Med. Mushrooms* **2021,** *23* (9), 15–27.

55. Zhu, F.; Du, B.; Xu, B. A Critical Review on Production and Industrial Applications of Beta-glucans. *Food Hydrocolloids* **2016,** *52* (2), 275–288.
56. Ahmad, A.; Anjum, F. M.; Zahoor, T.; Nawaz, H.; Dilshad, S. M. R. Beta-glucan: A Valuable Functional Ingredient in Foods. *Crit. Rev. Food Sci. Nutr.* **2012,** *52* (3), 201–212.
57. Chen, J.; Seviour, R. Medicinal Importance of Fungal β-(1→3), (1→6)-Glucans. *Mycol. Res.* **2007,** *111* (6), 635–652.
58. Mihailovic, M.; Arambasic Jovanovic, J.; Uskokovic, A.; Dinic, S.; Grdovic, N.; Markovic, J.; Vidakovic, M. β-Glucan Administration to Diabetic Rats Reestablishes Redox Balance and Stimulates Cellular Pro-survival Mechanisms. *J. Funct. Foods* **2013,** *5* (1), 267–278.
59. Mihailovic, M.; Arambasic, J.; Uskokovic, A.; Dinic, S.; Grdovic, N.; Markovic, J.; Vidakovic, M. β-Glucan Administration to Diabetic Rats Alleviates Oxidative Stress by Lowering Hyperglycaemia, Decreasing Non-enzymatic Glycation and Protein O-GlcNAcylation. *J. Funct. Foods* **2013,** *5* (3), 1226–1234.
60. Uskokovic, A.; Mihailovic, M.; Dinic, S.; Jovanovic, J. A.; Grdovic, N.; Markovic, J.; Vidakovic, M. Administration of a β-Glucan-Enriched Extract Activates Beneficial Hepatic Antioxidant and Anti-inflammatory Mechanisms in Streptozotocin-Induced Diabetic Rats. *J. Funct. Foods* **2013,** *5* (4), 1966–1974.
61. Zhu, K. X.; Nie, S. P.; Li, C.; Gong, D.; Xie, M. Y. *Ganoderma atrum* Polysaccharide Improves Aortic Relaxation in Diabetic Rats Via PI3K/Akt Pathway. *Carbohydr. Polym.* **2014,** *103*, 520–527.
62. Zhu, K.; Nie, S.; Li, C.; Lin, S.; Xing, M.; Li, W.; Xie, M. A Newly Identified Polysaccharide from *Ganoderma atrum* Attenuates Hyperglycemia and Hyperlipidemia. *Int. J. Biol. Macromol.* **2013,** *57*, 142–150.
63. Zheng, J.; Yang, B.; Yu, Y.; Chen, Q.; Huang, T.; Li, D. *Ganoderma lucidum* Polysaccharides Exert Anti-hyperglycemic Effect on Streptozotocin-Induced Diabetic Rats through Affecting β-Cells. *J. Theor. Comput. Chem.* **2012,** *15* (7), 542–550.
64. Ganeshpurkar, A.; Kohli, S.; Rai, G. Antidiabetic Potential of Polysaccharides from the White Oyster Culinary-Medicinal Mushroom *Pleurotus florida* (Higher Basidiomycetes). *Int. J. Med. Mushrooms* **2014,** *16* (3), 207–217.
65. Chen, Y. H.; Lee, C. H.; Hsu, T. H.; Lo, H. C. Submerged-Culture Mycelia and Broth of the Maitake Medicinal Mushroom *Grifolafrondosa* (Higher Basidiomycetes) Alleviate Type 2 Diabetes-Induced Alterations in Immunocytic Function. *Int. J. Med. Mushrooms* **2015,** *17* (6), 541–556.
66. Zhang, Y.; Hu, T.; Zhou, H.; Zhang, Y.; Jin, G.; Yang, Y. Antidiabetic Effect of Polysaccharides from *Pleurotus ostreatus* in Streptozotocin-Induced Diabetic Rats. *Int. J. Biol. Macromol.* **2016,** *83*, 126–132.
67. Zhou, S.; Liu, Y.; Yang, Y.; Tang, Q.; Zhang, J. Hypoglycemic Activity of Polysaccharide from Fruiting Bodies of the Shaggy Ink Cap Medicinal Mushroom, *Coprinus comatus* (Higher Basidiomycetes), on Mice Induced by Alloxan and Its Potential Mechanism. *Int. J. Med. Mushrooms* **2015,** *17* (10), 957–964.
68. Huang, H. Y.; Korivi, M.; Chaing, Y. Y.; Chien, T. Y.; Tsai, Y. C. *Pleurotus tuber-regium* Polysaccharides Attenuate Hyperglycemia and Oxidative Stress in Experimental Diabetic Rats. *Evid.-Based Compl. Alt. Med.* **2012,** 1–8. https://doi.org/10.1155/2012/856381

69. Kim, H.; Han, S.; Lee, C.; Lee, K.; Hong, D. Compositions Containing Polysaccharides from *Phellinus linteus* and Methods for Treating Diabetes Mellitus Using Same. U.S. Patent and Trademark Office: Washington, DC, 2004.
70. Yang, S.; Yan, J.; Yang, L.; Meng, Y.; Wang, N.; He, C.; Zhou, Y. Polysaccharides from Mushroom Fruiting Bodies Improve Insulin Resistance by Inhibiting Lipid Deposition Via Autophagy Enhancement. **2018**. Available at SSRN: https://ssrn.com/abstract=3248625 or http://dx.doi.org/10.2139/ssrn.3248625
71. Jeong, S. C.; Jeong, Y. T.; Yang, B. K.; Islam, R.; Koyyalamudi, S. R.; Pang, G.; Song, C. H. White Button Mushroom (*Agaricus bisporus*) Lowers Blood Glucose and Cholesterol Levels in Diabetic and Hypocholesterolemic Rats. *Nutr. Res.* **2010,** *30* (1), 49–56.
72. Gray, A. M.; Flatt, P. R. Insulin-releasing and Insulin-like Activity of *Agaricus campestris* (Mushroom). *J. Endocrinol.* **1998,** *157* (2), 259–266.
73. Kim, S. K.; Hong, U. P.; Kim, J. S.; Kim, C. H.; Lee, K. W.; Choi, S. E.; Park, K. H.; Lee, M. W. Antidiabetic Effect of *Auricularia auricula* Mycelia in Streptozotocin-Induced Diabetic Rats. *Nat. Prod. Sci.* **2007,** *13* (4), 390–393.
74. Ding, Z.; Lu, Y.; Lu, Z.; Lv, F.; Wang, Y.; Bie, X.; Zhang, K. Hypoglycaemic Effect of Comatin, an Antidiabetic Substance Separated from *Coprinus comatus* Broth, on Alloxan-Induced-Diabetic Rats. *Food Chem.* **2010,** *121* (1), 39–43.
75. Wang, J. C.; Hu, S. H.; Wang, J. T.; Chen, K. S.; Chia, Y. C. Hypoglycemic Effect of Extract of *Hericium erinaceus*. *J. Sci. Food Agric.* **2005,** *85* (4), 641–646.
76. Sun, J. E.; Ao, Z. H.; Lu, Z. M.; Xu, H. Y.; Zhang, X. M.; Dou, W. F.; Xu, Z. H. Antihyperglycemic and Antilipidperoxidative Effects of Dry Matter of Culture Broth of *Inonotus obliquus* in Submerged Culture on Normal and Alloxan-Diabetes Mice. *J. Ethnopharmacol.* **2008,** *118* (1), 7–13.
77. Xu, X.; Wu, Y.; Chen, H. Comparative Antioxidative Characteristics of Polysaccharide-Enriched Extracts from Natural Sclerotia and Cultured Mycelia in Submerged Fermentation of *Inonotus obliquus*. *Food Chem.* **2011,** *127* (1), 74–79.
78. Hwang, H. S.; Yun, J. W. Hypoglycemic Effect of Polysaccharides Produced by Submerged Mycelial Culture of *Laetiporus sulphureus* on Streptozotocin Induced Diabetic Rats. *Biotechnol. Bioprocess* **2010,** *15* (1), 173–181.
79. Yamac, M.; Kanbak, G.; Zeytinoglu, M.; Bayramoglu, G.; Senturk, H.; Uyanoglu, M. Hypoglycemic Effect of *Lentinus strigosus* (Schwein.) Fr Crude Exopolysaccharide in Streptozotocin-Induced Diabetic Rats. *J. Med. Food* **2008,** *11* (3), 513–517.
80. Cho, E. J.; Hwang, H. J.; Kim, S. W.; Oh, J. Y.; Baek, Y. M.; Choi, J. W.; Yun, J. W. Hypoglycemic Effects of Exopolysaccharides Produced by Mycelial Cultures of Two Different Mushrooms *Tremella fuciformis* and *Phellinus baumii* in Ob/Ob Mice. *Appl. Microbiol. Biot.* **2007,** *75* (6), 1257–1265.
81. Lo, H. C.; Tsai, F. A.; Wasser, S. P.; Yang, J. G.; Huang, B. M. Effects of Ingested Fruiting Bodies, Submerged Culture Biomass, and Acidic Polysaccharide Glucuronoxylomannan of *Tremella mesenterica* Retz.: Fr. on Glycemic Responses in Normal and Diabetic Rats. *Life Sci.* **2006,** *78* (17), 1957–1966.
82. Li, T. H.; Hou, C. C.; Chang, C. L. T.; Yang, W. C. Anti-hyperglycemic Properties of Crude Extract and Triterpenes from *Poria cocos*. *Evid.-Based Compl. Alt. Med.* **2010,** *8* (1), 1–8.

83. Li, N.; Li, L.; Fang, J. C.; Wong, J. H.; Ng, T. B.; Jiang, Y.; Wang, C. R.; Zhang, N. Y.; Wen, T. Y.; Qu, L. Y.; Lv, P. Y.; Zhao, R.; Shi, B.; Wang, Y. P.; Wang, X. Y.; Liu, F. Isolation and Identification of a Novel Polysaccharide–Peptide Complex with Antioxidant, Anti-proliferative and Hypoglycaemic Activities from the Abalone Mushroom. *Biosci. Rep.* **2012,** *32* (3), 221–228.
84. Wang, X. M.; Zhang, J.; Wu, L. H.; Zhao, Y. L.; Li, T.; Li, J. Q.; Liu, H. G. A Mini-review of Chemical Composition and Nutritional Value of Edible Wild-Grown Mushroom from China. *Food Chem.* **2014,** *151* (1), 279–285.
85. Zhang, C.; Liu, S.; Solomon, C. G.; Hu, F. B. Dietary Fiber Intake, Dietary Glycemic Load, and the Risk for Gestational Diabetes Mellitus. *Diabetes Care* **2006,** *29* (10), 2223–2230.
86. Jenkins, D. J.; Kendall, C. W.; Axelsen, M.; Augustin, L. S.; Vuksan, V. Viscous and Nonviscous Fibres, Nonabsorbable and Low Glycaemic Index Carbohydrates, Blood Lipids and Coronary Heart Disease. *Curr. Opin. Lipidol.* **2000,** *11* (1), 49–56.
87. Weickert, M. O.; Pfeiffer, A. F. Metabolic Effects of Dietary Fiber Consumption and Prevention of Diabetes. *J. Nutr.* **2008,** *138* (3), 439–442.
88. Asemi, Z.; Karamali, M.; Esmaillzadeh, A. Effects of Calcium–Vitamin D Co-supplementation on Glycaemic Control, Inflammation and Oxidative Stress in Gestational Diabetes: A Randomised Placebo-Controlled Trial. *Diabetologia* **2014,** *57* (9), 1798–1806.
89. Osorio-Yanez, C.; Qiu, C.; Gelaye, B.; Enquobahrie, D. A.; Williams, M. A. Risk of Gestational Diabetes Mellitus in Relation to Maternal Dietary Calcium Intake. *Public Health Nutr.* **2017,** *20* (6), 1082–1089.
90. Fujita, T.; Palmieri, G. M. Calcium Paradox Disease: Calcium Deficiency Prompting Secondary Hyperparathyroidism and Cellular Calcium Overload. *J. Bone Miner. Metab.* **2000,** *18* (3), 109–125.
91. Zemel, M. B; Nutritional and Endocrine Modulation of Intracellular Calcium: Implications in Obesity, Insulin Resistance and Hypertension. *Mol. Cell Biochem.* **1998,** *188* (1), 129–136.
92. Carneiro, A. A.; Ferreira, I. C.; Duenas, M.; Barros, L.; Da-Silva, R.; Gomes, E.; Santos-Buelga, C. Chemical Composition and Antioxidant Activity of Dried Powder Formulations of *Agaricus blazei* and *Lentinus edodes*. *Food Chem.* **2013,** *138* (4), 2168–2173.
93. Sun, L.; Niu, Z. A Mushroom Diet Reduced the Risk of Pregnancy-induced Hypertension and Macrosomia: A Randomized Clinical Trial. *J. Food Nutr. Res.* **2020,** *64*, 1–9.

CHAPTER 7

Role of Mushrooms in the Prevention of Glycation and Other Secondary Complications

VARSHA MAHESH MAYEKAR, HINA ALIM, AHMAD ALI, and NIMISHA PATEL*

Department of Life Sciences, University of Mumbai, Vidyanagari, Santacruz [East], Mumbai 400098, India

Corresponding author. E-mail: patelnimisha916@gmail.com

ABSTRACT

Diabetes mellitus is a chronic condition caused by beta cell dysfunction or a lack of insulin synthesis within our bodies. There are millions of people suffering from diabetes all over the world. Excessive intake of unhealthy foods and changes in the lifestyle have added to the increase in the number of cases. In the last one year many people suffering from diabetes have died due to comorbidity during this situation of COVID-19. Excess glucose leads to adverse biochemical events like glycation, a process in which reactivity of aldehyde group affects the amino group of proteins. This interaction generates a group of deleterious compounds commonly known as advanced glycation end products (AGEs). The presence of these products affects the function of biomolecules and leads to various pathophysiological conditions including diabetes, cataract, Alzheimer's, and Parkinson's. There are several approved and widely used antidiabetic agents available in the market today. However, most of these synthetic medicines have their own side effects and sometimes make

Therapeutic Mushrooms for Diabetes Mellitus: Current Evidences and Future Scope. Uzma Azeem, Khalid Rehman Hakeem, (Eds.)

the situation difficult for the people suffering from diabetes. On the other hand, drugs derived from natural products are being explored for effectiveness in preventing diabetes with few complications. Medicinal plants with antidiabetic properties have attracted much attention in recent times. Mushrooms have been used as medicinal plant since ancient times due to the presence of natural compounds. Mushrooms contain dietary fibers, polysaccharides, proteins, and a variety of other bioactive compounds. These biomolecules have shown to possess antioxidant, antidiabetic, antitumor, and antiaggregating activities that are helpful in the prevention of diabetes and other metabolic disorders. This book chapter deals with the brief description of the process of glycation, application of bioactive compounds in the treatment of glycation-induced metabolic disorders like diabetes and its secondary complications.

7.1 INTRODUCTION

Diabetes is a widespread chronic condition that affects millions of people throughout the world. This syndrome begins with a gradual increase in glucose levels in the body, but it can eventually reach toxic levels.[4] It was caused by an insulin imbalance in the body. According to the World Health Organization (WHO), it was the leading cause of death in humans. Diabetes can be caused due to the intake of high blood sugar, overweight, lack of exercise, unhealthy life style, genetics, or other factors. According to the pathogenesis, there are 3 types of diabetes: (a) Type 1 diabetes mellitus, (b) Type 2 diabetes mellitus, and (c) gestational diabetes mellitus.[5] Diabetes can go undiagnosed for a long time without causing major symptoms, but it can also lead to untreatable conditions such as coronary heart disease. As a result, early therapy is preferred to lessen the risk.[6] Insulin, rosiglitazone, troglitazone, phenformin, gliclazide, tolbutamide, and metformin are some of the chemical and biochemical antidiabetic medications that have been used in the treatment of diabetes and are helpful in managing hyperglycemia. However, some of them may have adverse side effects. As a result, natural diabetic medications extracted from medicinal plants are utilized to treat diabetes.[6] Glycation is a chemical reaction that occurs when free amino groups in biomolecules form a covalent connection with reducing sugar. Louise Camille Millard, a French scientist, was the first to discover it in 1912. As a result, the reaction is also known as the Millard reaction. This reaction is important from both a pathological and a physiological perspective.[9] Advanced glycation end products are a set of chemicallyheterogeneous groups of components composed of 2-[2-furoyl]-4 [5]-[2-furanyl]-1*H*-imidazole, crossline, pyrraline, pentosidine, carboxymethyl-hydroxylysine, carboxy-methyllysine, etc. These substances have the ability to cause oxidative damage to cells and change their activities. Its harmful effects are linked to oxidative stress and inflammation, two factors that contribute to cellular abnormalities in biological systems.[10] Mushrooms are eaten mostly for their flavor and appearance. They can be eaten fresh, dried, or processed through pickling, freezing, or canning.[1] Humans have consumed mush-rooms since ancient times, believing that they bring power in battle, and even the Romans acknowledged them as "food of the gods." They are regarded as healthful food in Chinese culture.[2] Auricularia auricular, often known as wood ear, has been cultivated in China. The button mushroom, which was first planted in France, has been farmed throughout Europe. There are 12,000 species of fungus utilized as mushrooms in the globe, but only 2000 species are edible. Around 200 species were collected from the woodland and used for their therapeutic properties. About 35 species have been cultivated commercially and 20 species have been cultivated on the basis of industrial scale.[3] Vitamins A, B, C, D, and K are abundant in edible mushrooms. They have a high protein and mineral content. However, they are low in saturated fat. They exhibit reactive oxygen species (ROS) scavengers as well as antioxidant activity, which is linked to their phenolic compounds.[7] Mushrooms have long been used in the treatment of diabetic wounds, as well as for blood glucose management and the modification of complications without causing harm. Their bioactive constituents, such as dietary fibers, terpenoids, polysaccharides, and protein complexes, as well as other components isolated from mushroom fruiting bodies, culture broth, and mycelium, have antihyperglycemic activity.[8] This chapter reviewed the importance of mushrooms and how they can be used to prevent Glycation and diabetes in great detail.

7.2 DIABETES MELLITUS

Diabetes mellitus is derived from the Greek word diabetes, which means "to syphon" or "to pass through," and the Latin word mellitus, which means "sweet." Apollonius coined the word sometime between 250 and 300 BC.[11] It is a metabolic disorder characterized by hyperglycemia as a result of the affected insulin secretion. Metabolic abnormality in protein, lipids, and carbohydrates results from the importance of the insulin as an anabolic hormone. Uncontrolled diabetes can cause coma, stupor or else patients can die due to the ketoacidosis.[12] Diabetes is a widespread chronic condition that affects millions of people throughout the world. This syndrome begins with a gradual increase in glucose levels in the body, but it can eventually reach toxic levels.[4] It was caused by insulin resistance and beta cell dysfunction. Kcnq1 is a gene that has been linked to impaired beta cell function as well as decreased insulin secretion. According to the World Health Organization, it was the leading cause of death in humans. Diabetes can be caused by excessive blood sugar intake, obesity, lack of exercise, a sedentary lifestyle, heredity, or other factors. It has been divided into three types:

(a) Type 1 diabetes mellitus (T1DM): Insulin-dependent diabetic mellitus is another name for it (IDDM). It is an immune system hereditary disease in which genes are responsible for the disease. There are also several other variables that cause the immune system to attack and destroy the β-cells in the pancreas that causes the insulin deficiency and type 1 diabetes mellitus. It can affect both adults and children, but it mostly affects children, which is why it is called "Juvenile diabetes."[13]

(b) Type 2 diabetes mellitus (T2DM): Non-insulin-dependent diabetic mellitus is another name for it (NIDDM). It was the most common form of the diabetes mellitus. It happens as a result of the interaction of genetics, behavioral, and environmental factors. It is the result of a combination of insulin insufficiency and insulin resistance.[14] Although it was largely noticed in youngsters with inactivity and obesity, this type of disease is most common in middle age or later life. According to certain studies, the number of adolescent and child cases with a combination of type 1 and type 2 diabetes is on the rise. As a result, this condition is referred to as "hybrid diabetes" or "double diabetes."[6]

(c) Gestational diabetes mellitus (GDM): During the pregnancy, it was the most common complication. According to the WHO, gestational diabetes mellitus (GDM) is defined as hyperglycemia that first appears during pregnancy.[15] Women with Gestational diabetes mellitus have a higher risk of developing Type 2 diabetes mellitus (T2DM), and their children have a higher risk of obesity and developing Type 2 diabetes mellitus (T2DM) early in life. Screening and diagnostic testing are used to determine the likelihood of having Gestational diabetes mellitus and to prevent its negative effects on both the mother and the kid.[16]

Specific pro-inflammatory cytokines trigger inflammatory reactions. Obesity and inflammation are linked, and both are linked to insulin resistance. By triggering mitochondrial stress and other reactions, pro-inflammatory cytokines promote beta cell death. In hyperglycemia, oxidative stress and inflammation can cause alterations in gene expression regulation, resulting in decreased insulin secretion and an increase in apoptosis.[66,67] Obesity is an inflammatory state. Adipose tissue is the main source of inflammation, with macrophage infiltration as the predominant source of cytokines in obese people. Insulin is secreted by beta cells to enhance glucose uptake into glucose-receiving tissues. Obesity is a risk factor for Type 2 diabetes mellitus because it deafens the glucose-receiving organs to insulin activity. Obesity can increase insulin demand, so the hyperfunction of the β-cells exhausts the β-cells, resulting in beta cell malfunction.[68]

7.3 GLYCATION

Glycation is a nonenzymatic event in which the free amino (–NH_3) group of macromolecules like nucleic acid or protein binds to lipids or carbohydrate's reducing sugar, forming Schiff base and more stable Amadori products. Then it undergoes through other processes like dehydration, rearrangement, and cyclization, before finally forming advanced glycation end products (AGEs).[17] Because both Amadori products and Schiff bases produce free radicals, which weaken antioxidant defense mechanisms, they can harm cellular organelles and enzymes.[18] It is divided into two stages: early stage and late stage. The interaction of the glucose amino group of proteins in the early stages creates the Schiff base, which is then rearranged to form ketoamine products. Then, after a few days, through rearrangement of these Schiff bases, Amadori products are generated.[18] As shown in Figure 7.1 these products are known as early glycation products. After then, this Amadori product goes through the last stage of glycation, which increases AGEs. The individual or combination reaction, which involves chemical rearrangement of the hydration and redox reactions, simplifies this. These advanced glycation end products (AGEs) constitute a persistent, nonhomogeneous set of molecules that contribute to abnormal intracellular activities via signaling pathways and cross linking of extracellular protein.[17] Glycation has been linked to a variety of ailments, including neurogenerative diseases, hypertrophy, myocardial infarction, ageing and associated disorders, and diabetes mellitus, according to several studies.[19] Oxidative stress is a physiological situation in which oxidative species prevail over antioxidant species, resulting in a loss of defense and inflammation. Because oxidation products are mostly present in the patient's plasma and cellular membrane, oxidative stress increases in renal failure. Glycation and lipoxidation pathways are aided by oxidized lipids and proteins, which participate in the generation of reactive carbonyl species.[69]

Type 2 diabetes mellitus (T2DM) is connected to increased oxidative stress, poor nutrition, and inflammation, which is preceded by insulin resistance. The advanced glycation end products (AGEs) degradation system and its receptor AGER1 counteract the effects of advanced glycation end products. SIRT1, an NAD-dependent deacetylase and factor, is linked to the actions of these receptors. SIRT1 has been shown to improve insulin effectiveness and fat mobilization, as well as to suppress inflammatory signals and boost adiponectin synthesis. Adipocytes and macrophages can transition to pro-oxidative stress, inflammatory phenotype, and early insulin resistance due to a lack of AGER1 and SIRT1 receptors.[62] Mushrooms are well known for their medicinal properties in traditional medicine, and they have also been used as culinary ingredients all across the world. There are numerous varieties of mushrooms that have been used to treat various diseases in various countries throughout history, including Korea, India, China, Japan, and others. Due to their biological components, medicine mushrooms have therapeutic agents against different ailments such as cancer, hypercholesterolemia, and hypertension, among others. In Table 7.1, we discussed about the various antidiabetic effects of different species of mushrooms. They are also employed in the cosmetic industry due to their therapeutic properties.[6] There is no distinction between edible and medicinal mushrooms because the majority of edible mushrooms have therapeutic properties. Edible mushrooms can be grown in a lab or found in the wild. Some of the most common mushrooms can be found

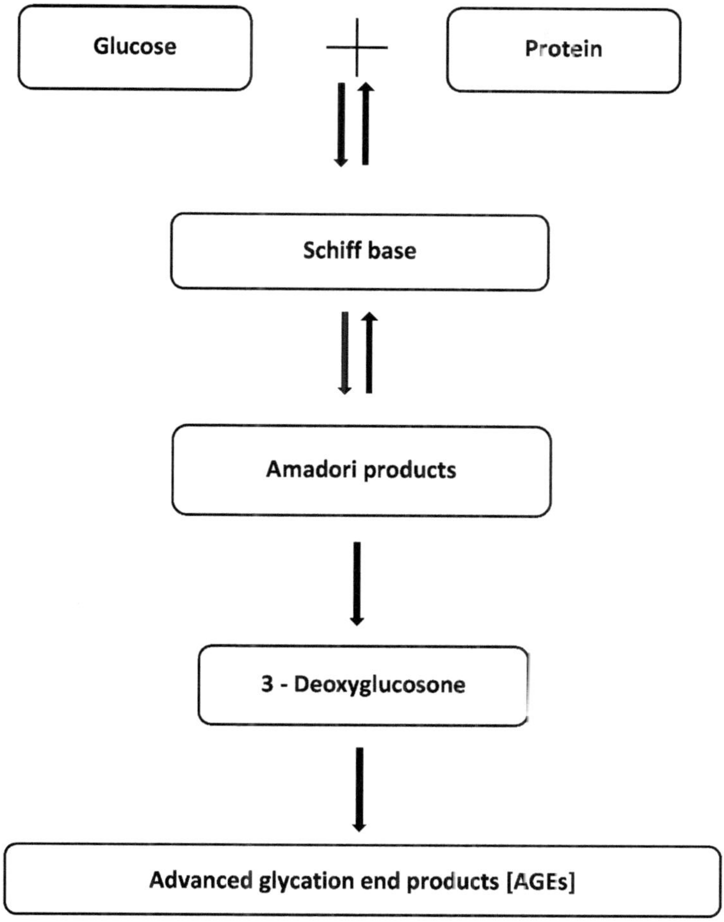

FIGURE 7.1 Glycation of protein and formation of advanced glycation end products (AGEs).

in supermarkets. Private gatherers collect ectomycorrhiza mushrooms in modest quantities. Mushrooms have a low glycemic index and a high mannitol content, making them beneficial to diabetes mellitus. It was high in B1, B2, B12, C, D, and E vitamins. They also have a high potassium level and a low nitrogen content. Mushrooms have long been utilized as home medicines in Asian countries to treat a variety of ailments caused by oxidative stress. Mushrooms have antioxidant, antiglycation, anti-cancer, immunological, immunostimulant, hepatoprotective, antidiabetic, anticoagulant, anticomplementary, antiviral, and other antimicrobial activities.[20] Button mushroom (*Agaricus bisporus*), Shiitake mushroom (*Lentinula edodes*), shaggymane mushroom (*Coprinus comatus*), nameko mushroom *(Pholiota microspora)*, White Jelly mushroom (*Tremella fuciformis*), Winter mushroom (*Flammulina velutipes*), Maitake mushroom (*Grifola frondosa*), Reishi (*Ganoderma lingzhi*), Wood ear mushroom (*Auricularia auricula-judae*) Pompom or Lion's head mushroom (*Hericium erinaceus*), Straw mushroom *(Volvariella volvacea*), Oyster mushroom (*Pleurotus ostreatus*), etc. are the most common mushrooms that can be grown in good conditions.[21] Consumption of these mushrooms helps to preserve cells from free radical damage and to slow down the ageing process. Mushrooms are natural sources of vitamin D and vitamin B12, which are produced through UV light-induced conversion of ergosterol to ergocalciferol. They are high in bioactive components like selenium, beta glucan, vitamin D, ergosterol, and ergothioneine, among others. Cognitive function, cancer, gastrointestinal health, bone density, blood pressure, lipid profile, weight management, glycemic control, and immunological function are all linked to these components.[22]

7.4 ANTIDIABETIC ACTIVITY OF VARIOUS MUSHROOMS

7.4.1 AGARICUS BISPORUS

Agaricus bisporus is a member of the Agaricaceae family. White button mushroom is the common name for this mushroom. The significance of the white button mushroom has been discussed in numerous studies. This mushroom sample has a high moisture content of 91–92 g/100 g and a high calorie content of 29–31 kcal/100 g. This mushroom also has 1.56% fat, 51.05% carbohydrate, and 29.14% protein.[40] It contains high content of dietary fibers, acidic polysaccharides, polyphenol, ergothioneine, folate, vitamin B12, C and Das shown in Figure 7.2. It possesses anti-inflammatory, hypercholesterolemic, and hypoglycemic effects.[41] The BSA (bovine serum albumin)/fructose assay was used to investigate *Agaricus bisporus*' antiglycation properties. It reflects the high antiglycation activity in the range of 500–550 mg AG/g fraction.[42] The efficacy of *Agaricus bisporus* on diabetes-induced dyslipidemia was investigated. They used hyperlipimidic rats to demonstrate the ingestion of it as a potential effective natural treatment against type 1 diabetes mellitus. They divided 32 rats into four

TABLE 7.1 Various Species of Mushrooms with Their Antidiabetic Effect.

Mushroom	Family	Common name	Mechanism of action	Reference
Agaricus bisporus	Agaricaceae	White button mushroom	Lower blood glucose level, cholesterol level	[22]
Antrodiacamphorate	Polyporaceae	Stout camphor fungus	Increase insulin secretion, protect from apoptosis, hypertension	[23]
Armillaria mellea	Physalacriaceae	Honey fungus	Decreases blood glucose level	[24]
Auriculariaauricular	Auriculariaceae	Wood ear mushroom	Reduce cholesterol and triglyceride level	[25]
Boletus edulis	Boletaceae	King mushroom	Removefree radicals for better hypoglycemic, improves glucose tolerance	[26]
Calvatia gigantea	Agaricaceae	Giant puffball	Inhibit the enzyme-α amylase, reduce glucose level	[27]
Coprinuscomatus	Agaricaceae	Shaggy mane	Lower blood glucose level, increase body insulin level, improves glucose tolerance	[28]
Cordyceps sinensis	Ophiocordycipitaceae	Caterpillar fungus	Diabetes-induced decreases in serum insulin concentration	[29]
Cyclocybe aegerita	Strophariaceae	Poplar mushroom, chestnut mushroom	Antidiabetic, manage blood pressure, cardiovascular disease	[30]
Flammulinavelutipes	Physalacriaceae	Enokitake	Scavenge-free radical and increase the response of antioxidant defense systemin OS	[31]
Ganoderma Lucidum	Ganodermataceae	Reishi mushroom	Decrease plasma sugar level, increase plasma insulin level	[32]
Grifola frondosa	Meripaceae	Maitake mushroom	Reduce the blood glucose level	[33]
Hericiumerinaceus	Hericiaceae	Pompomorlion's Head mushroom	Decrease cholesterol level, serum triglyceride level, and blood glucose level and improve free radical scavenging enzyme	[34]

TABLE 7.1 *(Continued)*

Mushroom	Family	Common name	Mechanism of action	Reference
Inonotus obliquus	Hymenochaetaceae	Chaga mushroom	Reduce glucose level, increase hepatic glycogen level, improve glucose tolerance	[35]
Lentinus edodes	Omphalotaceae	Shiitake mushroom	Decreases the level of ALT and AST, total cholesterol level, increase insulin level	[36]
Lepistanuda	Tricholomataceae	Wood blewit mushroom	Improve insulin tolerance, decreases the plasma glucose level, triglyceride level	[37]
Schizophyllum commune	Schizophyllaceae	Splitgill mushroom	Reduce blood glucose, TC, LDL and TG level decreases	[38]
Volvariellavolvacea	Pluteacea	Straw mushroom	Reduced blood glucose level, increase insulin level	[39]

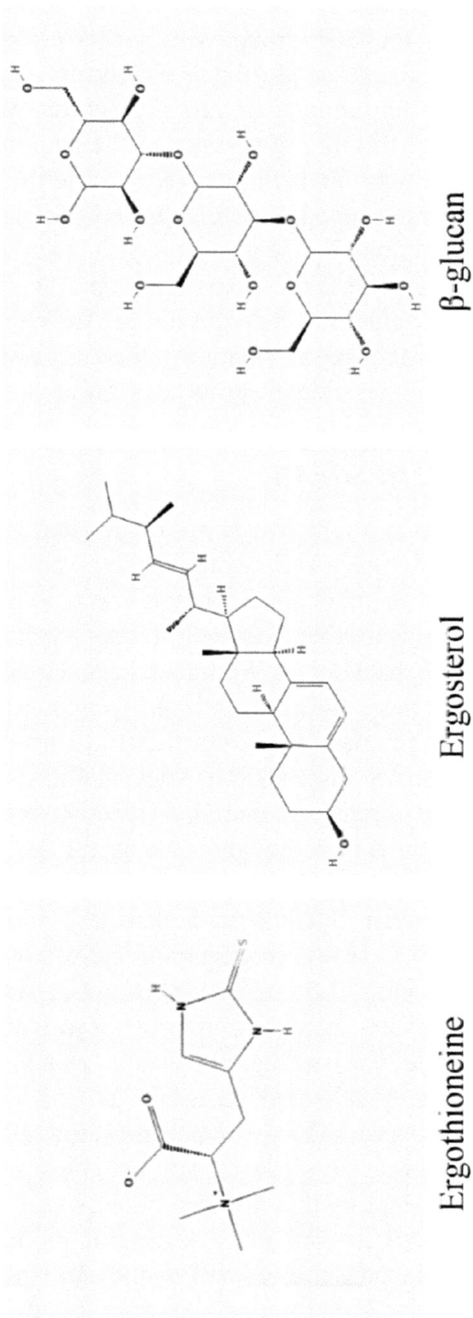

FIGURE 7.2 Bioactive compounds of *Agaricus bisporus*.

groups for this experiment. Group 1 is the control group, which received no drugs, group 2 is the ABP group, which received *Agaricus Bisporus* polysaccharides (ABP) 200 mg/kg body weight per day for the next 21 days orally, group 3 is the streptozotocin (STZ) group, which was injected with streptozotocin (STZ) 40 mg/kg once at the beginning, and group 4 is the ABP + STZ group, in which rats were injected with streptozotocin (STZ) at first, but then received *Agaricus Bisporus* polysaccharides (ABP) by orally around 200 mg/kg for the next 21 days. On day 22, blood samples and tissue specimens were taken from all groups. The results show that group 3 had a higher glucose concentration but their insulin levels were lower. According to all of the information gathered, *Agaricus bisporus* has antidiabetic and antihyperlipidemic properties that are linked to diabetes.[43]

7.4.2 ANTODIA CAMPHORATA

Antrodia camphorata is a rare Taiwanese fungus that has been used as a traditional medicine to treat a variety of ailments. It belongs to the Polyporaceae family. Stout camphor mushroom is the common name for this mushroom. Much work has been done on *A. camphorata* in an attempt to adapt this Oriental medicine into a Western-accepted treatment. Traditional Taiwanese medicine has long used A*ntrodia camphorata* to treat twisted muscles and muscle injuries, panic attacks, colds, headaches, flu, and a variety of other internal diseases. Diabetes mellitus, motion sickness, calenture, car sickness, influenza, and viral infection have all been treated with it. The mushroom is now thought to be useful in avoiding metabolic syndrome after years of use in Taiwan. It contains ergostatrien-3β-ol, dehydroeburicoic acid, antacin K compounds that have antidiabetic potential as shown in Figure 7.3. Many investigations have now revealed that its medicinal use extends much beyond its original use. As a result, the need for A-bearing fruit bodies has increased. In terms of availability, camphorata has surpassed.[23] Recently, it was suggested that *A. camphorata* may include peroxisome proliferator activated receptors gamma (PPAR-γ) ligands, which act as a junction rectifier for hypotriglyceride effects. Peroxisome proliferator activated receptors gamma (PPAR-γ) is a member of a large family of receptor receptors that are also expressed in β-cells and form heterodimers with RXR to bind PPRE to genetic promoters and employ genetic recordings. The presence of PPRE in the promoters of GLUT-2 and GLK, which are involved in hormone secretion, is consistent. In addition,

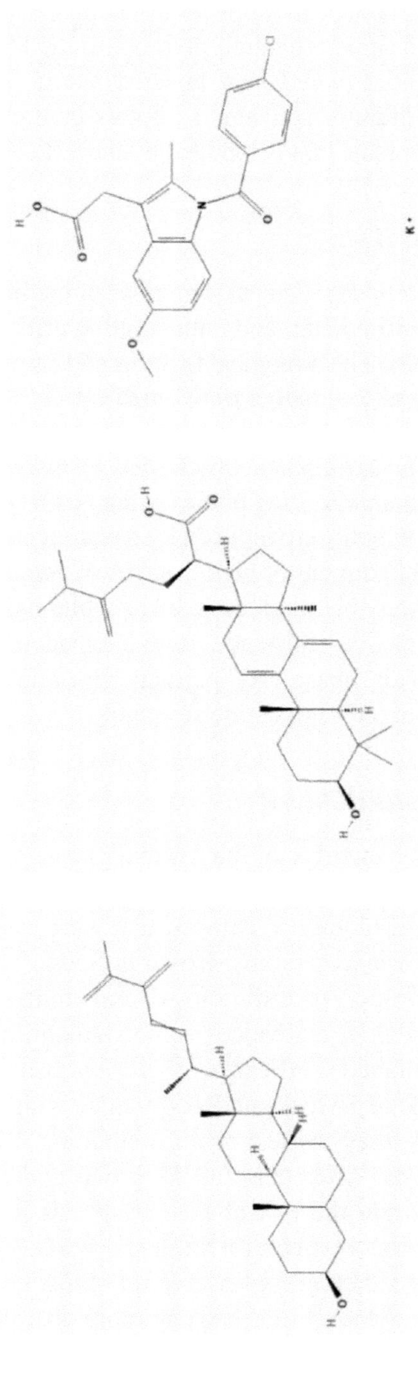

Antacin K

Dehydroeburicoic acid

Ergostatrien-3β-ol

FIGURE 7.3 Bioactive compounds of *Antrodia camphorata*.

several researchers investigated its impact on insulin secretion and apoptosis triggered by endoplasmic reticulum pressure in the MIN6 β-cell line. According to the findings, *A. camphorata* boosted insulin-dependent secretion by peroxisome proliferator activated receptors gamma (PPAR-γ) and protected cells from apoptosis that is induced by the ER stress.[44]

7.4.3 ARMILLARIA MELLEA

The edible fungus *Armillaria mellea* has a number of medicinal properties, including antidiabetic, antioxidant, and antiapoptotic effects. It belongs to the Physalacriaceae family. The biological features and components of these mushrooms could be used to create a novel medication. It contains fibrinolytic enzymes, steroids, sesquiterpene aryl esters, and polysaccharide, among other things.[45] The antidiabetic efficacy of *A. mellea* was examined by extracting the mushroom's fruiting bodies using NaOH solution. Type 2 diabetic rats were used, which were induced by dexamethasone and a high-fat diet. As a result, oral treatment of high dosages of associated migratory cell protein (AMCP) lowers blood glucose levels while increasing glucose tolerance capacity and insulin resistance. It also enhances the expression of the adipose triglyceride lipase (ATGL) and hormone sensitive lipase (HSL) and hence lowered the triglyceride serum.[46]

7.4.4 AURICULARIA AURICULAR

Auricularia auricular is a member of the Auriculariceae family. Wood ear mushroom is the popular name for this mushroom. It was macrofungi, which exhibit a variety of biological activity, that were used in traditional remedies for therapy. It was commonly grown in South, East, and Southeast Asia, as well as Europe. According to several studies, the extract of A. auricular has antidiabetic, anticancer, anticoagulant, and antioxidant properties.[25] The antidiabetic efficacy of *Auricularia auricular* was examined using 4 groups of 5-week-old KK-Ay mice with type 2 diabetes. For the next four weeks, they fed test meals containing 2[2F]%, 5[5F]%, 10[10F]%, and 20[20F]%. After that, the 5F group and half of the 20F group kept their diet, while the rest of the group was given a 20F diet with 5% mushroom hot water extract for another 3 weeks. The differences in body weight between diet groups were not statistically significant. Dietary intake declined as fatty foods became more prevalent, yet energy consumption differed dramatically between diet groups except the 20 FHWE group. Dietary fat content was shown to be substantially linked with blood glucose levels. Current findings in KK-Ay mice demonstrate that dietary fat levels control postprandial glycemia and that HWE's hypoglycemic effect is mostly attributable to lower food intake. It is primarily composed of carbohydrates.[47]

7.4.5 CALVATIA GIGANTEA

Calvatia gigantea is a member of the Agaricaceae family. It was named "big puffball mushroom" by locals. It was mostly recognized for its nutritional properties. These compounds such as gentisic acid, vanillic acid, protocatchuic acid have a variety of biological actions, including lowering blood glucose levels as shown in Figure 7.4. The traditional morphological method for identifying this mushroom has shown to be entirely ineffective. The in vivo activity and *in vitro*-amylase assay in alloxan-induced diabetic rats were utilized to identify the antidiabetic activity of the mushroom fruiting bodies. The [ITS] Internal Transcribed Spacers sequence analysis was used to identify the macrofungus. In vivo testing revealed that 400 mg/kg is the optimum activity for lowering blood glucose levels by 29.3% [27].

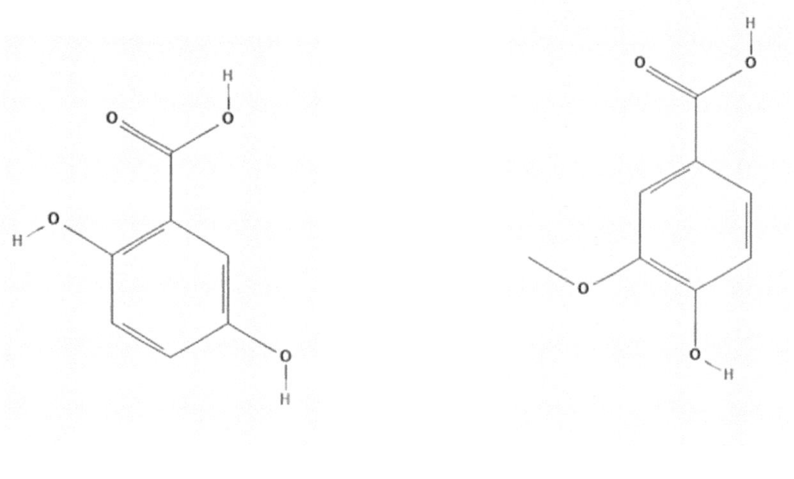

Gentisic acid Vanillic acid

FIGURE 7.4 Bioactive compounds of *Calvatia gigantea.*

7.4.6 *COPRINUS COMATUS*

C. comatus is a nutritionally dense edible fungus. It was a member of the Agaricaceae family. It has antidiabetic, antimutagenic, antitumor, and antioxidative characteristics. The hyperglycemic effect of this fungus, which contains vanadium and β-glucan, has been studied in several ways as shown in Figure 7.5. This component has the ability to mimic insulin and also has antidiabetic properties. In hyperglycemic mice, fermented *Coprinus comatus* rich in vanadium (CCRV) has the potential to lower blood glucose levels, insulin secretion, and gluconeogenesis inhibition.[6] According to a few studies, comatin (4,5-dihydroxy-2-methoxy-benzaldehyde) is responsible for the antidiabetic effect of this mushroom. Comatin is a nonenzymatic glycosylation process inhibitor. When mice with normal blood glucose levels are given 80 mg/kg comatin, their body weight drops from 5.14 mM to 4.28 mM in just three hours. It also lowered total cholesterol, triglyceride, and fructosamine levels. It was concluded that comatin could aid to maintain a low blood glucose level and enhance glucose tolerance.[48]

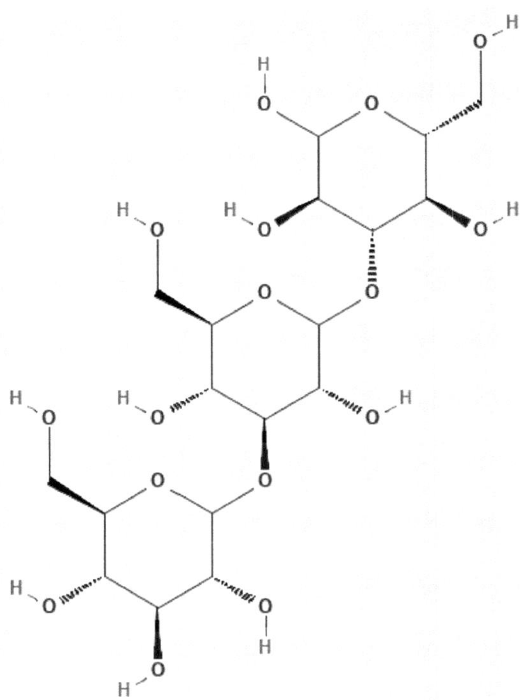

FIGURE 7.5 Bioactive components of *Coprinus comatus.*

7.4.7 CORDYCEP SINENSIS

Cordyceps sinensis is a highly prized fungus used in traditional Chinese medicine. It belongs to the Ophicordycipitaceae family. Caterpillar fungus mushroom is the popular name for this mushroom. It contains cordycepin, ciclosporin as major compounds as shown in Figure 7.6. According to recent research, this mushroom has the ability to alter immunological response, improve hyperglycemia and hyperlipidemia, and suppress tumor growth. According to certain reports, 95% of persons treated with 3 g/day *Cordyceps sinensis* mushroom show a reduction in plasma glucose level, whereas the other control group shows a 54% improvement with the treatment by using the other methods.[6] This mushroom contains vanadium, which has the ability to imitate the action of insulin, aiding in the increase of blood glucose levels while also having antidepressant properties. As a result, vanadium-enriched *Cordyceps sinensis* [VECS] has been proposed as a treatment for diabetes and depression.[29]

7.4.8 FLAMMULINA VELUTIPES

Flammulina velutipes is a widely cultivated edible fungus that may be found all over the world. It belonged to the family Physalacriaceae. It contains peptidoglycan as a major compound as shown in Figure 7.7. It has antiproliferative, immunomodulatory, and hepatoprotective effects. On Streptozotocin-induced diabetic rats, the antioxidant and renoprotective effects of En-RPS, Al-RPS, and Ac-RPS polysaccharide extracts of *F. velutipes* were investigated. The En-RPS extract from *F. velutipes* exhibits a significant antioxidant property, according to the results, which is also employed as a promising therapeutic drug for preventing diabetic neuropathy progression.[31]

7.4.9 GANODERMA LUCIDUM

Ganoderma lucidum is a member of the Ganodermataceae family. It was once thought to be a sacred fungus in ancient China, but it is now used for medicinal and spiritual purposes. It was mostly cultivated on a commercial scale. More than 400 bioactive substances are found in the basidiocarp, spore, and mycelia of this mushroom, including trace elements, protein,

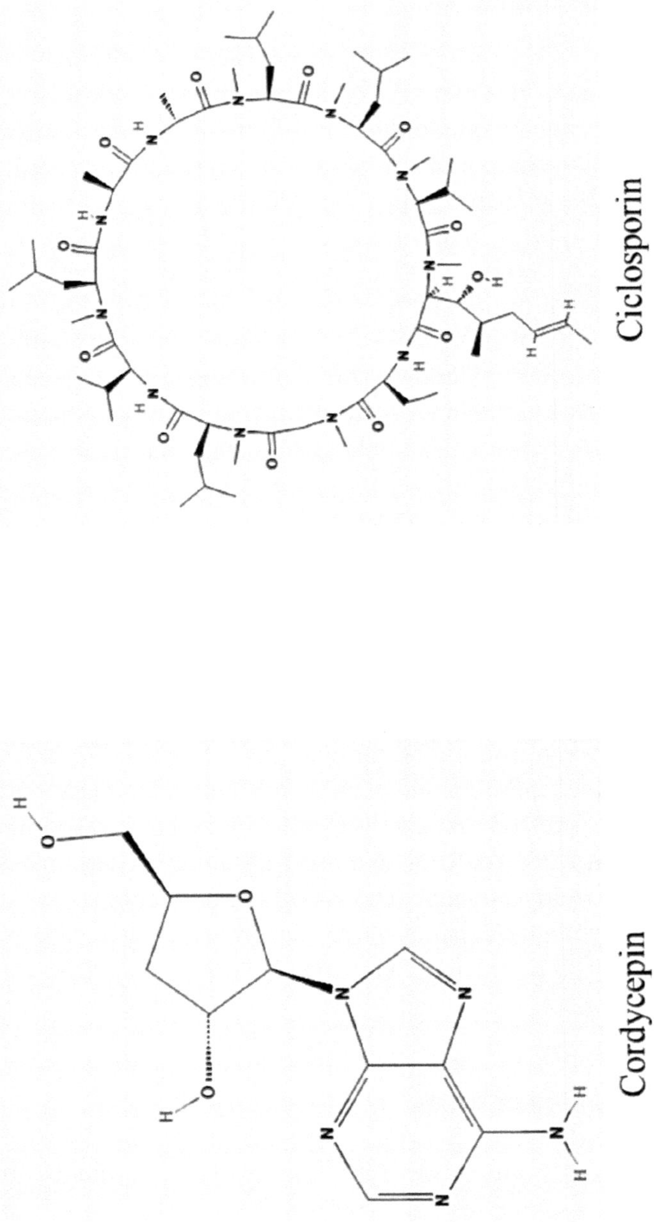

FIGURE 7.6 Bioactive components of *Cordyceps sinensis.*

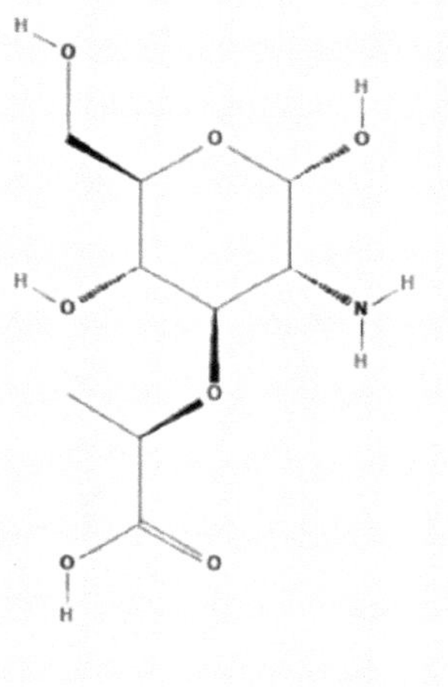

FIGURE 7.7 Bioactive compounds of *Flammulina velutipes.*

fatty acids, steroids, sterol, nucleotide, polysaccharides, and triterpenoids. This polysaccharide and triterpene can bind to the β-cells of the pancreas, causing insulin secretion to be stimulated while glucagon secretion is inhibited. The polysaccharides component of these mushrooms has hypolipidemic and hypoglycemic effects, according to various investigations. As a result, the oral glucose tolerance test (OGTT) aids in the lowering of blood glucose and insulin levels in diabetic rats.[49]

7.4.10 GRIFOLA FRONDOSA

The Meripaceae family included *Grifola frondosa*. Because of their therapeutic properties, it was mostly used in Japan, China, and Korea. The beneficial effects of this mushroom and its extract have been proven in numerous studies. It contains β-glucan and has antidiabetic effects as shown in Figure 7.8. Because it includes a glycosidase inhibitor, this mushroom aids in the reduction of blood glucose levels. This inhibitor is found in the aqueous methanol extract of these mushrooms.[6] The α-glucan 150–450 mg/kg was used to assess the antidiabetic efficacy of *Grifola frondosa* mushroom on diabetic mice. As a result, the levels of malondialdehyde, fatty acids, cholesterol, triglycerides, insulin, blood glucose, and body weight in the liver are reduced. It also raises glutathione peroxidase, superoxide dismutase, and hepatic glycogen levels, implying that glucan's action on insulin receptors leads to increased insulin sensitivity and insulin strengthening of the targeted external tissues.[50]

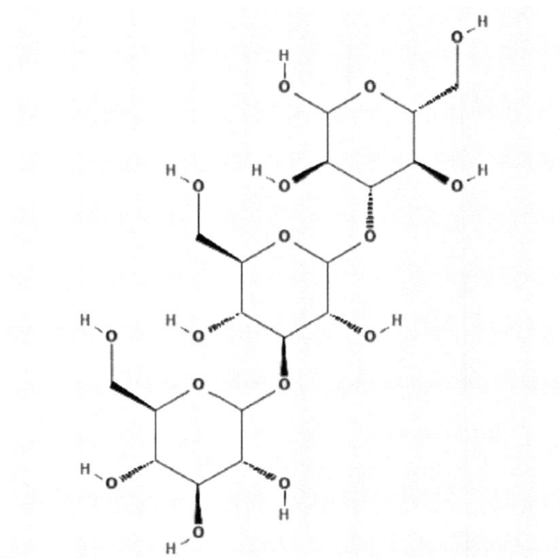

β-glucan

FIGURE 7.8 Bioactive components of *Grifola frondosa.*

7.4.11 HERICIUM ERINACEUS

Hericium erinaceus is a mushroom that is both edible and medicinal. Pom pom mushroom is a Hericiaceae mushroom that belongs to the Hericiaceae family. It has been utilized in Chinese traditional medicine for a long time. Antiaging, antioxidant, anticancer, immunomodulatory, antibacterial, and hemagglutinating activities were mostly found in mycelia and fruiting bodies. It has a variety of secondary components such as Erinacin, β-glucan as shown in Figure 7.9. Its fruiting bodies contain 6%, 14.3 mg/g weight amino acids, 7% ash, 5% fat, 61% carbs, and 20% proteins, whereas mycelia include 4%, 30.6 mg/g weight amino acids, 4% ash, 6% fat, 42% carbohydrates, and 42% proteins.[34] Streptozotocin-induced diabetes in rats was used to assess *H. erinaceus*'s antihyperglycemic efficacy. When

20–100 mg of extract per kg of body weight is added, total cholesterol, blood glucose, and serum triglyceride levels are reduced. It has a protective effect in a dose-dependent condition.[53] *H. erinaceus* is used as a food or medicine, and its therapeutic properties have led to its usage as a home remedy. It was primarily grown in Asia.[52] On streptozotocin (STZ)-induced diabetic mice, the hypolipidemic and hypoglycemic effects of aqueous extracts of this fungus were tested. The injection of 55 mg/kg body weight STZ resulted in diabetes. For four weeks, aqueous preparations of this fungus were given at doses of 100–200 mg/kg body weight. The extracts' effects on oxidative stress, lipids, blood, insulin, and glucose were studied. Rats' body weight was also measured at days 0, 14, and 28. On day 28, blood glucose levels were lower and insulin levels were increased. This extract also aids in the reduction of malondialdehyde (MDA) levels and increases the glutathione (GSH) level, glutathione peroxidase (gsh-px), superoxide dismutase (SOD), catalase (CAT) activity in liver tissue. In STZ-induced diabetic rats, the aqueous extracts of *Hericium erinaceus* were found to have antioxidant, hypolipidemic, and hypoglycemic properties.[51] This mushroom has an antidiabetic action and inhibits aldose reductase and glycosidase activity in a dose-dependent manner. As a result, it was discovered that glucose tolerance had improved and alloxan-induced diabetic mice administered *H. erinaceus* polysaccharides had lower blood glucose levels.[52]

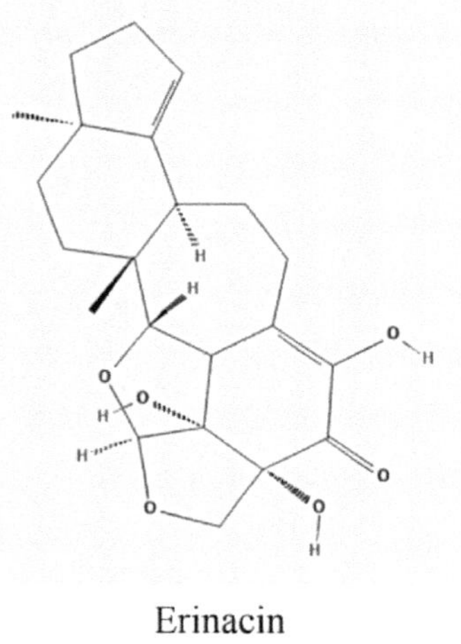

Erinacin

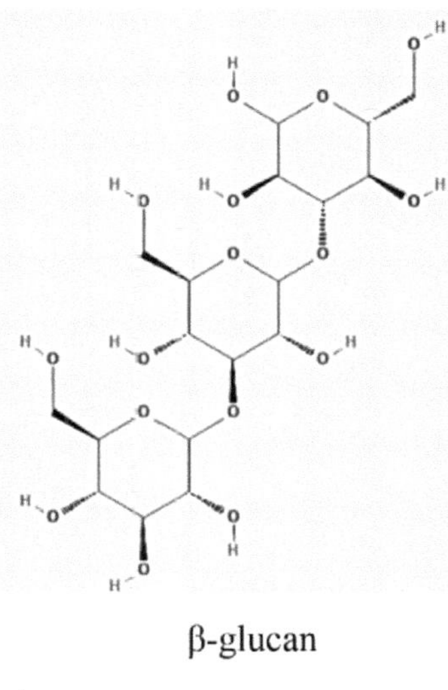

β-glucan

FIGURE 7.9 Bioactive compounds of *Hericium erinaceus*.

7.4.12 INONOTUS OBLIQUUS

The Hymenochaetaceae family includes *Inonotus obliquus*. It contains inotodiol and ergosterol as shown in Figure 7.10. The polysaccharides *Inonotus obliquus* (PIO) have antidiabetic action against Streptozotocin (STZ)-induced diabetes. PIO has been researched for its effects on body weight, blood glucose, beta-cell damage in the pancreas, oxidative stress, pro-inflammatory cytokines, and glucose metabolism in the liver. The findings suggest that administering a PIO can return abnormal oxidative activity indicators to normal levels. As a result, we came to the conclusion that the PIO is an effective advocate for STZ-induced diabetic rats and could be beneficial as an antihyperglycemic medication. The antidiabetic effect of *Inonotus obliquus* polysaccharides (IOPS) was investigated in diabetic rats caused by streptozotocin (STZ) and in high-fat diabetic mice. The findings show that taking Inonotus obliquus polysaccharides orally restores body and fat mass weight, improves insulin resistance and hepatic glycogen levels, improves glucose tolerance capacity, and lowers fasting blood glucose levels.[35]

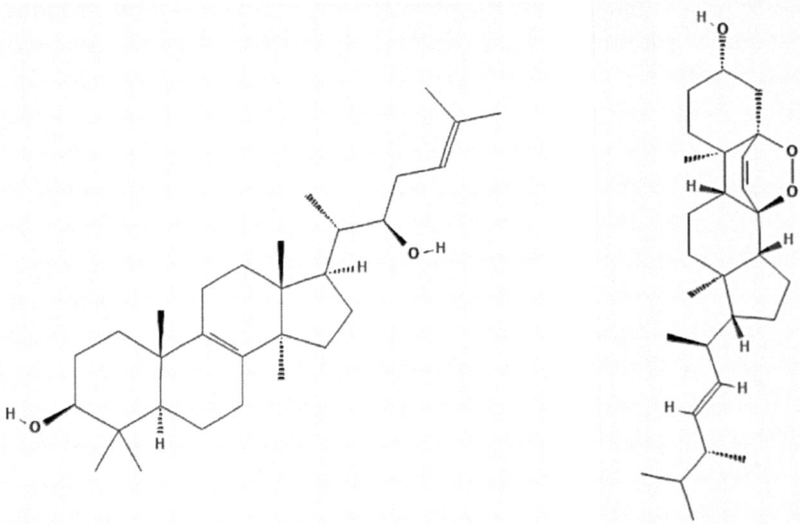

Inotodiol Ergosterol

FIGURE 7.10 Bioactive compounds of *Inonotus obliquus*.

7.4.13 *LENTINUS EDODES*

Lentinus edodes is a mushroom that is both therapeutic and appetizing. It was the second most popular edible mushroom, belonging to the Omphalotaceae family. It contains eritadenine, lectin, lentinan, ergosterol, vitamin B1, vitamin B2, vitamin C, minerals, fibers, carbohydrates, lipids, and proteins as shown in Figure 7.11.[49] Streptozotocin-induced diabetic mice were used to examine the hyperglycemic impact of *L. edodes*. As a result, the blood glucose level was reduced by 21.5%, the triglyceride level was reduced by 44.5%, the total cholesterol level was reduced by 25.1%, and the insulin level was increased by 22.1%. A glycoprotein with a molecular weight of 52 kDa includes 16 5% protein and 83.5% carbs. This mushroom aids in the destruction of β-pancreatic cells, the reduction of blood glucose levels, and the promotion of insulin synthesis.[55]

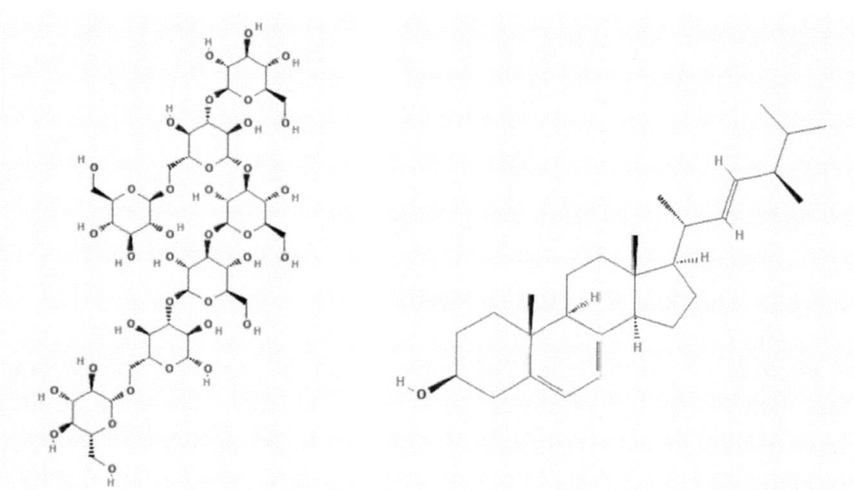

Lentinan Ergosterol

FIGURE 7.11 Bioactive components of *Lentinus edodes*.

7.4.14 *LEPISTA NUDA*

Clitocybe nuda (*Lepista nuda*) is an edible mushroom. It belongs to the Tricholomataceae family that is grown in Asia, Australia, the United States, Europe, Taiwan, the United Kingdom, the Holland, and France.

It has antibacterial as well as antioxidant properties. It contains 3-keto-drimenol component as shown in Figure 7.12. The antidiabetic properties of these mushrooms were investigated in STZ-induced diabetic mice. In mice the diabetes was induced by injecting the STZ. The mice were then separated into five groups and given 0.2, 0.5, or 1.0 g/kg body weight of mushrooms extract, vehicle, or metformin for 28 days. As a result, the lipid and blood glucose levels are reduced. Also, raise leptin and insulin levels.[56]

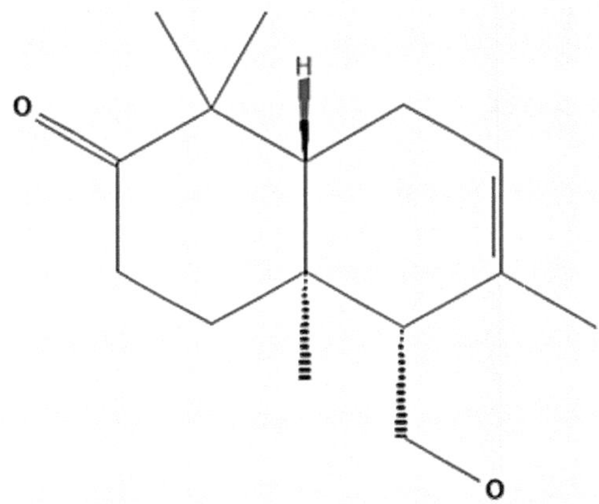

FIGURE 7.12 Bioactive compounds of *Lepista nuda.*

7.4.15 SCHIZOPHYLLUM COMMUNE

S. commune is inedible and Schizophyllaceae is a family of mushrooms that includes splitgill mushrooms. It was cultivated from dead wood. It has a variety of nutraceutical properties due to the presence of bioactive components such as schizophyllan, as shown in Figure 7.13. The antidiabetic effect of these mushrooms was determined using several extraction solvents. In comparison with ethanol extracts and hot water extracts, the methanol extract possesses antidiabetic effectiveness. As result, S. commune was determined to be a natural antidiabetic ingredient that is a better alternative to synthetic medicines.[57] The antidiabetic effect of an ethyl acetate extract of *S. commune* mushroom was reported in STZ-induced diabetic mice at two different doses. As a result, it aids in the reduction of blood glucose levels while also increasing body weight 14 days later. In mice, it restored renal parameters such as potassium level, sodium fractional excretion, blood urea nitrogen, and creatinine. As a result, the lipid profile and antioxidant parameters were both improved. In diabetic mice, homeostasis of liver enzymes was also enhanced. The medicinal potential of *S. commune* against diabetes was discovered as a result.[38]

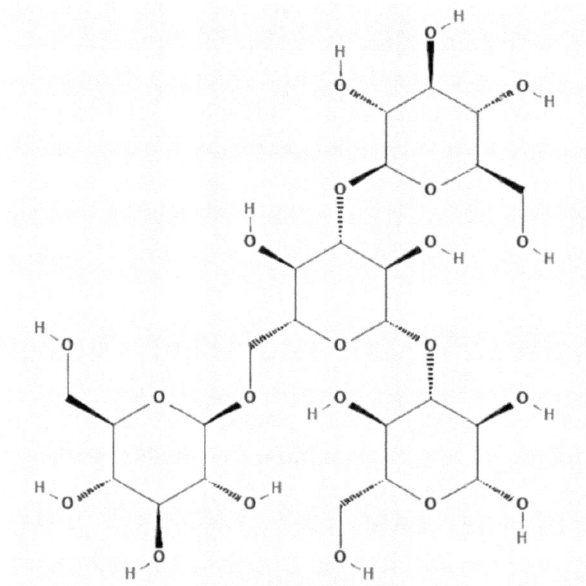

FIGURE 7.13 Bioactive compounds of *Schizophyllum commune.*

7.4.16 VOLVARIELLA VOLVACEA

Volvariella volvacea is an edible mushroom and it is a member of the Plutaceae family. It was mostly harvested in Asia's south and east. It was employed in human diets because of its nutritional value. By examining other vital profiles and glucose tolerance ability, the antidiabetic activity of *V. volvacea* mushroom was investigated against STZ-produced diabetic rats and normal rats. The mushroom sample was hydroalcoholic extracted, and then divided into two sections, each of which was lymphilized and dried in a hot air oven. Then it was administered into rats in various quantities to help diabetic animals lower their serum glucose levels. According to the findings, the lymphilization of this mushroom has a greater antidiabetic effect than the other parts.[39] In diabetic mice, the antidiabetic and other properties of the methanol extract of these mushrooms were investigated against oxidative stress. They were divided into six equal groups: group 1 was a control group, group 2 was a diabetic control group, group 3 was given glibenclamide, groups 4 and 5 were fed mushroom extract orally at 200 and 400 mg/kg for one month, and group 6 was given 40 mg/kg vitamin E. After therapy, mice were tested for nonenzymatic antioxidants, superoxide dismutase, catalase, glutathione-S transferase, glutathione peroxidase, reduced glutathione, advanced glycation end products, carbonyl end products, and lipid peroxide. As a result of the findings, it was discovered that this mushroom extract may be utilized to reduce advanced glycation end products, lipid peroxidase, protein carbonyl, as well as reverse the altered antioxidant enzymes and vitamin levels.[58]

7.5 ANTIGLYCATION ACTIVITY OF VARIOUS MUSHROOMS

Because advanced glycation end products (AGEs) can be found in a variety of foods, dietary consumption is a better predictor of advanced glycation end products (AGEs) production. However, foods rich in vitamin B6, vitamin D, polyphenols, and other minerals can help to reduce advanced glycation end products (AGEs). Autofluorescence is used to measure advanced glycation end products (AGEs) in the skin. As a result, the association between food intake and advanced glycation end products (AGEs), which involves ageing and related problems, was explored. A food consumption questionnaire was reported for those 39 people. Their advanced glycation end products (AGEs) were also determined in the skin using autofluorescence. As a result, the average skin AF was 2.1 AU, and the average mushroom intake was 15.7 g/day. As a result, the inverse relationship with mushroom skin AF and mushroom intake was concluded, implying that mushrooms should be consumed to lower advanced glycation end products (AGEs).[59] Commercially, *Boletus snicus* is the most important mushroom. The antiglycation effect of this fungus was studied using DEAE-cellulose and Sephadex G-100 column chromatography to extract two polysaccharides from its body. The average molecular weight of BSP-1b, a heteropolysaccharide with a significant quantity of glucose and a minor amount of arabinose, glucosamine hydrochloride, Mannose, and BSP-2b monosaccharide, which comprises arabinose, galactose, glucose, glucosamine hydrochloride, glucuronic acid, and Mannose. BSP-1b and BSP-2b have pyranose ring structures, and BSP-2b has a significant concentration of uronic acid, according to NMR and FTIR spectrum investigation. They both demonstrate high inhibitory effects on glycation and a dose-dependent response as a result. BSP-2b, on the other hand, has a stronger antiglycation activity than BSP-1b. As a result, BSP-2b appears to be capable of efficiently inhibiting the formation of advanced glycation end products (AGEs).[60] The effects of *Castanea sativa* and *Lactarius deterrimus* on oxidative stress (OS) and advanced glycation end products (AGEs)-mediated hepatorenal damage in Streptozotocin (STZ)-induced diabetic rats were investigated. For the next five days, experimental animals were given a 40 mg/kg Streptozotocin (STZ) solution. The extracts were administered intraperitoneally at a concentration of 60 mg/kg for 28 days following the Streptozotocin (STZ) injection. Improved hepatorenal function was linked to improved glycemic and lipid status, as well as inhibition of oxidative stress and hence oxidative damage to lipids and DNA in diabetic rats treated with the extracts. *In vitro*, both extracts suppress protein glycation and the generation of advanced glycation end products (AGEs), and in vivo, they aid in the reduction of nonenzymatic glycosylation in diabetic rats.[8] The suppression of advanced glycation end products (AGEs), fructosamine, and thiol groups, followed by the inhibition of protein carbonyl production, was used to assess *Ficus deltoidea's* antiglycation activity. The variant of this mushrooms extract reduced the development of fluorescence advanced glycation end products (AGEs) by 4.55–5.14 folds after 4 weeks of induction. This extract also reduces fructosamine levels by 47.0–86.5% while increasing thiol group levels by 64.3–83.7%. As a result of this research, the seven types of *Ficusdeltoidea* have the ability to suppress the development of advanced glycation end products (AGEs).[61] Natural antiglycation components have gotten a lot of attention in recent years because of their capacity to minimize and avoid chronic problems in diabetic patients. An annotation of the genome transcriptome from the tiger milk mushroom was carried out in one study to detect antiglycation and antidiabetic activities. This mushroom includes bioactive components that are responsible for antiglycation and diabetic complications management. The potential of antiglycation activity was investigated using the medium molecular weight fraction of a combination of sephadex G-50 gel chromatography and cold-water extract of tiger milk mushroom powder. It inhibits advanced glycation end products (AGEs), pentosidine, and lysine with an IC50 of 0.001 mg/ml, which is much lower than the positive control. As a result, it is believed that the mushroom's medium molecular weight fraction has the potential to become a glycation inhibitor.[10] To determine the antiglycation and antioxidant properties of polysaccharides isolated by ultrasonic assisted extraction from *Dictyophora rubrovolvata*. To acquire the two fractions of Pileus of *Dictyophora rubrovolvata-1* (DPP-1s) and Pileus of *Dictyophora rubrovolvata-2* (DPP-2s), this polysaccharide was separated and purified using DEAE-52 and sephadex G-100 column chromatography. As a result of the differences in uronic acid concentration and molecular weight, both fractions have substantial inhibitory effects on glycation and oxidation. Pileus of *Dictyophora rubrovolvata-1* (DPP-1s) also has lower bioactivity than DPP-2s. FTIR and UV spectra research indicated that Pileus of *Dictyophora rubrovolvata-2* (DPP-2s) lacks protein and instead contains a nuclear acid with a pyranose ring structure. Therefore, it is concluded that the Pileus of *Dictyophora rubrovolvata-2* (DPP-2s) can be used as a good source for antiglycation and antioxidant activity.[63] The nonenzymatic glycosylation reaction system of *Auricularia auricular* was used to test the inhibitory effects on the development of advanced glycation end products (AGEs). As a result, both AAPs-F and *Auricularia auricular* polysaccharides (AAPs) can suppress advanced glycation end products (AGEs) formation in both short- and long-term glycosylation in dose-dependent conditions as shown by UV and fluorospectrophotometry that shows activity against advanced glycation end products (AGE) at different concentrations.[64] *Ganoderma capense* was primarily utilized in Asia for therapeutic purposes, such as health promotion and the treatment of various chronic diseases, such as ageing, diabetes, and so on. Polysaccharides abound in this mushroom. Polysaccharides from *Ganoderma capense* were extracted *in vitro* to determine antiglycation and antiradical properties. This mushroom's dry powder was defatted. Then, using ethanol precipitation, extract with water or alkaline water and deproteinize. After that, we have four crude polysaccharides: *Ganoderma capense* 50, *Ganoderma capense* 70, *Ganoderma capense* 90. The antiglycation activity of all samples was initially investigated using a nonenzymatic glycation process. The antiradical capability of all samples was then assessed using the 1,1-diphenyl-2-picryhydazyl (DPPH) and hydroxyl radical assays. Polysaccharide content was also assessed using phenol sulfuric acid colorimetry. The results demonstrated that all samples have concentration-dependent hydroxyl radical and 1,1-diphenyl-2-picryhydazyl (DPPH) scavenging abilities. GC70 also has a better chance of preventing the production of advanced glycation end products (AGEs).[65]

7.6 CONCLUSION

Diabetes is a chronic condition caused by a shortage of insulin or insulin malfunction, which results in hyperglycemia. It has major adverse effects, such as cancer-related risk, cardiovascular danger, insulin resistance, and hyperglycemia. The rising impact of T2DM necessitates the development of safe and effective treatments, as well as prevention methods to lower disease prevalence and incidence. As a result of hyperglycemia, the generation of advanced glycation end products (AGEs) increases in diabetes. Increased glycation and glycated plasma protein buildup play a key role in a variety of illnesses. Many natural and pharmaceutical substances are being researched for their medicinal potential. Medicinal mushrooms have sparked interest as a potential new type of therapeutic and are appreciated for their potential healing properties. Mushroom bioactive compounds have been shown to have a controlling effect on diabetic patients by regulating seven pathophysiological pathways related to the diabetes. Because of their nutritional importance, several mushroom species are the best sources of bioactive components. Mushrooms used in the diet may be effective as dietary supplements.

KEYWORDS

- **diabetes mellitus**
- **glycation**
- **hyperglycemia**
- **insulin resistance**
- **mushrooms**

REFERENCES

1. Sharma, K. Mushroom: Cultivation and Processing. *Int. J. Food Process. Technol.* **2015,** *5*, 9–12.
2. Valverde, M. E.; Perez, T. H.; Lopez, O. P. Edible Mushrooms: Improving Human Health and Promoting Quality Life. *Int. J. Microbiol.* **2015,** *2015*, 376387.
3. Aida, F. M. N. A.; Shuhaimi, M.; Yazid; Maaruf, A. G. Mushroom as a Potential Source of Prebiotics: A Review. *Trends Food Sci. Technol.* **2009,** *20*, 567–575.
4. Kumar, D.; Ali, A. Antiglycation and Antiaggregation Potential of Thymoquinone. *NVEO* **2019,** *6*, 25–33.
5. Jiang, X.; Meng, W.; Li, L.; Meng, Z.; Wang, D. Adjuvant Therapy with Mushroom Polysaccharides for Diabetic Complications. *Front. Pharmacol.* **2020,** *11*, 1–12.
6. De, D. D.; Rapior, S.; Hyde, K. D. Medicinal Mushrooms in Prevention and Control of Diabetes Mellitus. *Fungal Divers.* **2012,** *56*, 1–29.
7. Mihailovic, M.; Jovanovic, J. A.; Uskokovic, A.; Grdovic, N.; Dinic, S.; Vidovic, S.; Poznanovic, G.; Mujic, I.; Vidakovic, M. Protective Effects of the Mushroom *Lactarius deterrimus* Extract on Systemic Oxidative Stress and Pancreatic Islets in Streptozotocin-induced Diabetic Rats. *J. Diabetes Res.* **2015,** *2015*, 1–10.
8. Jovanovic, J. A.; Mihailovic, M.; Uskokovic, A.; Grdovic, N.; Dinic, S.; Vidakovic, M. The Effects of Major Mushroom Bioactive Compounds on Mechanisms That Control Blood Glucose Level. *J. Fungi* **2021,** *7*, 58.
9. Pandey, R.; Kumar, D.; Ali, A. *Nigella sativa* Seed Extracts Prevent the Glycation of Protein and DNA. *Curr. Perspect. Med. Aroma Plant* **2018,** *1*, 1–7.
10. Yap, H. Y.; Tan, N. H.; Ng, S. T.; Tan, C. S.; Fung, S. Y. Inhibition of Protein Glycation by Tiger Milk Mushroom [*Lignosus rhinocerus (Cooke) ryvarden*] and Search for Potential Anti-diabetic Activity-related Metabolic Pathways by Genomic and Transcriptomic Data Mining. *Front. Pharmacol.* **2018,** *9*, 103.
11. Sapra, A.; Bhandari, P. Diabetes Mellitus. *StarPearls* **2021**. https://www.ncbi.nlm.nih.gov/books/NBK551501/
12. Kharroubi, A. T.; Darwish, H. M. Diabetes Mellitus: The Epidemic of the Century. *World J. Diabetes* **2015,** *6*, 850–867.
13. Guthrie, R. A.; Guthrie, D. W. Pathophysiology of Diabetes Mellitus. *Crit. Care Nurse Q.* **2004,** *27*, 113–125.
14. Olokoba, A. B.; Obateru, O. A.; Olokoba, L. B. Type 2 Diabetes Mellitus: A Review of Current Trends. *Oman Med J* **2012**, *27,* 269–273.
15. Alfadhli, E. M. Gestational Diabetes Mellitus. *Saudi Med. J.* **2015,** *36*, 399–406.
16. Kampann, U.; Madsen, L. R.; Skajaa, G. O.; Iversen, D. S.; Moeller, N.; Ovesen, P. Gestational Diabetes: A Clinical Update. *World J. Diabetes* **2015,** *6*, 1065–1072.
17. Ali, A.; Paramanya, A.; Prairna, M.; Doukani, K.; Zehtra, S. Antioxidants in Glycation Related Diseases. *Oxidative Stress and Antioxidant Defense: Biomedical Value in Health and Diseases*; Nova Science Publishers, Inc.: Hauppauge, NY, 2019; pp 465–488.
18. Ahmad, S.; Khan, M.; Akhter, F.; Khan, M. S.; Khan, A.; Ashraf, J. M. Glycoxidation of Biological Macromolecules: A Critical Approach to Halt the Menace of Glycation. *Glycobiology* **2014,** *24*, 979–990.

19. Singh, V. P.; Bali, A.; Singh, N.; Jaggi, A. S. Advanced Glycation End Products and Diabetic Complications. *Korean J. Physiol. Pharmacol.* **2014**, *18*, 1–14.
20. Kozarski, M.; Klaus, A.; Jakovljevic, D.; Todorovic, N.; Vunduk, J.; Petrovic P.; Niksic, M.; Vrvic, M. M.; Griensven, L. V. Antioxidant of Edible Mushrooms. *Molecules* **2015,** *20*, 19489–19525.
21. Caglarimak, N. Edible Mushrooms: An Alternative Food Item. *ICMBMP* **2011,** *5*, 548–554.
22. Blumfield, M.; Abbott, K.; Duve, E.; Cassettari, T.; Marshall, S.; Moore, F. F. Examining the Health Effects and Bioactive Components in *Agaricus bisporus* Mushrooms: A Scoping Review. *J. Nutr. Biochem.* **2020,** *84*, 108453.
23. Madamanchi, G.; Tzeng, Y. M. Review of Pharmacological Effects of *Antrodia camphorate* and Its Bioactive Compounds. *Evid. Based Complement. Altern. Med.* **2011,** *2011*, 212641.
24. Shengshu, A.; Lu, W.; Zhang, Y.; Yuan, Q.; Wang, D. Pharmacological Basis for Use of *Armillaria mellea* Polysaccharides in Alzheimer's Disease: Antiapoptosis and Antioxidation. *Oxid. Med. Cell Longev.* **2017,** *2017*, 4184562.
25. Mapoung, S.; Umsumarng, S.; Semmarath, W.; Arjsri, P.; Thippraphan, P.; Yodkeeree, S.; Limtrakul, P. Skin Wound-healing Potential of Polysaccharides from Medicinal Mushroom *Auricularia auricula-judae* (Bull.). *J. Fungi* **2021,** *7*, 247.
26. Xiao, Y.; Chen, L.; Fan, Y.; Yan, P.; Li, S.; Zhou, X. The Effect of *Boletus* Polysaccharides on Diabetic Hepatopathy in Rats. *Chem. Biol. Interact.* **2019,** *308*, 61–69.
27. Ogbole, O. O.; Nkumah, A. O.; Linus, A. U.; Falade, M. O. Molecular Identification, in Vivo and in Vitro Activities of *Calvatia gigantea* (Macro-fungus) as an Antidiabetic Agent. *Mycology* **2019,** *10*, 166–173.
28. Ratnaningtyas, N. I.; Hernayanti, H.; Ekowati, N.; Sukmawati, D.; Widianti, H. Chicken Drumstick Mushroom (*Coprinus comatus*) Ethanol Extract Exerts a Hypoglycaemic Effect in the *Rattus norvegicus* Model of Diabetes. *Biocatal. Agric. Biotechnol.* **2019,** *19*, 101050.
29. Guo, J. Y.; Han, C. C.; Liu, Y. M. A Contemporary Treatment Approach to Both Diabetes and Depression by *Cordyceps sinensis*, Rich in Vanadium. *Evid. Based Complement. Altern. Med.* **2009,** *7*, 387–389.
30. Petrovic, J.; Glamoclija, J.; Stojkovic, D.; Nikolic, M.; Ciric, A.; Fernandes, A.; Ferreira, I.; Sokovic, M. Bioactive Composition, Antimicrobial Activities and the Influence of *Agrocybe aegerita* (Brig.) Sing on Certain Quorum-sensing-regulated Functions and Biofilm Formation by *Pseudomonas aeruginosa*. *Food Funct.* **2014,** *5*, 3296–3303.
31. Lin, L.; Cui, F.; Zhang, J.; Gao, X.; Zhou, M.; Xu, N.; Zhao, H.; Liu, M.; Zhang, C.; Jia, L. Antioxidative and Renoprotective Effects of Residue Polysaccharides from *Flammulina velutipes*. *Carbohydr. Polym.* **2016,** *146*, 388–395.
32. Haou, T. M.; Jung, F. H.; Shui, T. C. Anti-diabetic Effects of *Ganoderma lucidum. Phytochemistry* **2015,** *114*, 1–5.
33. Hong, L.; Xun, M.; Wutong, W. Anti-diabetic Effect of an α-Glucan from Fruit Body of Maitake (*Grifola frondosa*) on Kk-Ay Mice. *Pharm. Pharmacol.* **2007,** *59* (4), 575–582.

34. Chaiyasut, C.; Sivamaruthi, B. S. Anti-hyperglycemic Property of *Hericium erinaceus*: A Mini Review. *Asian Pac. J. Trop. Biomed.* **2017,** *7* (11), 1036–1040.
35. Wang, J.; Wang, C.; Li, S.; Li, W.; Yuan, G.; Pan, Y.; Chen, H. Anti-diabetic Effects of *Inonotus obliquus* Polysaccharides in Streptozotocin-induced Type 2 Diabetic Mice and Potential Mechanism Via PI3K-Akt Signal Pathway. *Biomed. Pharmacother.* **2017,** *95*, 1669–1677.
36. Laurino, L. F.; Viroel, F. J. M.; Caetano, E.; Spim, S.; Pickler, T. B.; Castro, R. M. R.; Vasconcelos, E. A.; Jozala, A. F.; Hataka, A.; Grotto, D.; Gerenutti, M. *Lentinus edodes* Exposure before and after Fetus Implantation: Materno-fetal Development in Rats with Gestational Diabetes Mellitus. *Nutrients* **2019,** *11* (1), 1–14.
37. Chen, M. H.; Lin, C. H.; Shih, C. C. Antidiabetic and Antihyperlipidemic Effects of *Clitocybe nuda* on Glucose Transporter 4 and Amp-activated Protein Kinase Phosphorylation in High-fat-fed Mice. *Evid. Based Complement. Altern. Med.* **2014,** *2014*, 1–14.
38. Sharma, A.; Kaur, R.; Kaur, J.; Garg, S.; Bhatti, R.; Kaur, A. An Endophytic *Schizophyllum commune* Fr. Exhibits in-vitro and in-vivo Antidiabetic Activity in Streptozotocin Induced Diabetic Rats. *Amb. Express.* **2021,** *11* (1), 1–11.
39. Gupta, P. P.; Chandrakar, S.; Roy, A.; Verma, S.; Gupta, N.; Sahu, R. K. Assessment of Antidiabetic Activity of Hydroalcoholic Extract of *Volvariella volvacea. Eur. J. Mol. Clin. Med.* **2021,** *8* (3), 1499–1509.
40. Funda, A.; Owaid, M. N.; Shariati, M. A. The Nutritional and Medical Benefits of *Agaricus bisporus*: A Review. *J. Microbiol. Biotechnol. Food Sci.* **2017,** *7*, 281–286.
41. Jeong, S. C.; Jeong, Y. T.; Yang, B. K.; Islam, R.; Koyyalamudi, S. R.; Pang, G.; Cho, K. Y.; Song, C. H. White Button Mushroom (*Agaricus bisporus*) Lowers Blood Glucose and Cholesterol Levels in Diabetic and Hypercholesterolemic Rats. *Nutr. Res.* **2010,** *31* (1), 49–56.
42. Gallotti, F.; Lavelli, V. The Effect of UV Irradiation on Vitamin D2 Content and Antioxidant and Antiglycation Activities of Mushrooms. *Foods* **2020,** *9*, 1–10.
43. Zaid, O. A. R. A.; Sonbaty, S. M. El.; Hamam, M. A. Anti-diabetic Activity of *Agaricus Bisporus*: A Biochemical and Pathological Study. *Int. J. Pharm. Sci.* **2017,** *7* (2), 1740–1745.
44. Vong, C. T.; Tseng, H. H. L.; Kwan, Y. W.; Lee, S. M. Y.; Hoi, M. P. M. *Antrodia camphorate* Increases Insulin Secretion and Protects from Apoptosis in MIN6 Cells. *Front. Pharmacol.* **2016,** *7*, 1–10.
45. Gao, L. W.; Li, W. Y.; Zhao, Y. L.; Wang, J. W. The Cultivation, Bioactive Components and Pharmacological Effects of *Armillaria mellea. Afr. J. Biotechnol.* **2009,** *8*, 7383–7390.
46. Yang, S.; Meng, Y.; Yan, J.; Wang, N.; Xue, Z.; Zhang, H.; Fan, Y. Polysaccharide-enriched Fraction from *Amillariella mellea* Fruiting Body Improves Insulin Resistance. *Molecules* **2019,** *24*, *46.*
47. Takeujichi, H. P.; Mooi, L. Y. Reductive Effect of Hot-water Extracts from Woody Ear on Food Intake and Blood Glucose Concentration in Genetically Diabetic Kk-Ay Mice. *J. Nutr. Sci. Vitaminol.* **2004,** *50* (4), 300–304.
48. Ding, Z.; Lu, Y.; Lu, Z.; Lv, F.; Wang, Y.; Bie, X.; Wang, F.; Zhang, K. Hypoglycaemic Effect of Comatin, an Antidiabetic Substance Separated from *Coprinus comatus* Broth, on Alloxan-induced-diabetic Rats. *Food Chem.* **2010,** *121*, 39–43.

49. Lo, H. C.; Wasser, S. P. Medicinal Mushrooms for Glycemic Control in Diabetes Mellitus: History, Current Status, Future Perspective and Unlcved Problem (Review). *Int. J. Med. Mushrooms* **2011,** *13*, 401–426.
50. Friedman, M. Mushroom Polysaccharides: Chemistry and Antiobesity, Antidiabetes, Anticancer, and Antibiotic Properties in Cells, Rodents, and Humans. *Foods* **2016,** *5*, 80.
51. Liang, B.; Guo, Z.; Xie, F.; Zhao, A. Antihyperglycemic and Antihyperlipidemic Activities of Aqueous Extract of *Hericium erinaceus* in Experimental Diabetic Rats. *BMC Complement. Med. Ther.* **2013,** *13*, 1–7.
52. Wu, T.; Xu, B. Antidiabetic and Antioxidant Activities of Eight Medicinal Mushroom Species from China. *Int. J. Med. Mushrooms* **2015,** *17*, 129–140.
53. Wang, J. C.; Hu, S. H.; Wang, J. T.; Chen, K. S.; Chia, Y. C. Hypoglycemic Effect of Extract of *Hericium erinaceus. J. Sci. Food Agric.* **2005,** *85*, 641–646.
54. Liang, S.; Yongliang, Z. Preparation, Characterization and Antiglycation Activities of the Novel Polysaccharides from *Boletus snicus*. *Int. J. Biol. Macromol.* **2016,** *92*, 607–614.
55. Yang, B. K.; Kim, D. H.; JeJeong, S. C.; Das, S.; Choi, Y. S.; Shin J. S.; Lee, S. C.; Song, C. H. Hypoglycemic Effect of a *Lentinus edodes* Exo-polymer Produced from a Submerged Mycelial Culture. *Biosci. Biotechnol. Biochem.* **2002,** *66*, 937–942.
56. Shih, C. C.; Chen, M. H.; Lin, C. H. Validation of the Antidiabetic and Hypolipidemic Effects of *Clitocybe nuda* by Assessment of Glucose Transporter 4 and Gluconeogenesis and AMPK Phosphrylation in Streptozotocin Induced Mice. *Evid. Based Complement. Altern. Med.* **2014,** *2014*, 1–15.
57. Chandrawanshi, N. K.; Tandia, D. K.; Jadhav, S. K. Determination of Anti-diabetic Property of Organic and Non-organic Solvent Extracts of *Schizophyllum commune*. *NewBioWorld* **2019,** *1*, 5–8.
58. Punitha, S. C.; Muthu, R. Cardioprotective Effect of *Volvariella volvacea* in Streptozotocin Administered Rats. *Bangla. J. Pharmacol.* **2016,** *11*, 903–910.
59. Kawaguchi, Y.; Nirengi, S.; Kotani, K.; Somei, J.; Kawamoto, T.; Tsuzaki, K.; Yonei, Y.; Sakane, N. Mushroom Intake and Advanced Glycation End Products in the Skin among Community-dwelling Elderly Subjects: Preliminary Data. *J. Biomed.* **2017,** *2*, 8–11.
60. Liping, S.; Xuejiao, S.; Yongliang, Z. Preparation, Characterization and Antiglycation Activities of the Novel Polysaccharides from *Boletus snicus*. *Int. J. Biol. Macromol.* **2016,** *92*, 607–614.
61. Dom, N. S. M.; Yahaya, N.; Adam, Z.; Rahman, N. M.; Hamid, M. Antiglycation and Antioxidant Properties of *Ficus deltoidea* Varieties. *Evid. Based Complement. Altern. Med.* **2020,** *6374632*, 1–16.
62. Cai, W.; Ramdas, M.; Zhu, L.; Chen, X.; Striker, G. E.; Vlassara, H. Oral Advanced Glycation End Products (AGEs) Promote Insulin Resistance and Diabetes by Depleting the Antioxidant Defenses AGE Receptor-1 and Sirtuin 1. *Proc. Natl. Acad Sci.* **2012,** *109*, 15888–15893.
63. Sun, L.; Bao, C.; Chang, W.; Zhuang, Y. Preparation, Characteristics, Antioxidant and Antiglycation Activities of the Novel Polysaccharides from the Pileus of *Dictyophora rubrovolvata*. *Int. J. Food Sci. Technol.* **2016,** *52*, 161–170.

64. Shen, M.; Fang, Z.; Chen, Y.; Xiao, B.; Guo, L.; Xu, Y.; Wang, G.; Wang, W.; Zhang, Y. Hypoglycemic Effect of the Degraded Polysaccharides from the Wood Ear Medicinal Mushroom *Auricularia auricular judae* (Agaricomycetes). *Int. J. Med. Mushrooms* **2019,** *21*, 1033–1042.
65. Yan, C.; Kong, F.; Zhang, D.; Cui, J. Anti-glycated and Antiradical Activities *in Vitro* of Polysaccharides from *Ganoderma capense. Pharmacogn. Mag.* **2013,** *9*, 23–27.
66. Lin, C. Y.; Ni, C. C.; Yin, M. C.; Lii, C. K. Flavonoids Protect Pancreatic Beta-cells from Cytokines Mediated Apoptosis through the Activation of PI3-kinase Pathway. *Cytokines* **2012,** *59*, 65–71.
67. Gilbert, E. R.; Liu, D. Epigenetics: The Missing Link to Understanding β-Cell Dysfunction in the Pathogenesis of Type 2 Diabetes. *Epigenetics* **2012,** *7*, 841–852.
68. Cerf, M. E. Beta Cell Dysfunction and Insulin Resistance. *Front. Endocrinol.* **2013,** *4*, 1–12.
69. Bettiga, A.; Fiorio, F.; Marco, F. D.; Trevisani, F.; Romani, A.; Porrini, E.; Salonia, A.; Montorsi, F.; Vago, R. The Modern Western Diet Rich in Advanced Glycation End Products (AGEs): An Overview of Its Impact on Obesity and Early Progression of Renal Pathology. *Nutrients* **2019,** *11*, 1748.

CHAPTER 8

In Vitro Evaluation of the Antidiabetic Efficacy of Mushrooms

ASIF HAMID DAR, ABDUL HAMID WANI, MOHD YAQUB BHAT*, MEHRAJUD DIN TALIE, and NAYEEMA JAN

Plant Pathology, Mycology and Microbiology Laboratory, Department of Botany, University of Kashmir, Jammu and Kashmir 190006, India

**Corresponding author. E-mail: myaqub35@gmail.com*

ABSTRACT

Medicinal mushrooms have been valued as a traditional source of natural bioactive compounds over several decades and have been targeted as potential hypoglycemic and antidiabetic agents. A large number of in vitro studies have reported significant antidiabetic efficacy of a wide array of mushroom extracts and isolated mycoconstituents that impart their antidiabetic effects by modulating the activity of enzymes like α-glycosidase and aldose reductase; displaying insulin-like or insulin potentiating action; and DPPH-free radical scavenging activity that potentially neutralizes the oxidized "advanced glycated end products" (AGEs). The significant in vitro hypoglycemic effect and the corresponding in vivo antidiabetic activity exhibited by various mushrooms investigated emphasizes the fact that these macrofungi could potentially serve as a promising source of medicine and have the potential to serve as functional food and in addition the extract and its fractions may be explored for the development of natural product-based pharmaceuticals.

Therapeutic Mushrooms for Diabetes Mellitus: Current Evidences and Future Scope. Uzma Azeem, Khalid Rehman Hakeem, (Eds.)

8.1 INTRODUCTION

As per World Health Organization 2011 survey, diabetes results in 2.2% of the overall annual deaths globally and is one of the principal causes of mortality in human population.[1] Diabetes mellitus (DM) is the manifestation of multiple chronic ailments marked by elevated blood glucose level (BGL) and altered metabolism arising from either abnormal insulin release or action.[2] Among the 3 forms of diabetes (viz. type 1, type 2, and gestational diabetes), type 2 DM is most common. However, the term diabetes is often nontechnically categorized into two types, viz. diabetes insipidus and diabetes mellitus; however, in the current chapter the term signifies the later out of two. Studies acclaim that dietary pattern comprising of fruits and vegetables has diabetes-alleviating properties, and it improves many cardiovascular complications.[3–6] Medicinal mushrooms have been employed since the past in ethnomedicinal practices for curing various ailments, especially in countries like Japan, China, India, and Korea.[7–12] Extracts of medicinal mushrooms due to their health-boosting property are being increasingly used and it is well known that these extracts contain diverse biologically active compounds like glucans, polyphenols, fibers, alkaloids, terpenoids, proteins, lectins, polysaccharides, and sterols, which are responsible for these pharmacological activities.[13] Mushrooms owing to their low energy nature can be part of the health-conscious diet for diabetes patients, and it has been proven that consuming macrofungi markedly decreases the overall lipid content including bad cholesterol and elevates the level of good cholesterol.[14–17] In modern medicine, different types of diabetes are treated differently employing different approaches and different grades of antidiabetic pharmaceutical products, which exert their effect through various mechanisms, but these allopathic drugs pose drastic side-effects too. Therefore, to avoid potential side effects of pure chemical medications, natural antidiabetic agents have received a great deal of attention during the last two decades.[18–22] The two principal processes that take place during the onset of diabetes are decline in insulin hormone secretion and reduction in its sensitivity, and they are further aggravated by oxidative stress, which is manifested as an altered cell redox system, thereby modifying vital biomolecules like proteins, lipids, and nucleic acids. An abrupt surge in postprandial blood glucose level occurs due to digestion of polysaccharides by the pancreatic α-amylase and the subsequent breakdown of oligosaccharides and disaccharides into glucose by intestinal α-glucosidase.[23] Thus, inhibition of these enzymes represents an effective strategy for the type 2 diabetes amelioration.[24] Moreover, the nonenzymatic reaction of surplus glucose with plasma proteins leading to the generation of AGEs aggravates the problem by generating more ROS, thereby depleting nitric oxide/NO (an important gaseous chemical messenger) and enhancing inflammatory mediators, all of these factors reinforce diabetic complications and increase atherogenesis risk. Since it is known that excess BGL leads to ROS production; thus, proper management of FBGL and post-meal blood glycemic level is an efficient way to keep diabetic complications in check.[25] Looking at the molecular level, there are a number of molecules including protein kinase B (Akt), insulin receptor substrate-2 (IRS-2), and fork head transcription factor (Foxo 1) which mediate the insulin signaling inside the cell. Any kind of anomaly in these molecules is known to cause insulin resistance (IR). Modulation of Akt masks the c-Jun N-terminal kinase-1 (JNK1) activity, thereby enhancing the translocation of GLUT4 to plasma membranes of myocytes and adipocytes resulting in the enhanced uptake of glucose by these tissues leading to a congruent reduction of BGL. The IRS/PI3K signaling pathway performs the translocation of GLUT-4 transporter once insulin binds to its receptor. Foxo-1, a vital transcription factor, positively regulates IRS-2/insulin sensitivity; any interference to Foxo-1 affects peripheral insulin signaling leading to IR.[26] One more molecular phenomenon resulting in diabetes development is the insulin resistance (IR) caused by anomalous adenosine monophosphate-activated protein kinase (AMPK) signaling. AMPK, a serine/threonine kinase, on activation modulates the insulin response; therefore, it is also considered a potent target for the management of Type 2 DM.[27] Mushrooms not only serve for culinary purposes but also have been used as therapeutic foods for combating diseases like hypercholesterolemia, hypertension, diabetes, and cancer.[28,29] Medicinal mushrooms harbor ample proportion of important enzymes (laccase, superoxide dismutase, etc.), polysaccharides such as β-D-glucans, alkaloids, proteins, polyphenols, sterols, terpenoids, and lectins. These mycoconstituents are known to affect different metabolic pathways, thereby alleviating different health issues including improvement in insulin concentrations and reduction in BGL.[30,31] Mushrooms impart their antidiabetic effects by modulating various processes such as increase plasma insulin level, decrease ROS load, enhance sensitivity of IRS-2 by modulating AMPK signaling, modify gut microflora, and increase GLUT-4 translocation, which in turn decrease IR and enhance glucose uptake, and inhibit gut α-glucosidase thereby controling the post-prandial glycemic surge.[30,32]

Clinical trials of a drug can be done both in vivo and in vitro; however, for ethical considerations, it is always prudential to carry prior in vitro examination to avoid direct exposure of laboratory animals and humans to any potential mishap. Many researchers have elucidated the antidiabetic attributes of mushroom extracts and their isolated compounds and have performed in vitro studies to mark out their efficacy and to make advancements in the respective knowledge.

8.2 IN VITRO ANTIDIABETIC EFFICACY OF CRUDE MUSHROOM EXTRACTS

Ceddia et al.,[33] while analyzing the antidiabetic activity of methanolic extract of *Ganoderma lucidum* on L6 skeletal muscle cell line, reported that a dosage of 20 to 100 μg/ml resulted in considerable enhancement in percent glucose uptake. Glucose uptake increased with the magnitude of 183.4 ± 8.1, 195.3 ± 6.8, and 187.7 ± 9.4% at the doses of 20, 50, and 100 μg/ml, respectively, and this enhancement in glucose transport is reported to be at par with 100 nM insulin (increasing uptake by 180.4 ± 8.6%).[34] This increase in glucose uptake is thought to be mediated by PI3-Kinase as suggested by multifold increase in PI-3-phosphate (PI-3-P).[33] By employing densitometry analysis PI 3-kinase activities after 10, 30, and 60 min of the treatment increased by 5.8, 6.7, and 7.3-fold, respectively, much greater than that of 100 nM insulin treatment. Few studies also state that increase in glucose uptake after *G. lucidum* extract treatment is given to cells, could also be mediated by AMPK, Akt, and p38 MAPK (p38 mitogen activated protein-kinase) marked by the increase in phosphorylated forms of these proteins.[34,35] Phosphorylation level of AMPK α1 subunit by the said extract at 10, 30, and 60 minutes of treatment is elevated to the extent as it is phosphorylated by the drug, AICAR (5-aminoimidazole-4-carboxamide ribonucleoside). Though not as high a time-dependent increase in the phosphorylation level of AMPK α2 subunit has also been observed at 10, 30, and 60 minutes of treatment. Likewise, p38 MAPK phosphorylation was also reportedly increased. Keeping in view the results of the above study it could be inferred that *G. lucidum* extract may enhance glucose uptake by attenuation of PI 3-kinase, Akt, AMPK, and p38 MAPK signaling and could reset the glucose homeostasis. Hydroalcoholic extracts (100 mg/ml) of *Lenzites elegans*, *Ganoderma philippii*, and *Rigidoporus ulmarius*, when added to the in vitro starch digestion assay model employing enzymes α-glucosidase and α-amylase, inhibited the joint enzyme activity by 26.57% ± 0.68%, 40.22% ± 0.83%, and 65.54% ± 0.91%, respectively, as shown in Figure 8.1.[2]

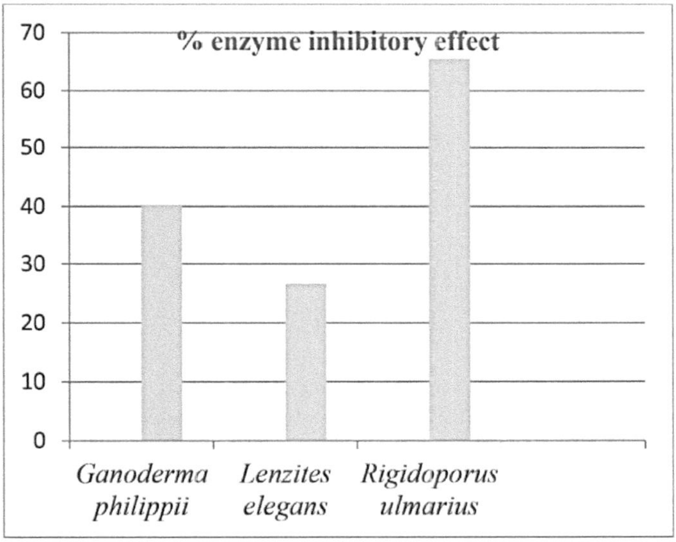

FIGURE 8.1 Percentage enzyme inhibition of hydroalcoholic extracts of three mushroom species.[2]

Huang et al.,[36] while employing methanol extract of *Antrodia cinnamomea* fruiting bodies and mycelia in α-glucosidase inhibitory bioassay, reported the high inhibition potency of 99% for fruitbody extract at a concentration of 1.2 mg/ml with a very low corresponding IC50 value (0.205 mg/ml); while mycelial extract showed less inhibition with a higher corresponding IC50 value (310 mg/ml). On the other hand, acarbose was found to exert a relatively lower inhibitory effect than that of the fruitbody extract, with maximum inhibition of 90.6% at a concentration of 2.5 mg/ml (IC50 of 0.278 mg/ml as depicted in Fig. 8.2). The authors of the aforementioned study also purified eight different compounds (dehydrosulphurenic acid, 25S-antcin I, 25S-antcin B, 25R-antcin B, 25S-antcin K, 25R-antcin K, dehydroeburicoic acid, and eburicoic acid) from *A. cinnamomea* sporocarps and subsequently evaluated these for α-glucosidase inhibitory activity. The relative inhibitory effect of these compounds on α-glucosidase is shown in Figure 8.3.

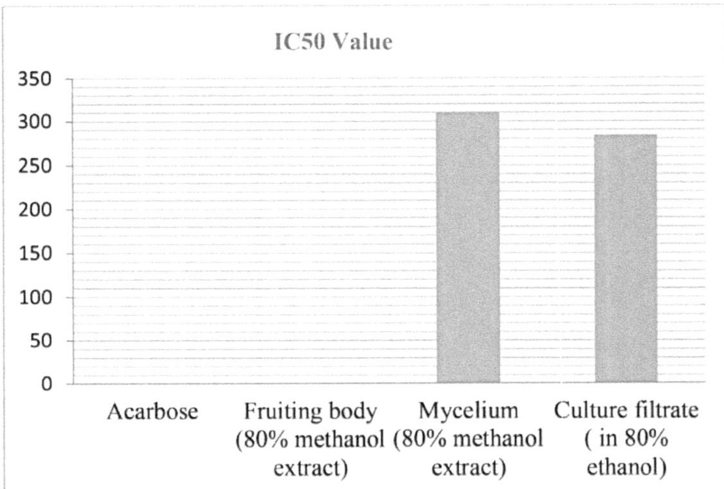

FIGURE 8.2 Methanol extracts of *Antrodia cinnamomea* sporocarps, mycelial and culture filtrates, their in vitro IC50 value against α-glucosidase compared to acarbose.[37]

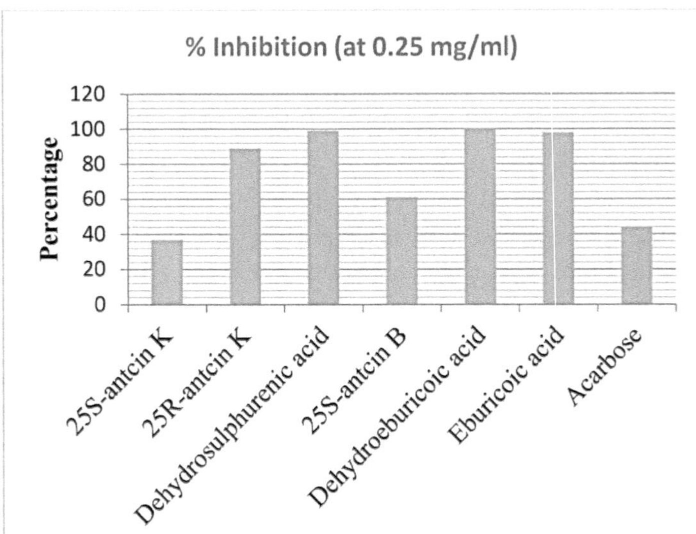

FIGURE 8.3 Different compounds from *Antrodia cinnamomea*, their in vitro EC50 values against α-glucosidase.[36]

Satria et al.[37] compared the α-glucosidase inhibitory effect of eight different growing stages of *Ganoderma lingzhi* and reported that ethanolic extracts of *G. lingzhi* at each stage exhibited higher α-glucosidase inhibition in comparison with positive control, acarbose. The average inhibitory effect of developmental stage 6 (IC50 = 40 ± 0.9 μg/ml) on α-glucosidase is found to be highest of all the eight stages, followed by stage 3 (IC50 = 47 ± 1.5 μg/ml), stage 7 (IC50 = 50 ± 1.7 μg/ml), stage 4 (IC50 = 51 ± 0.8 μg/ml), stage 5 (IC50 = 52 ± 1.2 μg/ml), stage 1 (IC50 = 59 ± 0.9 μg/ml), stage 2 (IC50 = 71 ± 3.8 μg/ml), and stage 8 (IC50 = 109 ± 4.6 μg/ml) with the lowest inhibitory effect on the given enzyme. Ogbole et al.[38] in their study pertaining to *Calvatia gigantea* reported that the crude extract obtained from the mushroom inhibited the enzyme α-amylase under in vitro conditions by 90 folds (IC50 = 0.46 μg/ml) as that of the standard drug, acarbose. The aforementioned work also stated that after fractionating the crude extract into fractions such as dichloromethane, ethyl acetate, butanol, and aqueous fraction, the IC50 value increased (inhibition potential decreased) to 5.3 μg/ml, 6.5 μg/ml, 5.7 μg/ml, and 6.2 μg/ml, respectively, though, still efficient than that of acarbose which showed IC50 of 45 μg/ml for α-amylase. Stojkovic et al.[39] studied the effects of methanolic extracts of *Coprinus comatus*, *Cordyceps militaris*, *Morchella conica*, *Phellinus linteus*, *Inonotus obliquus*, and *Agaricus blazei* on α-amylase and α-glucosidase enzymes. They reported that all of these mushroom species masked the activity of α-glucosidase with the highest inhibition achieved for *I. obliquus* (IC50 value of 220.31 μg/ml). However, α-amylase inhibited by *Agaricus blazei*, *Coprinus comatus*, *Inonotus obliquus*, and *Phellinus linteus* extracts only got significantly masked by *Coprinus comatus* extract (with an IC50 value of 714.45 μg/ml). Based on the above results, the antidiabetically effective lowest daily dose of mushroom powder was predicted to be 3 × 1.148 g/day for *I. obliquus*, and highest as 3 × 2.215 g/day for *Phellinus linteus*. Aqueous extracts and polysaccharide fractions of all the above-mentioned 6 mushroom species have been reportedly known to impart in vivo antidiabetic effects also.[39–41] The inhibitory effect of the extracts investigated[39] could be related to their chemical composition consisting of phenolic acids, organic acids, and fatty acids, and their specific combination for each species is predictive of their unique in vitro antidiabetic properties. Regarding *C. comatus*, organic acid profile displays five different acids viz citric, oxalic, quinic, malic, and fumaric acids and among phenolic acids dominant is p-hydroxybenzoic acid (0.09 mg/100 g) followed by p-coumaric acid and a related compound, cinnamic acid.[42] In *C. militaris* the organic acid found in higher amounts is citric acid 7.97 g/100 g DW[43] and *p*-hydroxybenzoic acid is the only phenolic acid reported in the species (0.02 mg/100 g DW).[39] Pandimeena et al.,[44] while performing in vitro assay of α-amylase, reported that the methanolic extract of *Pleurotus florida* at the concentrations of 0.5mg/ml and 1.0mg/ml reduced the enzyme's efficiency by 20.7% and 26.5%, respectively. A similar in vitro study[43] evaluated antidiabetic effects of *Pleurotus florida* using its methanol extract at 1000 μg/ml concentration against α-amylase and α-glucosidase enzymes. The said extract inhibited both α-amylase and α glucosidase with magnitudes of 94.93 ± 1.75% and 84.90 ± 0.42%, respectively. Su et al.[45] evaluated six medicinal mushroom species namely *Agaricus blazei*, *Ganoderma lucidum*, *Grifola frondosa*, *Hericium erinaceus*, *Coriolus versicolor*, and *Phellinus linteus* for their inhibitory activity on α-amylase and α-glucosidase enzymes under in vitro conditions. The results of their study depicted that n-hexane extracts of *C. versicolor* and *G. frondosa* displayed the strongest inhibition on α-amylase and α-glucosidase, with the corresponding IC50 values of 1.20 mg/ml and 0.0376 mg/ml, respectively. GC–MS analysis displayed that the said extract fraction possessed a significant quantity of unsaturated fatty acids especially linoleic and oleic acid and among these oleic acid exhibited the higher anti-α-glucosidase effect (IC50 = 0.0220 mg/ml) than that of linoleic acid (IC50 = 0.0327 mg/ml). Though both of these were more potent against α-glucosidase in comparison with acarbose, but their inhibition effect on α-amylase was weaker (IC50 > 1 mg/ml).[45] Azeem et al.[46] in their study while analyzing the hydroalcoholic extracts of six mushroom species belonging to *Inonotus* and *Phellinus* genera against α-amylase and α-glucosidase employing a starch assay setup reported that *P. fastuosus* showed the highest cumulative inhibitory effect on the enzymes with an IC50 value of 27.33 ± 1.45 mg/ml followed by *P. sanfordii* and *I. pachyphloeus* with their respective IC50 values of 30.33 ± 0.88 mg/ml and 52.00 ± 1.15 mg/ml. *P. allardii* with a considerably higher IC50 value of 98.00 ± 0.57 mg/ml as depicted in Figure 8.4 was found to be the least effective against these starch digesting enzymes.

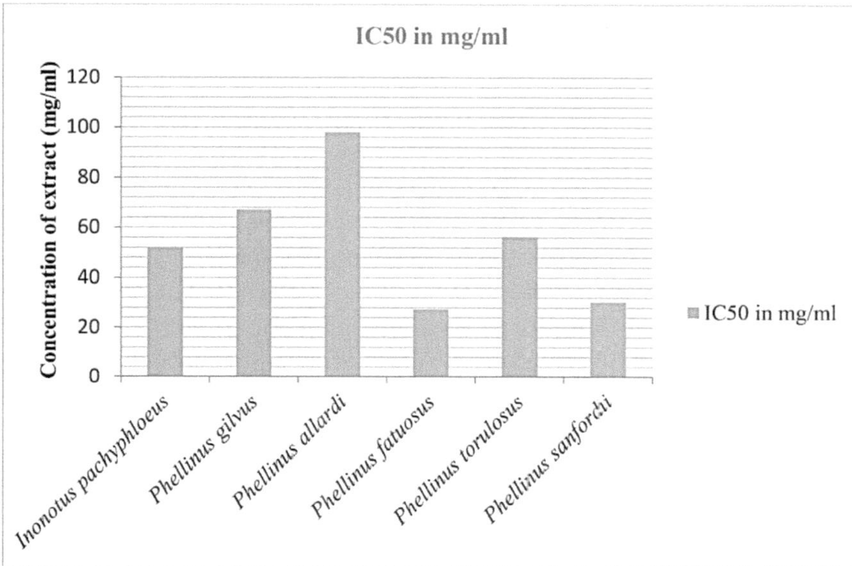

FIGURE 8.4 Hydroalcoholic extracts of *Inonotus* sp. and *Phellinus* spp. with their cumulative IC50 values against α-amylase and α-glucosidase.[46]

Liu et al.,[47] while evaluating *Stropharia rugosoannulata*, *Craterellus cornucopioides*, *Catathelasma ventricosum*, *Clitocybe maxima*, and *Laccaria amethystea* for their antihyperglycemic and antioxidant activity under in vitro conditions, reported that aqueous and ethanolic extracts of all the above-mentioned mushrooms showed considerable BGL lowering and antioxidant potential. Though ethanolic extracts manifested overall higher antihyperglycemic activity, but the aqueous extract of *C. ventricosum* exhibited the highest α-glucosidase inhibitory effect with an IC50 value of just 2.74 μg/ml, while the aqueous extract of *L. amethystea* showed the highest α-amylase inhibitory activity with an IC50 value of 4.37 μg/ml. Aqueous extracts of *L. amethystea* and *C. ventricosum* showed higher α-amylase and α-glucosidase inhibitory effects respectively compared to that of the positive control acarbose with much higher corresponding IC50 values of 36.04 μg/ml and 52.29 μg/ml against α-glucosidase and α-amylase. Among these mushrooms, the aqueous extract of *C. ventricosum* exhibited DPPH radical scavenging activity and reducing power very much similar to that of the positive control BHT (butylated hydroxytoluene), whereas the aqueous extract of *L. amethystea* showed the highest metal chelating activity similar to positive control EDTA (ethylenediamine tetraacetic acid) depicting the remarkable antidiabetic/nutriceutical potential of these mushroom species. Enzyme, protein tyrosine phosphatase 1B (PTP1B), is an important negative regulator of insulin receptor signaling and is responsible for decreasing the expression of insulin receptor β-subunit and is thus among the principal therapeutic targets in diabetes.[48,49] Teng et al.[50] evaluated seven fractions of *Ganoderma lucidum* against PTP1B in vitro and reported for the first time that proteoglycan from the said fungus potentially inhibit it. The aforementioned authors find out that proteoglycan-containing FYGL (Fudan-Yueyang-*G. lucidum*) fraction with percentage polysaccharide and protein content of 77 ± 3 and 16.8 ± 0.9, respectively, imparted the highest effect on PTP1B (IC50 = 5.12 ± 0.05 μg/ml), as shown in Figure 8.5.

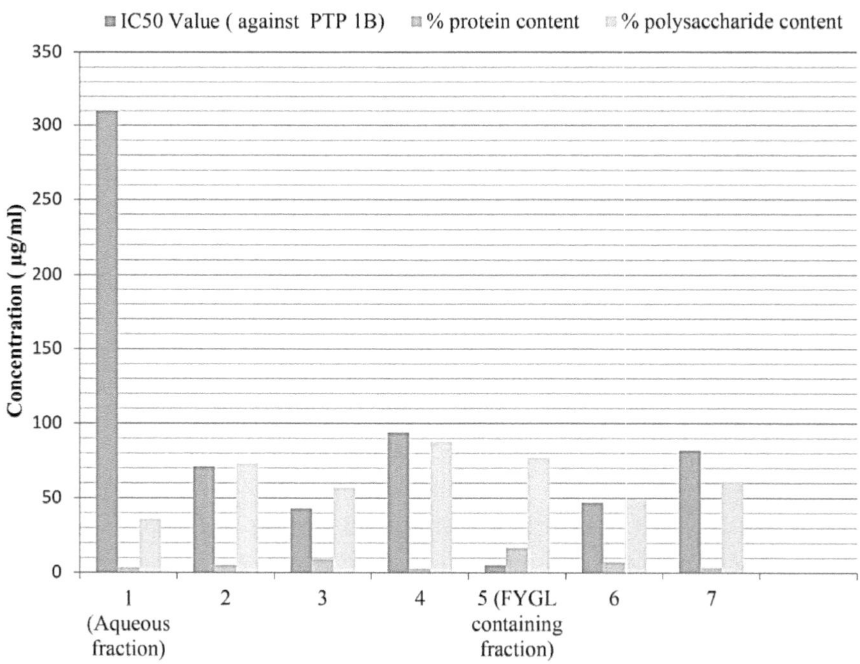

FIGURE 8.5 IC50 value against PTP 1B, percent protein content, and polysaccharide content of fractions (1–7).[50]

Xu and Wu[51] evaluated *Lentinula edodes*, *Grifola frondosa*, *Agrocybe aegerita*, *Auricularia auricula-judae*, *Hericium erinaceus*, *Russula sanguinea*, *Ganoderma lucidum*, and *Tremella fuciformis* for their antidiabetic activity making use of antioxidant activity assay and α-glycosidase and aldose reductase (AR) inhibitory assays. This study reported that amongst the tested mushrooms, the extract of *G. lucidum* exhibited the most significant dose-dependent inhibitory effect on α-glycosidase and aldose reductase with IC50 values of 4.88 mg/ml and 9.87 mg/ml, respectively. Moreover, it also showed the strongest DPPH scavenging activity (with an IC50 value of 3.66 mg/ml). In a recent study, the aforementioned eight mushroom species in combination with *Lentinula edodes* have remarkably alleviated the glucose intolerance and decreased the BGL in rats with gestational diabetes, inferring the potential of these mushroom species as nutraceuticals for the patients with gestational DM.[52] Yoshioka et al.[53] in their study evaluated the antidiabetic effect of *Grifola gargal* by making use of its low molecular weight fraction (GLF) of aqueous extract and examined its effects on glucose transport and GLUT4 movement in L6 myotubes. It was observed that glucose uptake got enhanced remarkably with the maximum absorption attained at 1000 μg/ml of GLF. The authors further fractionated the GLF by size-exclusion chromatography and GLF-E fraction was shown to induce glucose uptake more significantly than parental GLF fraction at a relatively lower concentration of 200 μg/ml, inferring that GLF-E possessed the active principle "adenosine" which enhanced the GLUT4 translocation and glucose transport in L6 myotubes. The signaling mechanism of GLUT4 translocation in L6 myotubes involved the binding of adenosine to A1AR protein which thereby triggers downstream phosphotidyl inositol 3-kinase/protein kinase-B and AMPK pathways and in turn facilitates the GLUT4 translocation to the plasma membrane.

8.3 IN VITRO ANTIDIABETIC EFFICACY OF MUSHROOM TERPENES

Ying et al.[54] in their study revealed that terpenoids from *Inonotus obliquus* act as inhibitors of the intestinal enzyme α-glucosidase. Kim et al.[55] have reported that the aqueous extract obtained from the mushroom *Cordyceps militaris* inhibited the enzyme α-glucosidase with the magnitudes of 45.77% at 0.1 mg/ml concentration, 54.76% at 0.25 mg/ml, 58.74% at 0.5 mg/ml, and 60.5% at 1.0 mg/ml concentration. Ying et al.[56] reported the isolation of two triterpenoids having α,β-dimethyl, α,β-unsaturated δ-lactone side chains from *Inonotus obliquus* and their study also revealed that these triterpenoids suppressed α-glucosidase activity more effectively as compared to the positive control, acarbose. Fatmawati et al.[57] tested the chloroform extract of *Ganoderma lucidum* sporocarp against α-glucosidase while performing in vitro inhibitory assay and found that the neutral fraction of the $CHCl_3$ extract had a greater inhibitory effect (with an IC50 value of 88.7 μg/ml) on the enzyme than that of the standard drug, acarbose as illustrated in Figure 8.6. The neutral fraction of the $CHCl_3$ extract was subjected to chromatographic separation to elute out the active principle, (3β, 24E)-lanosta-7, 9(11),24-trien-3,26-diol (referred to as ganoderol-B). The pure ganoderol-B had been found to have a higher inhibitory activity (IC50 = 48.5 μg/ml) than that of the extract as a whole. This is the first report of lanostane triterpenoids as potent inhibitors of α-glucosidase.

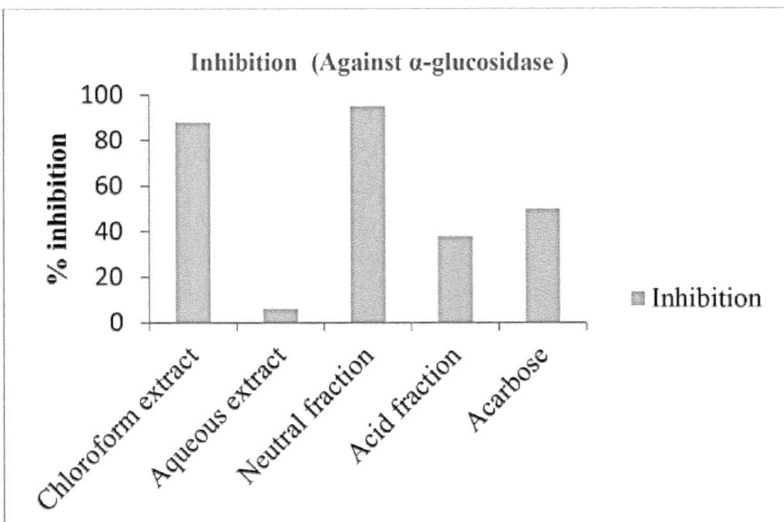

FIGURE 8.6 *Ganoderma lucidum* aqueous extract, chloroform extract, its acidic and neutral fraction, and their α-glucosidase inhibitory activity.[57]

Source: Reprinted with permission from Ref. [57]. © 2011 Elsevier.

Ganoderic acid-Df (GA-Df), a lanostane triterpenoid that is obtained from sporocarps of *Ganoderma lucidum*, has shown significant in vitro inhibition against aldose reductase (an IC50 value of 22.8 μM),[58] whereas its methyl ester produced relatively less inhibition (IC50 > 200 μM) indicating that carboxyl group in the side chain is vital for the inhibitory activity as is supported by El-Kabbani et al.[59] stating that the AR inhibitory compound possessing a carboxyl group shows electrostatic complementation with the oppositely charged domain of aldose reductase enzyme, thus facilitating the inhibition. Fatmawati et al.,[60] while working on stereomeric requirements of lanostane-type triterpenoids for potent α-glucosidase inhibition, isolated 15 bioactive ganoderma acids from the acidic fraction and 3 ganoderma alcohols from the neutral fraction of *Ganoderma lingzhi* chloroform extract. Ganoderol-B, a ganoderma alcohol, produced the strongest inhibitory effect having an IC50 value 5 fold slower than that of acarbose (IC50 = 521.5 μM), whereas ganoderma alcohols, namely ganoderiol-F and ganodermanontriol, showed IC50 values three times lower than and equal to that of acarbose, respectively. Among the ganoderma acids only few showed considerable inhibition on α-glucosidase, with ganoderic acid-Df having IC50 value almost 2.5 times lower than positive control; ganoderenic acid-A and ganoderic acid-B with IC50 lower than control; and ganoderic acid-A showing IC50 equal to acarbose as shown in Figure 8.7. Although ganoderol-B and ganoderiol-F have almost similar structures, the former possessed higher α-glucosidase inhibitory activity and the only structural difference between these two alcohols is at C-3 with ganoderol-B having a hydroxyl group at C-3, while the later do not possess this group. Ganoderol-B and ganoderiol-F showed their respective IC50 values 5 and 3 times lower than that of ganodermanontriol. The structural difference between these compounds is that the former two have double bonds at C24 and C25, whereas ganodermanontriol does not have these double bonds in its structure. Therefore, from the structure–activity relationship of ganoderma alcohols it has become clear that hydroxyl group at C-3 and double bonds at C24 and C25 are vital for potent α-glucosidase inhibition.[60]

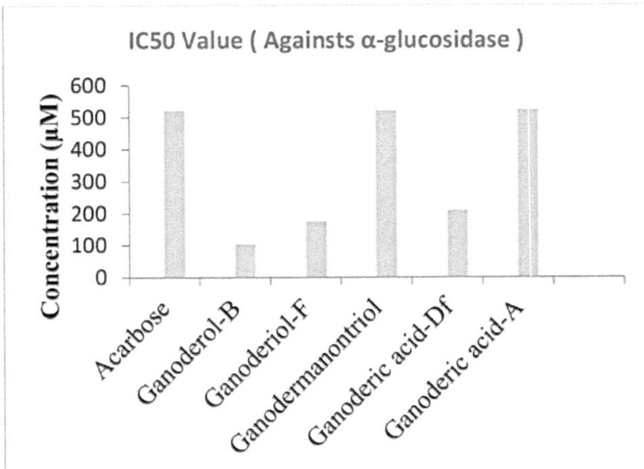

FIGURE 8.7 Lanostane triterpenoids from the acidic and neutral fraction of the chloroform extract of *Ganoderma lingzhi* and their inhibitory potential in terms of IC50 value.[60]

Ganoleuconin-E, ganoleuconin-M, ganoleuconin-N, ganoleuconin-P, and ganoderone-A from *Ganoderma leucocontextum* have reportedly shown a remarkable inhibitory effect on yeast α-glucosidase in vitro showing IC50 values of 12.7, 13.6, 2.5, 5.9, and 13.7 µM, respectively, as depicted in Figure 8.8. The presence of farnesyl hydroquinone moiety imparted stronger α-glucosidase inhibition of ganoleuconins M, N, and P than the positive control acarbose (IC50 = 273.1 ± 30.5).[61]

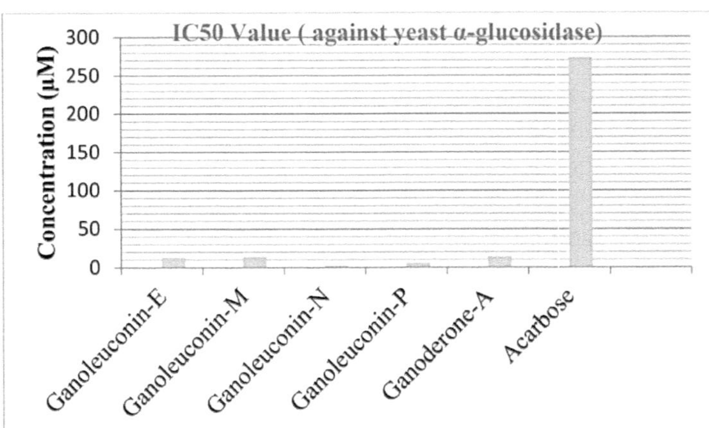

FIGURE 8.8 Lanostane triterpenoids from *Ganoderma leucocontextum* with their IC50 value against α-glucosidase.[61]

Polycyclic meroterpenoids, namely, spirolingzhine-A, spirolingzhine-B, spirolingzhine-D, Ganoleucin-D, spiroapplanatumine-K, spiroapplanatumine-L, isolated from sporocarps of *Ganoderma leucocontextum*, have been reported to show significant inhibitory effects against bovine lens aldose reductase, with spirolingzhine-D showing most potent inhibition having a much lower IC50 value of 9.4 μM as compared to positive control epalrestat (IC50 = 17.5 μM) as depicted in Figure 8.9.[62]

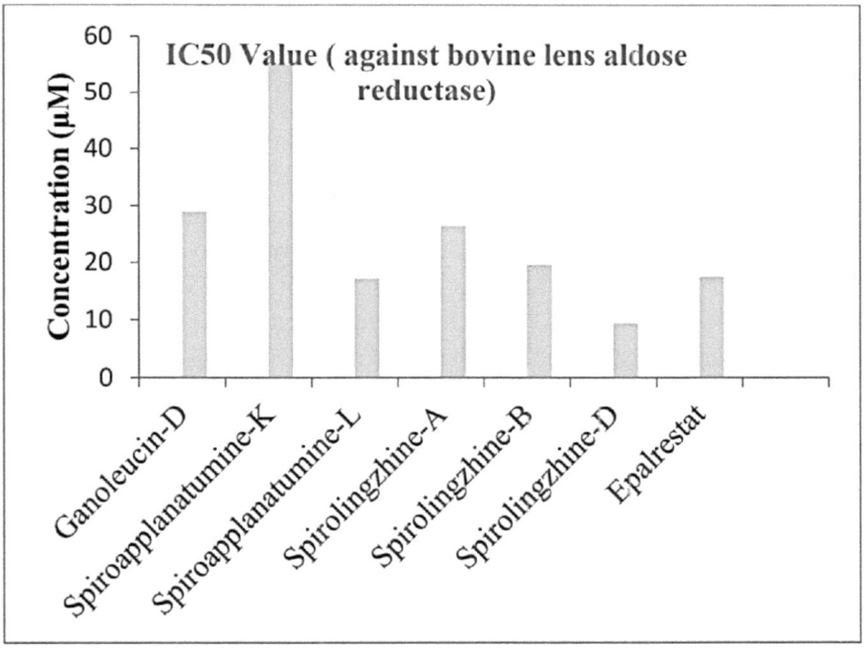

FIGURE 8.9 Meroterpenoids from *Ganoderma leucocontextum* and their IC50 value against bovine lens aldose reductase.[62]

The acidic fraction of the chloroform extract of *Ganoderma lucidum* yielded 13 different ganoderma acids and their corresponding methyl esters. Among the ganoderma acids, ganoderic acid Df (GA-Df) exhibited the most potent inhibition on aldose reductase with an IC50 of 22.8 μM, whereas its corresponding methyl ester imparted very low inhibition with a higher IC50 value of 189.4 μM.[59] Similarly, ganoderic acid-C2 (GA-C2) and ganoderenic acid-A showed considerable inhibition with the corresponding IC50 values of 43.8 and 119.2 μM, respectively; whereas methyl ganoderate-C2 (IC50 >183.9 μM) and methyl ganoderenate A (IC50 >183.9 μM) were found to show very less inhibition than their corresponding acids as depicted in Figure 8.10. Therefore, the presence of carboxyl group in the chemical structure of ganoderma acids is responsible for their potent aldose reductase inhibition.[59,63] The carboxyl (COOH) hydrophilic moiety behaves like polar groups of many pharmaceutical agents such as tolrestat and zopolrestat used for aldose reductase inhibition, and it potentially binds with aldose reductase in the carboxylate (COO^-) form.[63] Ganoderic acid-Df when compared with ganoderic acid-C1 (GA-C1) with a much higherIC50 value of 194.4 μM than GA-Df suggested that the presence of –OH group at C-11 of GA-Df is meant for its higher inhibition capacity since the presence of this moiety at C-11 is the only structural difference between these two. Similarly, aldose reductase inhibition capacity of GA-C2 (IC50 = 43.8 μM) was found to be much higher than that of ganoderenic acid-A (IC50 > 193.5 μM). GA-C2 possess an extra –OH group at C-3, which differentiates it from ganoderenic acid A. In the same way, the comparison of GA-C2 (having OH at C-7) with ganolucidic acid B (with IC50 >199.2 μM) revealed that much less inhibitory activity of the later could be assigned to its structural difference of having H2 moiety as the C-7 functional group. Likewise, the stereomeric difference between GA-C2 and ganoderic acid-B (IC50 >193.5 μM) is only at C-15 functional group with former having OH and later having C=O, respectively. Comparative analysis of the structure of ganoderenic acid-A (IC50 = 119.2 μM) and ganoderic acid-A (IC50 >193.5 μM) revealed that the only difference between these two compounds is the double bond at C-20 and C-22 in the former. This comparative analysis suggested that –COOH in the side chain and –OH group at C-11 remarkably enhances AR inhibitory activity of GA-Df. In the same way –OH substituents at C-3, C-7, and C-15 of ganoderic acid-C2 are responsible for its unexpectedly high AR inhibitory property; on the other hand, double bonds at C-20 and C-22 of ganoderenic acid-A make it a potent aldose reductase inhibitor.

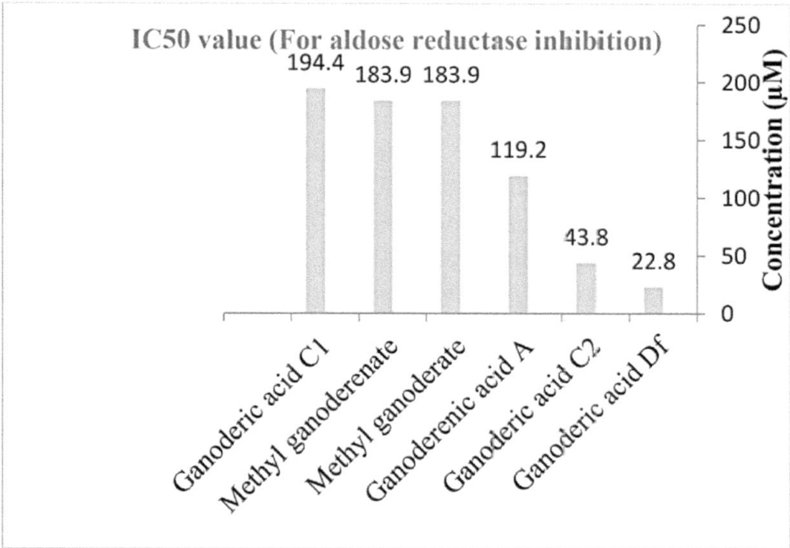

FIGURE 8.10 Ganoderma acids, their methyl esters from *Ganoderma lucidum*, and their inhibition on aldose reductase in terms of IC50 value.[63]

Similarly, for ganoderma acids the α-glucosidase inhibitory effect of ganoderenic acid-A is higher than that of positive control and ganoderic acid-A has almost the same IC50 value as that of acarbose. The only difference between these acids is the presence of double bonds in the chemical structure of the former at C20 and C22, whereas the latter is devoid of them. Likewise, the IC50 value of ganoderic acid-B is significantly lower than that of ganoderic acid-A; the only structural difference between them is that the former possess a hydroxyl group at C-3, whereas the latter has a carbonyl group instead of this. Thus, for ganoderma acids to show potent inhibition on α-glucosidase their chemical structure should harbor a carboxyl group in the side chain, double bonds at C20 and C22 and hydroxyl group at C-3.[59,60]

8.4 IN VITRO ANTIDIABETIC EFFICACY OF MUSHROOM POLYSACCHARIDES

In a study the mushroom exopolysaccharides considerably reduced the blood glucose level of diabetic mice and quenched the superoxide and hydroxyl radicals in vitro.[63] *Hericium erinaceus*, a highly scrutinized edible and medicinal mushroom when tested on liver tissue, reportedly decreased the lipid level and improved the catalytic activity of SOD and glutathione peroxidase.[65–67] Cai et al.[68] isolated and administered a *Hericium erinaceus* polysaccharide, namely HEP-C in streptozotocin rats at a dosage of 150 and 300 mg/kg/bw and observed remarkable improvement in FBG and antioxidant enzyme actions. These effects are thought to be facilitated by the activation of PI3K/Akt signaling pathway. Polysaccharides derived from *Hericium erinaceus* and *Phellinus linteus* remarkably reduced the BGL and improved glucose intolerance by modulating Foxo-1 signaling pathway.[69,70] Kim et al.[71] in their study while examining the impact of *Phellinus linteus* derived polysaccharide PLP on nonobese diabetic (NOD) mice and found that BGL dropped from 499 mg/dl to 110 mg/dl. Wang et al.[72] analyzed *Inonotus obliquus* polysaccharide (IOPS) and its chromium-III complex ligated form (IOPC) for their antidiabetic effects on liver L-02 cell line. The authors of the aforementioned study came with results that both the IOPS and IOPC showed a remarkable DPPH quenching activity. IOPC showed a considerable α-amylase and α-glucosidase inhibitory effect as compared with IOPS inferring its presumed use for postprandial BGL regulation. Moreover, AGE the formation is considerably masked by both IOPS and its complex. Ying et al.[73] isolated polysaccharides from sporocarps of 6 mushroom species *Armillaria mellea* (AM), *Hypsizygus marmoreus* (HM), *Gomphidius rutilus* (GR), *Agrocybe cylindracea* (AC), *Pleurotus eryngii* (PE), and *Pleurotus ostreatus* (PO), and fractionated them into alkaline, neutral, and acidic fractions. On the evaluation of their antidiabetic activity on fatty acid-induced insulin resistant Hepa1–6 cell line, alkali-soluble polysaccharides AAMP, AGRP, and AACP remarkably increased glucose transport at very low concentration (0.01 mg/ml) similar to that of 20 μM metformin suggesting that these alkali-soluble polysaccharides could attenuate insulin sensitivity. Among neutral fraction of polysaccharides, AAMP-N and AGRP-N also enhanced glucose transport remarkably at 0.01 mg/ml, and by screening their monosaccharide monomer composition AAMP-N and AGRP-N appeared to have a similar galactoglucan domain, inferring that galactoglucan may be involved in insulin sensitization. Autophagy is associated with the maintenance of insulin function in mammalian cells. Polysaccharides from various mushroom species have been shown to induce autophagy,[74] and likewise polysaccharides from *Armillaria mellea* were found to activate autophagy after 3 h of treatment in HeLa cell line stably expressing GFP-tagged LC3 puncta, an autophagosome marker. According to the number of LC3 puncta, the autophagy-inducing capacities of polysaccharides were AAMP-N > AAMP > AAMP.[75] The antagonizing effect of *Armillaria mellea* polysaccharides on fatty acid-induced insulin resistance evaluated in Hepa1–6 cell line has shown that 0.1 mg/ml of AAMP and AAMP-N and 20 μM of MET treatment intensified phosphorylation of insulin receptor and its downstream protein kinase-B. Many studies[74,75] have reported that fatty acid treatment suppressed autophagy in Hepa1–6 cells; however, fatty acid treatment immediately followed by the addition of 0.1 mg/ml of AAMP-N dramatically restores the autophagy marked by increased LC3-II/LC3-Puncuta expression and increased p62 protein destruction. Based on the results of insulin resistance and autophagy assays, it is inferred that *Armillaria mellea* polysaccharides, especially the neutral fraction AAMP-N, increases autophagy and insulin-mediated glucose absorption.[73] *Auricularia auricula-judae* polysaccharides (AAPs) and their acid hydrolyzed fraction (AAPs-F) at 0.5 mg/ml and 0.2 mg/ml respectively inhibited advanced glycated end product (AGE) formation in a nonenzymatic glycosylation reaction setup. Moreover, AAPs-F at 0.5 mg/ml remarkably increased the glucose absorption in HepG2 human cell line by a magnitude of 24.4% in a dose-dependent fashion and has significantly extended the lifespan of *Caenorhabditis elegans* by 32.9% under high sugar stress conditions.[76] Cao et al.[77] isolated polysaccharides from *Coprinus comatus* as two separate fractions of intracellular polysaccharides (ICPs) and extracellular polysaccharide (ECPs) and tested them for in vitro antioxidant and α-amylase inhibitory activities and reported that the ICPs exhibit the strongest total antioxidant (6.34 ± 0.33 U/ml) and DPPH radical scavenging (63.78 ± 0.38%) activities at the concentration of 10 mg/ml. The authors of the aforementioned study have also reported that both the ICPs and ECPs and their deproteinized fractions at a concentration of 10 mg/ml impart significant inhibition on α-amylase with the highest effect reported for ICPs with the magnitude of 87.15 ± 0.99%. Zhang et al.[78] isolated *Ganoderma lucidum* polysaccharide (*Gl*-PS) and investigated its in vitro protective effect on alloxan-treated pancreatic islets. This study also reported that isolated pancreatic cells, when treated with alloxan for 4.5 h, experienced dose-dependent toxicity, with 3.2 mM and 6.4 mM alloxan reducing viability of the islets by 50% and 80%, respectively, however, preincubation of islets with 100 μg/ml *Gl*-PS for

12 h partly protected the islets from alloxan-induced toxicity. However, by extending the preincubation time to 24 h *Gl*-PS showed a protective effect in a concentration-dependent manner. Treatment with *Gl*-PS at the concentrations of 25 μg/ml and 100 μg/ml improved the alloxan caused cell viability loss from 47.87% to 70.3% and 80.15%, respectively. Using ROS fluorescent probe and with the aid of confocal microscopy, the aforementioned workers[78] observed constant fluorescence intensity in the normal pancreatic islets; however, in the alloxan control group, fluorescence of free radicals began to increase after 10 minutes of alloxan addition and attained peak after 30 minutes with the increase in fluorescence by 4.5 folds as that of normal cells. Though, the addition of 100 μg/ml *Gl*-PS together with alloxan still caused enhancement in fluorescence intensity; however, when the islets were preincubated with 100 μg/ml *Gl*-PS for 24 h fluorescence of free radicals was completely inhibited.

8.5 IN VITRO ANTIDIABETIC EFFICACY OF MUSHROOM STEROLS AND STEROL DERIVATIVES

Wu et al.[79] isolated bioactive compound, ergosterol peroxide (EPO), from *Grifola frondosa* fruiting bodies and examined its antidiabetic effects on palmitate (PA)-induced C2C12 skeletal muscle cell line under in vitro conditions and astonishingly found that EPO upregulated glucose absorption and increased cell viability to a great extent. The most optimal concentration of EPO to improve cell viability and to enhance glucose uptake was found to be 5 μM. The EPO treatment at this concentration has also been found to scavenge reactive oxygen species, and to modulate phosphotidyl inositol 3-kinase/protein kinase-B, MAPK, and GLUT-4 signaling pathways. Moreover, EPO at this concentration enhanced the expression of PI3K, Akt, p-Akt, IRS-1, p-IRS-1, and GLUT-4 proteins, while p-JNK and p-p38 expression was downregulated. Interestingly, the enhancement in glucose absorption at 5 μM EPO treatment was at par to insulin treatment, and apart from this GLUT-4 siRNA treatment was also reversed. This aforementioned research work also reported that EPO below 10 μM does not show any cytotoxic effect on C2C12 cells and is sufficient to enhance glucose uptake. Though the palmitate treatment on the C2C12 cell line reduced cell viability to about 81.43%, but co-treatment of cells with 0.5–5 μM EPO displayed absolute protection against palmitate-induced toxicity and increased the glucose absorption up to a remarkable extent. Xiang et al.[80] observed that ergosterol isolated from *Pleurotus ostreatus*, when applied to "L6 rat myoblast cell line," upregulated GLUT-4 expression and enhanced the phosphorylation of protein kinase-C (PKC) and protein kinase-B (Akt) which thereby increased the glucose uptake up to a remarkable extent. Lee et al.,[81] while performing bioassay-guided fractionation of the dichloromethane extract of *Ganoderma applanatum*, isolated eight novel compounds for the first time and they were subsequently tested in vitro for the aldose reductase inhibitory activity. Among these ergosterol peroxide (EPS) showed the highest inhibitory effect with an IC50 value of 15.4 μg/ml at par with positive control TMG (tetramethylene glutaric acid; IC50 = 0.6 μg/ml), as shown in Figure 8.11, while the rest of these compounds showed a relatively insignificant inhibitory effect with IC50 values greater than 100 μg/ml.

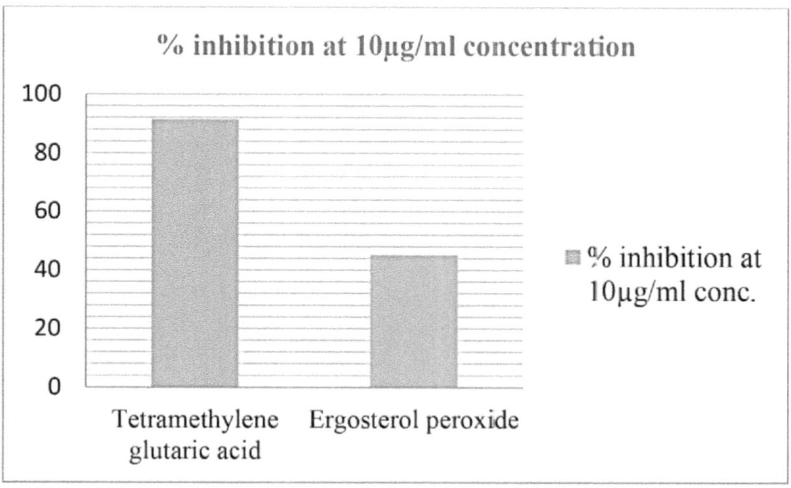

FIGURE 8.11 Percentage inhibition imparted by EPS on rat lens aldose reductase.[81]

8.6 CONCLUSION

Mushrooms being rich in numerous bioactive constituents like dietary fibers, proteins, polyphenols, glucans, flavonoids, alkaloids, terpenoids, polysaccharides, lectins, sterols are known for their antidiabetic effects since ancient times. Several in vitro studies have demonstrated the antidiabetic activity of different extract fractions and purified mycoconstituents obtained from various mushroom species. These extracts and myco-constituents impart in vitro antidiabetic effects by modulating various enzymes associated with polysaccharide metabolism; by attenuating the insulin signaling; by triggering DPPH-free radical scavenging and anti-oxidant activity, etc. The significant in vitro antidiabetic activity and the corresponding in vivo hypoglycemic effect exhibited by various mushrooms emphasize the fact that these macrofungi could potentially serve as a promising source of natural antidiabetic medicine.

KEYWORDS

- **mushrooms**
- **antidiabetic**
- **in vitro studies**
- **diabetes**
- **cholesterol**

REFERENCES

1. Whiting, D. R.; Guariguata, L.; Weil, C.; Shaw, J. IDF Diabetes Atlas: Global Estimates of the Prevalence of Diabetes for 2011 and 2030. *Diabetes Res. Clin. Pract.* **2011,** *94* (3), 311–321.
2. Kaur, A.; Dhingra, G. S.; Shri, R. Evaluation of Carbohydrate Metabolism Inhibition by Some Species of Medicinal Mushrooms from India. *Int. J. Med. Mushrooms* **2015,** *17* (4), 351–360.
3. Bazzano, L. A.; Li, T. Y.; Joshipura, K. J.; Hu, F. B. Intake of Fruit, Vegetables, and Fruit Juices and Risk of Diabetes in Women. *Diabetes Care* **2008,** *31* (7), 1311–1317.
4. Kanazawa, K. Bioavailability of Non-nutrients for Preventing Lifestyle-related Diseases. *Trends Food Sci. Technol.* **2011,** *22* (12), 655–659.
5. Mirmiran, P.; Noori, N.; Zavareh, M. B.; Azizi, F. Fruit and Vegetable Consumption and Risk Factors for Cardiovascular Disease. *Metab. Clin. Exp.* **2009,** *58* (4), 460–468.
6. Gallagher, A. M.; Flatt, P. R.; Duffy, G. A. W. Y.; Abdel-Wahab, Y. H. A. The Effects of Traditional Antidiabetic Plants on *in Vitro* Glucose Diffusion. *Nutr. Res.* **2003,** *23* (3), 413–424.
7. Hobbs, C. *Medicinal Mushrooms: An Exploration of Tradition, Healing and Culture*. Botanica Press: Santa Cruz, CA, 1995; 252 p.

8. Hobbs, C. Medicinal Value of *Lentinus edodes* (Berk.) Sing. (Agaricomycetideae). A Literature Review. *Int. J. Med. Mushrooms* **2000,** *2* (4), 287–302.
9. Hobbs, C. Medicinal Value of Turkey Tail Fungus *Trametes versicolor* (L.: Fr.) Pilát (Aphyllophoromycetideae). A Literature Review. *Int. J. Med. Mushrooms* **2004,** *6* (3), 195–218.
10. Hobbs, C. The Chemistry, Nutritional Value, Immunopharmacology, and Safety of the Traditional Food of Medicinal Split-gill Fungus *Schizophyllum commune* Fr.: Fr. (Schizophyllaceae). A Literature Review. *Int. J. Med. Mushrooms* **2005,** *7* (2), 127–140.
11. Chang, S. T. Global Impact of Edible and Medicinal Mushrooms on Human Welfare in the 21st Century: Nongreen Revolution. *Int. J. Med. Mushrooms* **1999,** *1* (1), 1–8.
12. Mizuno, T. The Extraction and Development of Antitumor-active Polysaccharides from Medicinal Mushrooms in Japan. *Int. J. Med. Mushrooms* **1999,** *1* (1), 9–29.
13. Popovic, V.; Zivkovic, J.; Davidovic, S.; Stevanovic, M.; Stojkovic, D. Mycotherapy of Cancer: An Update on Cytotoxic and Antitumor Activities of Mushrooms, Bioactive Principles and Molecular Mechanisms of Their Action. *Curr. Top. Med. Chem.* **2013,** *13* (21), 2791–2806.
14. Mattila, P.; Salo-Vaananen, P.; Konko, K.; Aro, H.; Jalava, T. Basic Composition and Amino Acid Contents of Mushrooms Cultivated in Finland. *J. Agric. Food Chem.* **2002,** *50* (22), 6419–6422.
15. Smiderle, F. R.; Olsen, L. M.; Ruthes, A. C.; Czelusniak, P. A.; Santana-Filho, A. P.; Sassaki, G. L.; Gorin, P. A. J.; Iacomini, M. Exopolysaccharides, Proteins and Lipids in *Pleurotus pulmonarius* Submerged Culture Using Different Carbon Sources. *Carbohydr. Polym.* **2012,** *87* (1), 368–376.
16. Kim, D. H.; Yang, B. K.; Jeong, S. C.; Hur, N. J.; Surajit, D.; Yun, J. W.; Choi, J. W.; Lee, Y. S.; Song, C. H. A Preliminary Study on the Hypoglycemic Effect of the Exo-polymers Produced by Five Different Medicinal Mushrooms. *J. Microbiol. Biotechnol.* **2001,** *11* (1), 167–171.
17. Wani, B. A.; Bodha, R. H.; Wani, A. H. Nutritional and Medicinal Importance of Mushrooms. *J. Med. Plant Res.* **2010,** *4* (24), 2598–2604.
18. Andujar-Plata, P.; Pi-Sunyer, X.; Laferrere, B. Metformin Effects Revisited. *Diabetes Res. Clin. Pract.* **2012,** *95* (1), 1–9.
19. BARI 2D Study Group. A Randomized Trial of Therapies for Type 2 Diabetes and Coronary Artery Disease. *N. Engl. J. Med.* **2009,** *360* (24), 2503–2515.
20. Eurich, D. T.; McAlister, F. A.; Blackburn, D. F.; Majumdar, S. R.; Tsuyuki, R. T.; Varney, J.; Johnson, J. A. Benefits and Harms of Antidiabetic Agents in Patients with Diabetes and Heart Failure: Systematic Review. *Br. Med. J.* **2007,** *335* (7618), 497.
21. Kirkham, S.; Akilen, R.; Sharma, S.; Tsiami, A. The Potential of Cinnamon to Reduce Blood Glucose Levels in Patients with Type 2 Diabetes and Insulin Resistance. *Diabetes Obes. Metab.* **2009,** *11* (12), 1100–1113.
22. Yeh, G. Y.; Eisenberg, D. M.; Kaptchuk, T. J.; Phillips, R. S. Systematic Review of Herbs and Dietary Supplements for Glycemic Control in Diabetes. *Diabetes Care* **2003,** *26* (4), 1277–1294.
23. Gray, G. M. Carbohydrate Digestion and Absorption: Role of the Small Intestine. *N. Engl. J. Med.* **1975,** *292* (23), 1225–1230.
24. Krentz, A. J.; Bailey, C. J. Oral Antidiabetic Agents. *Drugs* **2005,** *65* (3), 385–411.

25. Ighodaro, O. M. Molecular Pathways Associated with Oxidative Stress in Diabetes Mellitus. *Biomed. Pharmacother.* **2018,** *108*, 656–662.
26. Saini, V. Molecular Mechanisms of Insulin Resistance in Type 2 Diabetes Mellitus. *World J. Diabetes* **2010,** *1* (3), 68–75.
27. Coughlan, K. A.; Valentine, R. J.; Ruderman, N. B.; Saha, A. K. AMPK Activation: A Therapeutic Target for Type 2 Diabetes. *Diabetes Metab. Syndr. Obes.* **2014,** *7*, 241–253.
28. Bobek, P.; Galbavy, S. Hypocholesterolemic and Antiatherogenic Effect of Oyster Mushroom (*Pleurotus ostreatus*) in Rabbits. *Nahrung* **1999,** *43* (5), 339–342.
29. Bobek, P.; Ozdin, L.; Kuniak, L. The Effect of Oyster Mushroom (*Pleurotus ostreatus*), Its Ethanolic Extract and Extraction Residues on Cholesterol Levels in Serum, Lipoproteins and Liver of Rat. *Nahrung* **1995,** *39* (1), 98–99.
30. Higaki, M.; Eguchi, F.; Zhang, J.; Kikukawa, T.; Abe, C.; Kato, K.; Hasegawa, K.; Watanabe, Y. Improvement of Pancreatic β-Cells by Hot Water Extract from Cultured *Agaricus blazei* (CJ-01) Fruiting Bodies in GK Rats. *J. Tradit. Med.* **2000,** *17* (5), 205–214.
31. Gulati, V.; Singh, M. D.; Gulati, P. Role of Mushrooms in Gestational Diabetes Mellitus. *AIMS Med. Sci.* **2019,** *6* (1), 49–66.
32. Sedan, A. The Significance of *in Vitro* Studies. *Quintessen. Int. (Berlin, Germany: 1985)* **2007,** *38* (1), 13–14.
33. Ceddia, R. B.; Somwar, R.; Maida, A.; Fang, X.; Bikopoulos, G.; Sweeney, G. Globular Adiponectin Increases GLUT4 Translocation and Glucose Uptake But Reduces Glycogen Synthesis in Rat Skeletal Muscle Cells. *Diabetologia* **2005,** *48* (1), 132–139.
34. Fujita, T.; Funako, T.; Hayashi, H. 8-Hydroxydaidzein, an Aldose Reductase Inhibitor from Okara Fermented with *Aspergillus* sp. HK-388. *Biosci. Biotechnol. Biochem.* **2004,** *68* (7), 1588–1590.
35. Sato, S.; Kador, P. F. Inhibition of Aldehyde Reductase by Aldose Reductase Inhibitors. *Biochem. Pharmacol.* **1990,** *40* (5), 1033–1042.
36. Huang, H. T.; Wang, S. L.; Nguyen, V. B.; Kuo, Y. H. Isolation and Identification of Potent Antidiabetic Compounds from *Antrodia cinnamomea*—An Edible Taiwanese Mushroom. *Molecules* **2018,** *23* (11), 2864.
37. Satria, D.; Tamrakar, S.; Suhara, H.; Kaneko, S.; Shimizu, K. Mass Spectrometry-based Untargeted Metabolomics and α-Glucosidase Inhibitory Activity of Lingzhi (*Ganoderma lingzhi*) During the Developmental Stages. *Molecules* **2019,** *24* (11), 2044.
38. Ogbole, O. O.; Nkumah, A. O.; Linus, A. U.; Falade, M. O. Molecular Identification, in Vivo and *in Vitro* Activities of *Calvatia gigantea* (Macro-fungus) as an Antidiabetic Agent. *Mycology* **2019,** *10* (3), 166–173.
39. Stojkovic, D.; Smiljkovic, M.; Ciric, A.; Glamoclija, J.; Van-Griensven, L.; Ferreira, I. C.; Sokovic, M. An Insight into Antidiabetic Properties of Six Medicinal and Edible Mushrooms: Inhibition of α-Amylase and α-Glucosidase Linked to Type-2 Diabetes. *S. Afr. J. Bot.* **2019,** *120* (1), 100–103.
40. Qin, D. W.; Gu, Z.; Guo, J. Y. Medicinal Mushroom for Prevention of Disease of Modern Civilization. *Evid.-Based Complement. Altern. Med.* **2015,** *2015*. https://doi.org/10.1155/2015/812725

41. Zhao, C.; Liao, Z.; Wu, X.; Liu, Y.; Liu, X.; Lin, Z.; Huang, Y.; Liu, B. Isolation, Purification, and Structural Features of a Polysaccharide from *Phellinus linteus* and Its Hypoglycemic Effect in Alloxan-induced Diabetic Mice. *J. Food Sci.* **2014,** *79* (5), 1002–1010.
42. Bizarro, A.; Ferreira, I. C.; Soković, M.; Van-Griensven, L. J.; Sousa, D.; Vasconcelos, M. H.; Lima, R. T. *Cordyceps militaris* (L.) Link Fruiting Body Reduces NCI-H460 Cellular Viability through a Mechanism Involving p53 and p21. *Molecules* **2015,** *20* (8), 13927–13940.
43. Prabu, M.; Kumuthakalavalli, R. Antidiabetic Potential of the Oyster Mushroom *Pleurotus florida* (Mont.) Singer. *Int. J. Curr. Pharm. Res.* **2017,** *9* (4), 51–54.
44. Pandimeena, M.; Prabu, M.; Sumathy, R.; Kumuthakalavalli, R. Evaluation of Phytochemicals and *in Vitro* Anti-inflammatory, Anti-diabetic Activity of the White Oyster Mushroom, *Pleurotus florida*. *Int. Res. J. Pharm. Appl. Sci.* **2015,** *5* (1), 16–21.
45. Su, C. H.; Lai, M. N.; Ng, L. T. Inhibitory Effects of Medicinal Mushrooms on α-Amylase and α-Glucosidase-Enzymes Related to Hyperglycemia. *Food Funct* **2013,** *4* (4), 644–649.
46. Azeem, U.; Shri, R.; Dhingra, G. S. *In Vitro* and In Vivo Antihyperglycemic Activities of Medicinal Mushrooms (Agaricomycetes) from India. *Int. J. Med. Mushrooms* **2021,** *23* (2), 29–41.
47. Liu, Y. T.; Sun, J.; Luo, Z. Y.; Rao, S. Q.; Su, Y. J.; Xu, R. R.; Yang, Y. J. Chemical Composition of Five Wild Edible Mushrooms Collected from Southwest China and Their Antihyperglycemic and Antioxidant Activity. *Food Chem. Toxicol.* **2012,** *50* (5), 1238–1244.
48. Combs, A. P. Recent Advances in the Discovery of Competitive Protein Tyrosine Phosphatase 1B Inhibitors for the Treatment of Diabetes, Obesity, and Cancer. *J. Med. Chem.* **2010,** *53* (6), 2333–2344.
49. Feldhammer, M.; Uetani, N.; Miranda-Saavedra, D.; Tremblay, M. L. PTP1B: A Simple Enzyme for a Complex World. *Crit. Rev. Biochem. Mol. Biol.* **2013,** *48* (5), 430–445.
50. Teng, B. S.; Wang, C. D.; Yang, H. J.; Wu, J. S.; Zhang, D.; Zheng, M.; Fan, Z. H.; Pan, D.; Zhou, P. A Protein Tyrosine Phosphatase 1B Activity Inhibitor from the Fruiting Bodies of *Ganoderma lucidum* (Fr.) Karst and Its Hypoglycemic Potency on Streptozotocin-Induced Type 2 Diabetic Mice. *J. Agric. Food Chem.* **2011,** *59* (12), 6492–6500.
51. Wu, T.; Xu, B. B. Antidiabetic and Antioxidant Activities of Eight Medicinal Mushroom Species from China. *Int. J. Med. Mushrooms* **2015,** *17* (2), 129–140.
52. Laurino, L. F.; Viroel, F. J.; Pickler, T. B.; Gerenutti, M. Functional Foods in Gestational Diabetes: Evaluation of the Oral Glucose Tolerance Test (OGTT) in Pregnant Rats Treated with Mushrooms. *Reprod. Toxicol* **2017,** *72* (1), 1–12.
53. Yoshioka, Y.; Harada, E.; Ge, D.; Imai, K.; Katsuzaki, H.; Mishima, T.; Gabazza, E. C. O.; Ashida, H. Adenosine Isolated from *Grifola gargal* Promotes Glucose Uptake Via PI3K and AMPK Signalling Pathways in Skeletal Muscle Cells. *J. Funct. Foods* **2017,** *33*, 268–277.
54. Ying, Y. M.; Zhang, L. Y.; Zhang, X.; Bai, H. B.; Liang, D. E.; Ma, L. F.; Shan, W. G.; Zhan, Z. J. Terpenoids with Alpha-glucosidase Inhibitory Activity from the Submerged Culture of *Inonotus obliquus*. *Phytochemistry* **2014,** *108* (5), 171–176.

55. Kim, D. J.; Kang, Y. H.; Kim, K. K.; Kim, T. W.; Park, J. B.; Choe, M. Increased Glucose Metabolism and Alpha-glucosidase Inhibition in *Cordyceps militaris* Water Extract-treated HepG2 cells. *Nutr. Res. Pract.* **2017,** *11* (3), 180–189.
56. Liu, S. Y.; Chen, L.; Li, X. C.; Hu, Q. K.; He, L. J. *Lycium barbarum* Polysaccharide Protects Diabetic Peripheral Neuropathy by Enhancing Autophagy Via mTOR/p70S6K Inhibition in Streptozotocin-induced Diabetic Rats. *J. Chem. Neuroanat.* **2018,** *89*, 37–42.
57. Fatmawati, S.; Shimizu, K.; Kondo, R. Ganoderol B: A Potent α-Glucosidase Inhibitor Isolated from the Fruiting Body of *Ganoderma lucidum. Phytomedicine* **2011,** *18* (12), 1053–1055.
58. Fatmawati, S.; Shimizu, K.; Kondo, R. Ganoderic Acid Df, a New Triterpenoid with Aldose Reductase Inhibitory Activity from the Fruiting Body of *Ganoderma lucidum. Fitoterapia* **2010,** *81* (8), 1033–1036.
59. El-Kabbani, O.; Wilson, D. K.; Petrash, M.; Quiocho, F. A. Structural Features of the Aldose Reductase and Aldehyde Reductase Inhibitor-binding Sites. *Mol. Vis.* **1998,** *4* (4), 19.
60. Fatmawati, S.; Kondo, R.; Shimizu, K. Structure–Activity Relationships of Lanostane-type Triterpenoids from *Ganoderma lingzhi* as α-Glucosidase Inhibitors. *Bioorg. Med. Chem. Lett.* **2013,** *23* (21), 5900–5903.
61. Wang, K.; Bao, L.; Xiong, W.; Ma, K.; Han, J.; Wang, W.; Yin, W.; Liu, H. Lanostane Triterpenes from the Tibetan Medicinal Mushroom *Ganoderma leucocontextum* and Their Inhibitory Effects on HMG-CoA Reductase and α-Glucosidase. *J. Nat. Prod.* **2015,** *78* (8), 1977–1989.
62. Zhang, J.; Ma, K.; Chen, H.; Wang, K.; Xiong, W.; Bao, L.; Liu, H. A Novel Polycyclic Meroterpenoid with Aldose Reductase Inhibitory Activity from Medicinal Mushroom *Ganoderma leucocontextum. J. Antibiot.* **2017,** *70* (8), 915–917.
63. Fatmawati, S.; Shimizu, K.; Kondo, R. Structure–Activity Relationships of *Ganoderma* Acids from *Ganoderma lucidum* as Aldose Reductase Inhibitors. *Bioorg. Med. Chem. Lett.* **2011,** *21* (24), 7295–7297.
64. Mao, Y.; Mao, J.; Meng, X. Extraction Optimization and Bioactivity of Exopolysaccharides from *Agaricus bisporus. Carbohydr. Polym.* **2013,** *92* (2), 1602–1607.
65. Rahman, M. A.; Abdullah, N.; Aminudin, N. Inhibitory Effect on *in Vitro* LDL Oxidation and HMG Co-A Reductase Activity of the Liquid–Liquid Partitioned Fractions of *Hericium erinaceus* (Bull.) Persoon (Lion's Mane Mushroom). *Biomed. Res. Int.* **2014,** *2014*, 828149.
66. Samberkar, S.; Gandhi, S.; Naidu, M.; Wong, K. H.; Raman, J.; Sabaratnam, V. Lion's Mane, *Hericium erinaceus* and Tiger Milk, *Lignosus rhinocerotis* (Higher Basidiomycetes) Medicinal Mushrooms Stimulate Neurite Outgrowth in Dissociated Cells of Brain, Spinal Cord, and Retina: An *in Vitro* Study. *Int. J. Med. Mushrooms* **2015,** *17* (11), 1047–1054.
67. Liang, B.; Guo, Z.; Xie, F.; Zhao, A. Antihyperglycemic and Antihyperlipidemic Activities of Aqueous Extract of *Hericium erinaceus* in Experimental Diabetic Rats. *BMC Complement. Altern. Med.* **2013,** *13* (1), 1–7.

68. Cai, W. D.; Ding, Z. C.; Wang, Y. Y.; Yang, Y.; Zhang, H. N.; Yan, J. K. Hypoglycemic Benefit and Potential Mechanism of a Polysaccharide from *Hericium erinaceus* in Streptozotoxin-induced Diabetic Rats. *Process Biochem.* **2020,** *88* (1), 180–188.
69. Chaiyasut, C.; Sivamaruthi, B. S. Anti-hyperglycemic Property of *Hericium erinaceus*—A Mini Review. *Asian Pac. J. Trop. Biomed.* **2017,** *7* (11), 1036–1040.
70. Feng, H.; Zhang, S.; Wan, J. M. F.; Gui, L.; Ruan, M.; Li, N.; Zhang, H.; Wang, H. Polysaccharides Extracted from *Phellinus linteus* Ameliorate High-fat High-fructose Diet Induced Insulin Resistance in Mice. *Carbohydr. Polym.* **2018,** *200* (36), 144–153.
71. Kim, H. M.; Kang, J. S.; Kim, J. Y.; Park, S. K.; Kim, H. S.; Lee, Y. J.; Yun, J.; Hong, J. T.; Kim, Y.; Han, S. B. Evaluation of Antidiabetic Activity of Polysaccharide Isolated from *Phellinus linteus* in Non-obese Diabetic Mouse. *Int. Immunopharmacol.* **2010,** *10* (1), 72–78.
72. Wang, C.; Gao, X.; Santhanam, R. K.; Chen, Z.; Chen, Y.; Xu, L.; Wang, C.; Ferri, N.; Chen, H. Effects of Polysaccharides from *Inonotus obliquus* and Its Chromium(III) Complex on Advanced Glycation End-products Formation, α-Amylase, α-Glucosidase Activity and H_2O_2-induced Oxidative Damage in Hepatic L02 Cells. *Food Chem. Toxicol.* **2018,** *116* (12), 335–345.
73. Ying, Y. M.; Zhang, L. Y.; Zhang, X.; Bai, H. B.; Liang, D. E.; Ma, L. F.; Shan, W. G.; Zhan, Z. J. Terpenoids with Alpha-glucosidase Inhibitory Activity from the Submerged Culture of *Inonotus obliquus*. *Phytochemistry* **2014,** *108* (5), 171–176.
74. Yang, S.; Yan, J.; Yang, L.; Meng, Y.; Wang, N.; He, C.; Fan, Y.; Zhou, Y. Polysaccharides from Mushroom Fruiting Bodies Improve Insulin Resistance by Inhibiting Lipid Deposition Via Autophagy Enhancement. *Lancet* **2018.** http://dx.doi.org/10.2139/ssrn.3248625
75. Li, X.; Gong, H.; Yang, S.; Yang, L.; Fan, Y.; Zhou, Y. Pectic Bee Pollen Polysaccharide from *Rosa rugosa* Alleviates Diet-induced Hepatic Steatosis and Insulin Resistance Via Induction of AMPK/mTOR-mediated Autophagy. *Molecules* **2017,** *22* (5), 699.
76. Shen, M.; Fang, Z.; Chen, Y.; Chen, Y.; Xiao, B.; Guo, L.; Xu, Y.; Wang, G.; Wang, W.; Zhang, Y. Hypoglycemic Effect of the Degraded Polysaccharides from the Wood Ear Medicinal Mushroom *Auricularia auricula-judae* (Agaricomycetes). *Int. J. Med. Mushrooms* **2019,** *21* (10), 1033–1042.
77. Cao, H.; Ma, S.; Guo, H.; Cui, X.; Wang, S.; Zhong, X.; Wu, Y.; Zheng, W.; Wang, H.; Yu, J.; Ma, L.; Chun-Chao, H. Comparative Study on the Monosaccharide Compositions, Antioxidant and Hypoglycemic Activities *in Vitro* of Intracellular and Extracellular Polysaccharides of Liquid Fermented *Coprinus comatus*. *Int. J. Biol. Macromol.* **2019,** *139* (4), 543–549.
78. Zhang, H. N.; He, J. H.; Yuan, L.; Lin, Z. B. *In Vitro* and in Vivo Protective Effect of *Ganoderma lucidum* Polysaccharides on Alloxan-Induced Pancreatic Islets Damage. *Life Sci.* **2003,** *73* (18), 2307–2319.
79. Wu, S. J.; Tung, Y. J.; Ng, L. T. Anti-diabetic Effects of *Grifola frondosa* Bioactive Compound and Its Related Molecular Signaling Pathways in Palmitate-induced C2C12 Cells. *J. Ethnopharmacol.* **2020,** *260*, 112962.
80. Xiong, M.; Huang, Y.; Liu, Y.; Huang, M.; Song, G.; Ming, Q.; Ma, X.; Yang, J.; Deng, S.; Wen, Y.; Shen, J. Antidiabetic Activity of Ergosterol from *Pleurotus ostreatus* in KK-Ay Mice with Spontaneous Type 2 Diabetes Mellitus. *Mol. Nutr. Food Res.* **2018,** *62* (3). doi: 10.1002/mnfr.201700444.

81. Lee, S. H.; Shim, S. H.; Kim, J. S.; Kang, S. S. Constituents from the Fruiting Bodies of *Ganoderma applanatum* and Their Aldose Reductase Inhibitory Activity. *Arch. Pharm. Res.* **2006,** *29* (6), 479–483.

CHAPTER 9

In Vivo Appraisal and Clinical Trials of the Antidiabetic Potential of Mushrooms

ASHRAFALSADAT HATAMIAN-ZARMI[1*], HALE ALVANDI[1], SOHEIL KIANIRAD[1], ELHAM ANSARI[1], BAHMAN EBRAHIMI-HOSEINZADEH[1], and ZAHRA BEAGOM MOKHTARI HOSSEINI[2]

[1]*Department of Life Science Engineering, Faculty of New Sciences and Technologies, University of Tehran, Tehran, Iran*

[2]*Department of Chemical Engineering, Faculty of Petroleum and Petrochemical Engineering, Hakim Sabzevari University, Sabzevar, Iran*

**Corresponding author. E-mail: hatamian_a@ut.ac.ir*

ABSTRACT

Diabetes is one of the leading causes of death, characterized by elevated blood glucose levels, leading to serious health problems. According to World Health Organization, about 422 million people worldwide have diabetes, increasing the prevalence every year. Type 2 diabetes, the most common type, occurs when the body becomes resistant to insulin, and in type 1 diabetes, insulin production is insufficient. Currently, there are several drugs to control the disease, but their inefficacy and side effects are a cause of concern. Therefore, natural components such as fungi and their metabolites to treat diabetes have emerged recently. Medicinal mushrooms

Therapeutic Mushrooms for Diabetes Mellitus: Current Evidences and Future Scope. Uzma Azeem Khalid Rehman Hakeem, (Eds.)

have been used in traditional medicine in Asia for thousands of years and have various advantages such as antioxidant, antidiabetic, hypolipidemic, and antitumor properties. There are about 35 species grown commercially, and 20 of them are on an industrial scale. Numerous works have been done to investigate the antidiabetic activity of medicinal mushrooms, and several in vivo and clinical studies have further approved their efficiency. However, more studies are needed to confirm their effects on humans. This chapter provides an overview of different medicinal mushrooms with antidiabetic activity and discusses their efficacy on animal models and humans.

9.1 INTRODUCTION

Diabetes is a chronic disease that causes many health problems.[1] According to the World Health Organization, about 380 million people worldwide will have diabetes by 2030.[2,3] Diabetes refers to a set of metabolic disorders that cause high blood glucose levels over a long period. The disease is caused by the inability of pancreatic cells to produce enough insulin, or the body's cells do not respond to the insulin produced. There are different types of diabetes.[4,5] In type 1 diabetes, insulin production is insufficient, and in type 2 diabetes, the cells are resistant to insulin absorption and inadequate insulin production.[6] Diabetic retinopathy, nephropathy, and cardiovascular disease are common complications of diabetes. About 85% of all diabetic patients eventually develop diabetic retinopathy.[2] Several drugs are used to control diabetes with different mechanisms of action. Still, due to side effects and lack of appropriate therapeutic effects, the focus has shifted from chemical to natural drugs derived from herbs and fungi.[1,5] Fungi and their metabolites are a rich source of bioactive compounds. The use of medicinal fungi has been practiced in traditional East Asian medicine for thousands of years. So far, about 35 species of mushrooms have been grown commercially and 20 species on an industrial scale, including edible and medicinal mushrooms.[7] Fungi and their metabolites have been used to treat various diseases such as migraines, heart disease, gastrointestinal disorders, and cancers.[1] Recent studies show that fungal metabolites have anti-inflammatory, antioxidant, antidiabetic, and immune-enhancement properties.[8,9] In addition, studies show that flavonoids, terpenoids, alkaloids, and polyphenols in medicinal fungi can have antidiabetic effects.[1] Various studies have examined the antidiabetic effect of medicinal fungi on animal models. Different fungi products such as fruit bodies, mycelium, and polysaccharides have been used in these studies. In most of these studies, streptozotocin was used to induce diabetes in animals. It causes irreversible damage to pancreatic β-cells, resulting in degranulation and loss of insulin secretion.[10,11] In this chapter, we review the studies on the effects of medicinal fungi on animal models. We will also discuss the clinical effect of these fungi and the differences in the effectiveness of different fungal compounds.

9.2 MEDICINAL FUNGI WITH ANTIDIABETIC PROPERTIES

9.2.1 AGARICUS BISPORUS

Agaricus bisporus (white button mushroom) has the highest production in the world.[12] This fungus has high amounts of dietary fiber (19%), vitamins C, D, B12, folate, and polyphenols, useful for cardiovascular disease and diabetes.[13] Thiobarbituric acid reactive substances (TBARS) are a reagent in the measurement of malondialdehyde (MDA). There is a significant correlation between MDA and blood glucose levels in diabetic patients. The amount of TBARS in diabetic mice is 1.78 ± 0.03 nmol/mg proteins, and consumption of *A. bisporus* for two weeks reduces it to 1.29 ± 0.01.[14,15] Clinical studies show that the levels of SOD and GPx antioxidant enzymes are significantly reduced in patients with type 2 diabetes. As the disease progresses, the antioxidant content is depleted, and oxidative stress increases. Therefore, antioxidative therapies are critical in preventing and controlling diabetes.[16] This fungus has a high phenolic content, and its consumption significantly increased the activity of antioxidant enzymes in the serum, liver, and heart of mice.[17] Treatment of diabetic rats with *A. bisporus* (200 mg/kg body weight) for three weeks significantly reduced triglyceride (TG) and plasma glucose concentrations to 39.1% and 24.7%, respectively. Also, liver gain weight, aspartate aminotransferase, and alanine aminotransferase increased to 15.7% and 11.7%, respectively.[13] Treatment of streptozotocin-induced diabetic rats with *A. bisporus* (200 mg/kg body weight/day) for 21 days caused them to gain weight compared to the control group. This fungus lowers blood glucose, cholesterol, TG, and MDA levels. Studies show that high cholesterol can affect the metabolism and function of β-cells. The high dietary fiber of this fungus plays an important role in lowering cholesterol.[1,18] *A. bisporus* stimulates insulin secretion and G6PD activity in rats by repairing pancreatic β-cells.[18] It also has a lectin-like molecule that stimulates insulin secretion and glucagon in islet cells.[19] Vishvakarma et al. investigated the effect of *A. bisporus* on glucose uptake in 3T3-L1 fat cells. This fungus stimulates the absorption of glucose by adipocytes, like rosiglitazone. Also, its antioxidant activity has a protective effect on cells and is nontoxic.[20] Treatment of alloxan-induced diabetic rats with 500 mg/kg of *A. bisporus* extract reduces blood glucose by 50% after 14 days. The flavonoids of this fungus with antioxidant activity prevent the oxidation of DNA of pancreatic β-cells. Flavonoids are also inhibitors of GLUT2 and reduce the absorption of glucose and fructose from the intestine. *A. bisporus* also stimulates insulin secretion by increasing the uptake of Ca^{2+} ions by pancreatic β-cells.[21,22] Studies show that taking 100 g of *A. bisporus* for 16 weeks can benefit 37 pre-diabetics adults. Consumption of this fungus increases antioxidant markers ORAS (oxygen radical absorption capacity) and anti-inflammatory hormones. It significantly reduces oxidative stress factors, carboxymethyl lysine, and methylglyoxal in serum.[23]

9.2.2 AGARICUS BLAZEI

Agaricus blazei Murill (ABM) is a basidiomycetes brown fungus. This fungus belongs to the Agaricaceae family.[24] *A. blazei* is also known as *Agaricus brasiliensis*, *Agaricus subrufescens,* or Almond mushroom.[1] *Agaricus blazei* Murrill is widely cultivated in Japan to its medicinal properties. This fungus has been used in traditional medicine to treat hepatitis, diabetes, and many clinical studies have been performed to evaluate its anticancer properties.[25,26] ABM contains β-glucan, an immune stimulant and enhancer of insulin production. The control of diabetes by this fungus may be related to the activity of its polysaccharides. These polysaccharides cause the development of plasma insulin (decrease in pancreatic glucagon) and increase insulin sensitivity. They reduce the breakdown and absorption of carbohydrates by controlling the activity of α-glycosidase enzymes in the gut. They also increase peripheral tissues' hepatic glycogen and glucose utilization and inhibit free radicals (lipid peroxidation).[24] This fungus can lower blood glucose by containing isoflavonoids such as genistein, genistin, and daidzein.[1] Studies show that the type and volume of solvent for the preparation of medicinal fungal extracts can alter its biological properties.[27] Wei et al. evaluated the antioxidant and antidiabetic properties of the fruit body extract of *A. blazei* Murill; the results showed that ethyl acetate extract significantly inhibited the activity of DPPH, ABTS, and hydroxyl radicals more than ethanolic extract. Analysis of glucose uptake by HepG2 cells showed that the *A. blazei* ethyl acetate extract had significant glucose-lowering activity and was comparable to metformin. *A. blazei* controls blood sugar after eating by improving glucose uptake by HepG2 cells.[28] Animal and pilot studies have shown the beneficial effect of this fungus in type 2 diabetes.[29] This fungus causes the reproduction of Langerhans islet cells in healthy and diabetic mice.[30] *A. blazei* can increase insulin blockage in patients with type 2 diabetes mellitus.[31] Hsu et al. conducted clinical studies on the antidiabetic effect of *A. blazei* Murill fruiting body extract on diabetic patients between 20 and 75 years. For more than one year, these patients had type 2 diabetes and used gliclazide and metformin for more than six months. Patients received the *A. blazei* supplement 1500 mg daily for 12 weeks. The results showed that the HOMA-IR index was significantly reduced in patients who used the ABM extract supplement (from 4.8 to 3.6) and was much lower than the control group (from 6.3 to 6.6). Glycosylated hemoglobin (HbA1c), which is associated with insulin resistance, also decreases. Plasma adiponectin levels also increased after 12 weeks of treatment, and this extract had no side effects on liver function.[29] Vitak et al. observed that consumption of *A. brasiliensis* mycelium could improve anemia in addition to its antidiabetic effect.[32] A mixture of *A. brasiliensis* and *G. lucidum* mycelium decreased blood glucose and HbA1c concentration in diabetic rats after 14 days.[33]

9.2.3 *CORDYCEPS SPP.*

About 800 kinds of *Cordyceps* spp. are known in the world. *Cordyceps militaris* has been one of China's three most important medicines, with metabolites such as cordycepin, which is now used as a functional food.[34] This fungus lowers blood sugar in diabetic rats, improves liver function, and activates enzymes in glucose metabolism in the liver.[35,36] The *C. militaris* water extract stimulates the expression of HNF-1α in HepG2 cells, thus increasing glucose uptake by increasing GLUT2. By studying the mechanism of PI3k, Akt, and GSK-3β and measuring glycogen content, Kim et al. found that *C. militaris* increase glucose storage in the liver as glycogen. The extract of this fungus inhibits the α-glucosidase better than acarbose.[34] *C. militaris* polysaccharides can lower blood glucose, TG, and cholesterol levels in diabetic rats after seven days of consumption (50 mg/kg body weight).[37] Dong et al.[38] found an extract of *C. militaris* increases glucose metabolism in Sprague-Dawley diabetic rats after three weeks. Patel and Ingalhalli[39] suggested that cordycepin controls diabetes by inactivating NF-κB. In vivo, cordycepin (50 mg/kg) had no significant effect on blood glucose in diabetic mice after 3 days; after 7 days, blood glucose decreased significantly.[40] The exact mechanism of action of cordycepin is not fully understood, but possible routes have been suggested.[41] Yun et al. stated that cordycepin modulates the immune system by reducing nitric oxide production and reducing the proliferation of T-lymphocytes. As a result, pancreatic β-cells are protected from damage.[40] It also prevents the production of pro-inflammatory cytokines such as TNF-α, IL-1β, IL-6 in macrophages.[42] Cordycepin improves serum glutamic oxaloacetic transaminase (sGOT) and serum glutamic pyruvic transaminase (sGPT) activity. This metabolite can act as an immune modulator and inhibitor of the immune system in type 1 diabetes, which functions similarly to sulfonylureas.[40] The effect of cordycepin on diabetic nephropathy has also been reported; Cordycepin inhibits cell apoptosis, renal fibrosis, and autophagy in diabetic nephropathy rats.[43] Also, P-AKT and P-GSK-3β returned to normal in all diabetic rats after cordycepin treatment.[44] *Cordyceps cicadae* are known in traditional Chinese medicine as "Chan Hua" and have been used to treat palpitations, dizziness, and malaria. Alloxan-induced diabetic rats were treated with *C. cicadae* polysaccharides for 30 days. The polysaccharides of this fungus improve the weight and function of antioxidant enzymes in rats. 400 mg/kg of these polysaccharides reduce blood sugar by 45% after 10 days.[45] *Cordyceps taii* polysaccharides reduce fasting blood glucose, HOMA IR, TG, and LDL-C in streptozotocin-induced diabetic mice.[46] *Cordyceps sinensis* polysaccharides stimulate insulin secretion from the pancreatic islets and reduce their metabolism.[47] In one randomized trial, the blood sugar level of patients treated with *C. sinensis* (3 g/day) decreased significantly.[1,48] The extract of this fungus survives β-cells, increases renal NKA activity, and can treat diabetes.[49]

9.2.4 FOMES FOMENTARIUS

Fomes fomentarius, also known as tinder fungus, has been used for thousands of years to treat gastrointestinal disorders, liver cirrhosis, inflammation, and various cancers.[50] This fungus is of great ecological and economic importance due to its many nutritional and medicinal compounds. The antiproliferative activity of polysaccharides of this fungus on different cancer cell lines has been investigated.[50,51] This fungus is rich in β-glucans and terpenoids.[52] Recent studies have shown that *F. fomentarius* have antioxidant, antidiabetic, and lipid-lowering activity.[53] Studies show that diabetes reduces SOD and CAT activities and increases MDA synthesis. Oxidative stress in diabetic patients causes dysfunction of red blood cells and the immune system. *F. fomentarius* extract is a rich source of polyphenols, has antioxidant activity, and can repair catalase activity. The amount of SOD in the diabetic mice group treated with *F. fomentarius* increased more than 2.5 times than the control and reached 260.60 ± 9.97 U/ml blood.[14,50] Culture composition and physicochemical conditions can affect antioxidant properties in this fungus. By optimizing the culture medium of the *F. fomentarius*, its polysaccharides antioxidant activity increased to 16.11%.[50] One of the important metabolites of this fungus is fumentariol, which has antidiabetic properties. It also suppresses ROS production in RAW264.7 cells.[54,55] Table 9.1 summarizes the anti-diabetic effects of some medicinal mushroom species.

9.2.5 GANODERMA LUCIDUM

Ganoderma lucidam belongs to the family Ganodermataceae, the most famous fungus in traditional East Asian medicine. *G. lucidam* is known as "Lingzhi" in China and "Reishi" in Japan. This fungus has antimicrobial, anti-inflammatory, antioxidant, and antidiabetic properties. It improves the function of the immune system.[69–71] Decoction of *G. lucidum* has been used as a potent medicine to treat diabetes.[10] Studies show that the antidiabetic properties of this fungus are due to various compounds in the extract of the fruit body, mycelium extract, polysaccharides, proteoglycans, and terpenoids. The molecular structure and properties of these compounds were investigated. It was determined that in each gram of *G. lucidum* extract, there was 97.2 mg of β-glucan, 25.80 mg of alpha-beta glucan, 0.75 mg

TABLE 9.1 Some Medicinal Mushroom Species with Reported Antidiabetic Effects.

Mushroom	Animal model	Administration	Bioactive compound	Antidiabetic effects	Reference
Agaricus bisporus	STZ-induced diabetic mice	200 mg/kg body weight, orally for 2 weeks	Powder of methanolic extract	Reduction of TBARS	[14]
	STZ-induced diabetic rats	200 mg/kg body weight, orally for 3 weeks	Powder of fruiting body	Reduced TG and plasma glucose concentrations, liver gain weight, increased aspartate aminotransferase, and alanine aminotransferase	[13]
	Kunmig mice	300, 600, 1200 mg/kg body weight, 30 days	Ethanolic extract of fruiting body	Enhanced antioxidant activity enzymes (SOD, CAT, and GSH-Px) in serum, liver, and heart of mice	[17]
	STZ-induced diabetic rat	200 mg/kg body weight, 21 days	Powder of fruiting body	Decreased in glucose concentration, cholesterol, TG, LDL, MDA level. Increased in insulin level and G6PD activity, HDL level, CAT, GPx, SOD activities and GSH level. Increased in body weight, and repaired pancreatic tissue damage in islets of Langerhans	[18]
Schizophyllum commune	Alloxan-induced diabetic rat	500 mg/kg body weight, 14 days	Ethanolic extract of fruiting body	Decreased blood glucose and MDA levels, as well as increased SOD activity in diabetic rats	[21]
	STZ-induced diabetic rat	100 mg/kg body weight, 14 days	Ethyl acetate extract of mycelium	Restoration of renal parameters including creatinine, blood urea nitrogen, fractional excretion of sodium and potassium level. Improvement in lipid profile and level of antioxidant parameters. Reduced glutathione, TBARS, and superoxide anion generation. More pronounced improved liver enzymes (serum glutamic pyruvic transaminase, serum glutamic-oxaloacetic transaminases, and alkaline phosphatase) homeostasis at higher concentration of *S. commune*	[56]

TABLE 9.1 *(Continued)*

Mushroom	Animal model	Administration	Bioactive compound	Antidiabetic effects	Reference
	Mice	3,5 g/kg body weight of *Schizophyllum* spp. derived β-glucan, orally 12 weeks	*Schizophyllum* spp. derived β-glucan	Increased in the length of small intestine compared to the control group. Dietary fiber consumption enhanced goblet cell density along with mucosal layer thickness	[57]
Coprinus spp.	Alloxan-induced diabetic mice	150 mg/kg body weight, 20 days	Se-polysaccharide (SPS) isolated from selenium-enriched mycelia of *C. comatus*	Decrease in blood glucose levels. Decreased serum TC, TG, and LDL levels and increased HDL concentration. Decrease in the level of MDA, increase in the activities of enzymic antioxidants and the levels of non-enzymic antioxidants in liver and kidney of diabetic mice. Effects of SPS was more potent than that of polysaccharide from the mycelia of *C. comatus* at the same dose	[58]
Pleurotus florida	Alloxan induced diabetic rat	200 mg/kg body weight, 14 days	Methanolic extract of fruiting body	Inhibition of α-amylase and α-glucosidase activity in a dose dependent manner. Antidiabetic activity comparable to Glibenclamide, a standard antidiabetic drug	[3]
Cordyceps militaris	STZ-induced diabetic mice	50 mg/kg (CCCA and CMESS), 0.2 mg/kg cordycepin, 10 days	CCCA (crude cordycepin containing adenosine) and CMESS (ethanol soluble supernatant) fractions of cordyceps, cordyceps fruiting body	CMESS reduced blood glucose level by 35.5 after 3 days. Reduced blood glucose level in long-term usage (7 days). CCCA with high cordycepin contents (0.656 mg/4 mg) did not influence the blood glucose levels. The proliferation of T-lymphocyte was significantly decreased, while NO production was increased more than two-fold to STZ control in the cordycepin-administered group. The proliferation of macrophages and NO production were significantly decreased in CMESS administered group	[40]

TABLE 9.1 *(Continued)*

Mushroom	Animal model	Administration	Bioactive compound	Antidiabetic effects	Reference
	STZ-induced diabetic rats	0.5, 1, 2 mg/kg body weight, 4 weeks	Fruiting body	Decreases in plasma glucose, food, and water intake, and urine output. Normalization of total cholesterol, TG, and HCL in diabetic rats. Renal protective activity by inhibitory effects on albuminuria, creatinine, urea nitrogen, and n-acetyl-β-d glycosaminidase. Exertion of beneficial modulation of inflammatory factors and oxidative enzymes. Compared to untreated diabetic rats, CM decreased the expression of phosphor-AKT and phosphor GSK-3β in the kidneys	[44]
	STZ-induced diabetic rat	0.05 and 2 g/kg, orally for 3 weeks	Water or alcohol extract	Significant reduction in blood glucose levels by promoting glucose metabolism and strongly suppressed total cholesterol and TG concentration in serum. Antioxidative effects indicated by normalized superoxide dismutase and glutathione peroxidase levels. The inhibitory effects on blood urea nitrogen, creatinine, uric acid, and protein revealed the protection of *C. militaris* extracts against diabetic nephropathy	[38]
Hericium erinaceus	STZ-induced diabetic rats	100 and 200 mg/kg body weight, 28 days	Aqueous extract of *H. erinaceus*	Decrease in serum glucose level and a significant rise in serum insulin level. Attenuation of lipid disorders. Increased in CAT, SOD, GSH-Px, and GSH level activities significantly reduced MDA level in the liver tissue	[59]
Inonotus obliquus	Alloxan-induced diabetic mice	500 mg/kg body weight, 20 days	Total extract, and ethyl acetate fraction	Significant decrease in blood glucose level, and the total cholesterol level in serum, increase in glutathione peroxidase activity, and improvement in the physiological growth characteristics. Decrease in the levels of triglyceride and MDA and increase in the HDL level	[60]

TABLE 9.1 *(Continued)*

Mushroom	Animal model	Administration	Bioactive compound	Antidiabetic effects	Reference
	STZ-induced diabetic mice	900 mg/kg body weight, 4 weeks	*I. obliquus* polysaccharide	Improved glucose tolerance ability and increased hepatic glycogen level in diabetic mice. Also, the expression of PI3K-p85, p-Akt (ser473), GLUT was increased in diabetic mice	[61]
Trametes versicolor	STZ-induced diabetic mice	500, 1000, 1500 mg/kg body weight, 21 days	Methanol extract	Significant reductions in serum glucose, TG, and ALT levels in treatment groups compared to the control group. Pathology studies showed lower destruction of liver tissue in these groups	[62]
	STZ, nicotinamide-induced diabetic rats	0.1 g/kg body weight, 28 days	Extracellular polysaccharopeptides of LH-1 strain of *T. versicolor*	Lowered postprandial blood sugar. Increase in proximal tibia volume, trabecular number, and femoral bone strength	[63]
Lentinus edodes	STZ-induced diabetic rats	400 mg/kg for 21 days	Extracellular polysaccharopeptides of *T. versicolor*	Decreased blood glucose, TC, TG, and LDL levels and increased HDL concentration	[9]
	Alloxan-induced diabetic mice	50 mg/kg body weight β-glucan, 14 days	Β-glucan of shiitake mushroom	Decreased in blood glucose level of 55.87%. IC50 value were 64.31 μg/ml	[64]

TABLE 9.1 *(Continued)*

Mushroom	Animal model	Administration	Bioactive compound	Antidiabetic effects	Reference
	Pancreatectomized (Px) rats	0.5 (AGM-L) and 1 (AGM-H) g/kg body weight AGM, 12 weeks	Freeze-dried aronia, red ginseng, ultraviolet-irradiated Shiitake and nattokinase (AGM; 3.4:4.1:2.4:0.1)	AGM prevented bone mineral density in the lumbar spine and femur and lean body mass in the hip and leg of Px rats. Lower decrease of visceral fat mass compared to control group. AGM improved glucose metabolism by potentiating insulin secretion and reducing insulin resistance in insulin-deficient type 2 diabetic rats. AGM alleviated body composition changes and prevented the modulation of the gut microbiome	[65]
Pleurotus pulmonarius	Mice	0.1 mg/ml, 28 days	Water extract, 50% ethanol extract, and ethanol extract of *L. edodes* (LEE)	LEE inhibited glucose intake through the monolayer of differentiated Caco-2 cells; however, neither water nor the 50% (v/v) ethanol extract affected glucose transport through these cells at the same concentration. LEE reduced plasma glucose levels by 64.0% in the high fat diet-fed mice	[66]
	STZ, nicotinamide-induced diabetic rats	200 and 400 mg/kg body weight, orally 4 weeks	Water extract	Significant reduction in blood sugar in diabetic Wistar albino rats after 4 weeks. This fungus controls the activity of the α-amylase and repairs the pancreas, liver, and kidney tissues	[67]
Pleurotus ostreatus	Sucrose-induced diabetic *Drosophila Melanogaster* (Fruit-Fly)	100, 250, 500 mg/10 g fly diet, 28 days	Fruiting body	Prolonged the survival time of fruit flies and significantly reduced the amount of circulating glucose. Catalase activity is also significantly increased in the *P. ostreatus* treated group	[68]

of protein, and 1.35 mg of glucuronic acid.[71,72] The extract of this fungus in doses up to 5000 mg/kg has no toxic effect on mice.[10] *G. lucidum* polysaccharides increase plasma insulin levels and decrease plasma glucose levels in mice. In addition, *G. lucidum* polysaccharides increase hepatic glucokinase, phosphofructokinase, and glucose-6-phosphate dehydrogenase activities. These polysaccharides also inhibit glycogen synthetase activity, thereby reducing hepatic glucose production, preventing high blood sugar.[72–74] Studies show that these polysaccharides can also affect the expression of mRNA involved in glycogenolysis. Studies show that the structure and molecular weight of fungal polysaccharides can affect their function. Low molecular weight *G. lucidum* polysaccharides can protect pancreatic cells from apoptotic by regulating Bcl-2 (anti-apoptotic protein).[27,72] Streptozotocin treatment significantly increased lipid peroxides. It also decreased nonenzymatic antioxidant levels and antioxidant enzyme activity in the plasma and liver of rats. *G. lucidum* polysaccharides with antioxidant activity prevent the pancreatic islets from damage. These polysaccharides increase superoxide dismutase, catalase, and glutathione peroxidase activities in the plasma and liver of rats.[2] *G. lucidum* polysaccharides significantly reduce MDA levels in rabbits and protect the liver against oxidative damage.[75] In addition to increasing GSH-Px, SOD, and CAT, the polysaccharides of this fungus prevent the production of ROS in vascular endothelial cells by reducing NOX expression.[76,77] The effect of *G. lucidum* polysaccharides on different animal models such as Wistar rats, SD rats, pregnant rats, and Kunming species mouse has been studied. In all experiments, the consumption of polysaccharides of this fungus reduces blood glucose.[77] *G. lucidum* polysaccharides (100 mg/kg) reduce the blood sugar of hyperglycemia mice, and 200 mg/kg polysaccharides reduce the blood sugar of normal mice.[77] Zhang et al. observed that polysaccharides recover β-cells, stimulate insulin secretion, and improve liver glucokinase activity in diabetic mouse.[77] Studies show that *G. lucidum* reduces serum glucose levels by suppressing the hepatic PEPCK gene.[78] It can also increase glucose uptake into L6 skeletal muscle cells by stimulating PI 3-kinase and AMPK.[79] Huang et al. investigated the antidiabetic activity of submerged medium and mycelium of *G. lucidum*. After five weeks, weight and TG decreased in rats, and HDL increased. *G. lucidum* downregulated hepatic acetyl-CoA carboxylase, fatty acid synthase, and lipoprotein lipase.[80] The antidiabetic activity of proteoglycans of this fungus has also been investigated in rats and mice. FYGL is a homogeneous and acidic proteoglycan composed of glucose, galactose, and rhamnose units. Its molecular weight is 100.2 kDa and it can interact with PTP1B after entering the bloodstream causing a significant reduction in PTP1B in the skeletal muscle of diabetic rats.[81,82] *G. lucidum* triterpenoids are also aldose reductase and α-glucosidase inhibitors.[72] *G. lucidum* can prevent diabetic wound inflammation in rats by inhibiting the NF-κB and AP-1 signaling pathways.[83] Consumption of 1 g/kg/day of dried mycelium of *G. lucidum* for two weeks reduces blood sugar in diabetic rats. Studies show that intensifying the pathways of glucose polyol degradation leads to the accumulation of osmotically active metabolites such as sorbitol and fructose. This can cause hemolysis of red blood cells. *G. lucidum* improves the function of red blood cells by balancing blood glucose levels.[32] *G. lucidum* polysaccharides facilitate Ca^{2+} influx in β-pancreatic cells and increase insulin secretion.[84] In a clinical study, patients with type 2 diabetes consumed *G. lucidum* polysaccharides three times daily for 12 weeks (1800 mg). This treatment reduced fasting blood glucose, HbA1c significantly and *G. lucidum* is safe to use.[85] Aqueous extract of *G. lucidum* can alter the composition of the gut microbiota. The extract of this fungus has high molecular weight polysaccharides (>300 kDa) and is not digested in the stomach or small intestine. By digestion of these polysaccharides by bacteria in the large intestine, they produce short-chain fatty acids (SCFAs) that stimulate the secretion of GLP-1 by intestinal cells. In addition to regulating liver function, GLP-1 can induce β-cell proliferation.[86,87] The effect of *G. lucidum* in the treatment of diabetic wounds has also been studied. The cream containing the polysaccharides of this fungus heals the wounds of diabetic rats in the posterior neck region.[88]

9.2.6 *GRIFOLA FRONDOSA*

Grifola frondosa is also known as Maitake, which belongs to the Polyporaceae family.[89] It is one of the most popular edible mushrooms in China and is widely cultivated for its medicinal properties. *G. frondosa* polysaccharides have antidiabetic properties and improve immune function, and the structure of some of them is known.[90] GC-MS analysis showed that *G. frondosa* is a rich source of oleic acid which can inhibit α-glucosidase activity. Inhibitors of this enzyme can help lower blood sugar by prolonging the digestion of carbohydrates in the intestinal.[91] The polysaccharides of this fungus (900 mg/kg day) significantly decrease TG and LDL-C levels and increase hepatic glycogen levels ($p < 0.05$).[92] Treatment of diabetic mice with 150 mg/kg body weight polysaccharides significantly reduces HbA1c after four weeks. These polysaccharides increase choroid structure and improve inflammation. *G. frondosa* also increases the expression of IRS1 and PI3K mRNAs, which are involved in the insulin signaling pathways. Studies show that the population of Firmicutes and Proteobacteria increases in the intestines of diabetic mice. *G. frondosa* polysaccharides alter the gut microflora and significantly increase the population of Bacteroidetes.[89] The ratio of Bacteroidetes to Firmicutes plays an important role in regulating blood glucose.[93] The polysaccharides of this fungus cause a significant increase in *Porphyromonas gingivalis*, which affects glycemic levels in diabetes.[89,94] *G. frondosa* also increases *Alistipes*, which plays an important role in glucose and fat metabolism.[92] In diabetic rats, serum BUN, Scr, NAG levels, and urinary albuminuria are very high, which are nephropathy symptoms. Treatment of diabetic rats with *G. frondosa* polysaccharides reduces these factors after four weeks. They also regulated IL-2, IL-6, TNF-α, IFN-α levels.[95] *G. frondosa* contains Vanadium and an α-glucose inhibitor; Vanadium is a cofactor for enzymes involved in insulin signaling and regulates glucose metabolism in diabetes. It also regulates the production of inflammatory cytokines.[11] Studies have shown that *G. frondosa* α-glucan has an antidiabetic effect in mice by improving immune function and eliminating factors that damage pancreatic β-cells.[6]

9.2.7 *HERICIUM ERINACEUS*

Hericium erinaceus is also known as "Lion's Mane" and "Monkey's Mushroom," one of the major producers of terpenoids. The polysaccharides of this fungus have high antioxidant activity and strengthen the immune system by increasing the production of TNF-α.[27] The antidiabetic activity of the fruit body and mycelium of this fungus has been proven.[96] D-threitol, D-arabinitol, and α-D-glucan in this fungus hypoglycemic in diabetic rats.[96,97] Aqueous extract of *H. erinaceus* (100 and 200 mg/kg BW) reduces serum glucose in diabetic rats after 28 days. This extract significantly increases insulin levels and enzyme activity (AT, SOD, GSH-Px, and GSH level).[59] *H. erinaceus* ethanolic extract (200 mg/kg body weight) reduced LDL-C by 45.5% and increased HDL-C by 31.1%

in diabetic rats after four weeks.[98] The polysaccharides of this fungus reduce fasting blood glucose, increase glucose tolerance, improve lipid metabolism, and inhibit lipid peroxidation. They are also involved in activating PI3K/Akt signaling pathway.[99] More studies in the animal and clinical phases are needed to evaluate its antidiabetic effect despite the many properties of this fungus.

9.2.8 *INONOTUS OBLIQUUS*

Inonotus obliquus has been used to treat heart disease, cancer, and diabetes in Russia and Europe since the 16th century.[100] This fungus prevents DNA damage by inhibiting free radicals.[1] *I. obliquus* polysaccharides significantly increase the concentration of antioxidant enzymes in diabetic mice and repair pancreatic tissue.[101] Treatment of alloxan-induced diabetic rats with the *I. obliquus* polysaccharides (150 and 300 mg/kg body weight) reduces blood glucose levels by more than 35% after 21 days. Consumption of these polysaccharides increases insulin levels and hepatic glycogen content in diabetic mice and can repair the damaged pancreas tissue in these mice.[102] *I. obliquus* extract can inhibit α-glucosidase activity (IC50=220.31 μg/ml).[103] This effect is comparable with acarbose.[104] 93.3 μg/ml polysaccharides with a molecular weight of 1.7×10^4 Da also inhibit α-glucosidase activity up to 50%.[105] Treatment of alloxan-induced diabetic mice with ethyl acetate extract of *I. obliquus* significantly ($p < 0.05$) reduces their water and food intake. This extract lowers blood sugar, TG, MDA and increases HDL and hepatic glycogen levels. The compounds lanosterol, inotodiol, trametenolic acid, and ergosterol peroxide in this fungus inhibit α-amylase activity.[60] The dry matter of culture broth of *I. obliquus* (500 mg/kg) reduces blood glucose level by 30% after 3 weeks in diabetic mice. It also increased HDL, insulin level, and liver glycogen level.[106] Wang et al. found that *I. obliquus* polysaccharides (900 mg/kg) significantly ($p < 0.01$) improved glucose tolerance ability and increased hepatic glycogen levels in diabetic mice. Also, the expression of PI3K-p85, p-Akt (ser473), GLUT was increased in diabetic mice.[61] The pyran-type polysaccharides of this fungus improve glucose uptake in HepG2 cells.[107] Vanadium-enriched *I. obliquus* also has metabolites with hypoglycemic activity and is not toxic to animals.[1]

9.2.9 *LENTINUS EDODES*

Lentinus edodes, also known as Shiitake mushroom, have been used in traditional Chinese and Japanese medicine for over 2000 years to treat diseases. This fungus is still widely used today due to its good taste and properties such as anti-inflammatory, antitumor, and antidiabetic.[108] One of the most well-known secondary metabolites of Shiitake is lentinan. Lentinan (400–800 kDa) prevents apoptosis of pancreatic β-cells by inhibiting ROS production.[107] The antidiabetic activity of this fungus, along with other medicinal plants and fungi, has also been extensively studied. Among the important compounds produced by the fungus Shitake and *Saccharomyces cerevisiae* is β-glucan, which lowers blood glucose levels. Afiati et al. investigated the effect of β-glucans of these two fungi on diabetic mice. Commercial β-glucans also reduced blood glucose levels by 32.31%. Treatment with β-glucans from Shiitake and *S. cerevisiae* reduced blood glucose levels by 55.87% and 58.00%, respectively (this difference was insignificant). Studies show that the structural similarity of fungal β-glucans, which have β-(1.3) and β-(1.6) bonds, causes them to function similarly and control the glucose uptake rate. β-Glucans also prevent the absorption of excessive cholesterol in the stomach and intestines.[64] Shiitake can improve glucose and lipid metabolism by changing the gut microbiome population of diabetic Wistar rats and reduce diabetic problems such as cardiovascular disease.[65] The effect of the fruit body extract of *L. edodes* on Caco-2 cells, which are used as a model for intestinal glucose transport, has also been investigated. The extract of this fungus inhibits glucose transfer up to 37.2%. *L. edodes* significantly reduced adipose tissue accumulation in the intestine and reduced plasma glucose levels by up to 64% in high-fat rats.[66,109] It is estimated that 90 grams of Shiitake mushroom powder per day can increase the excretion of fat in the stool, prevent weight gain, and reduce TG.[110] Kim et al. observed that treatment of streptozotocin-induced diabetic rats with *L. edodes* polysaccharides for 7 days (50 mg/kg body weight) could significantly reduce blood glucose, TG, and cholesterol levels ($p < 0.05$).[37] In another study, diabetic rats were treated with a mixture of *G. lucidum* and *L. edodes* fungi. This compound lowers blood glucose and can also be used for patients with gestational diabetes.[111] Some studies show that Shiitake polysaccharides stimulate the growth of beneficial bacteria in the gut.[86]

9.2.10 *PHELLINUS SPP.*

Phellinus linteus has been used to treat diabetes and obesity in traditional Chinese, Korean, and Japanese medicine.[112] The polysaccharides of this fungus reduce fasting blood glucose after four weeks, change the metabolism of hepatic phospholipids, and modify the insulin signaling pathway by affecting the FOXO signaling pathway in diabetic rats.[113] The *P. linteus* polysaccharides also suppress the production of inflammatory cytokines such as TNF-α.[114] It reduced plasma glucose and cholesterol by 49% and 32%, respectively.[1] Oral administration of it (100 mg/kg body weight/day) reduces blood glucose by up to 35% in diabetic mice ($p < 0.05$).[6] The polychlorinated compound of *Phellinus ribis* improves diabetes by acting on PPAR-gamma.[1] *Phellinus baumii* polysaccharides consisting of mannose, xylose, and fucose have been used in traditional medicine to improve glucose tolerance.[6] Ethyl acetate extract of this fungus increases glucose uptake in insulin-resistant HepG2 cells. The high phenolic content of this fungus can prevent oxidative damage to β-cells.[115] Consumption of its fruitbody extract (50, 100, 150 mg/kg of body weight) also reduces blood glucose in diabetic mice and improves glycolipid metabolism. This extract can also activate the IRS1/PI3K/AKT pathway and be used as a supplement in the treatment of diabetes.[116] A mix of mushrooms *Ganoderma* spp. and *P. baumii* regulates diabetes by inhibiting PTP1B.[117] *Phellinus merrillii* ethanolic extract reduces α-glucosidase and aldose reductase activity.[1]

9.2.11 *PLEUROTUS SPP.*

The genus *Pleurotus*, also known as the oyster mushroom, is edible and has about 40 species. This fungus is a good source of prebiotics due to its high fiber content.[118] One of the most important edible fungi economically is *Pleurotus florida*. It is nontoxic to mice by up to 4000 mg/kg body weight. This fungus is beneficial for human health due to its protein and various biological properties, including antioxidant, antimicrobial, anti-inflammatory, antitumor, and antidiabetic activities. One treatment mechanism in type 2 diabetes is inhibiting carbohydrate-hydrolyzing enzymes such as α-amylase and α-glucosidase, which reduce glucose uptake. 1000 μg/ml methanolic extract of the fruiting body of oyster mushroom inhibits α-amylase and α-glucosidase by 94.93% and 84.90%, respectively. The fruiting bodies of these fungi contain phenols, flavonoids, saponins, tannins, and terpenoids, which are thought to inhibit these enzymes. 200 mg/kg body weight of the extract of this fungus significantly reduces blood glucose, serum cholesterol, serum TG, and LDL levels in diabetic rats. It causes a significant increase in HDL levels.[3,6] Li et al. investigated the antidiabetic effect of *Pleurotus eryngii* on alloxan-induced hyperglycemic mice. Consumption of this extract (100 and 200 mg/kg) for 5 weeks significantly reduces blood glucose ($p < 0.05$) and HbA1c levels ($p < 0.01$) and significantly increases insulin secretion ($p < 0.05$). *Pleurotus eryngii* also increases the concentration of hepatic glycogen and recovers damaged β-cells.[102,119] The polysaccharide–protein complex of *Pleurotus abalonus* protects the damaged pancreatic tissue in diabetic mice with its antioxidant properties, increased insulin expression, and decreased circulating glucose levels.[120] *P. ostreatus* extract increases the expression of the catalase gene and improves the activity of the antioxidant system in rats.[121] It also increases GLUT 4 expression in L6 cells. *P. ostreatus* prevents β-cells damage in Wistar mice.[112,122] *Pleurotus ferulae* polysaccharides increase antioxidant enzymes and HDL-C activity in hyperglycemic rats and decrease LDL-C levels.[112] Omale et al. (2020) investigated the effect of *P. ostreatus* fruit body on sucrose-induced type-2 diabetic *Drosophila melanogaster*. This extract prolongs the survival time of fruit flies and significantly reduces circulating glucose ($p < 0.05$). Catalase activity is also significantly ($p < 0.05$) increased in *P. ostreatus*-treated group.[68] In clinical studies, a mixture of *P. ostreatus* and *Pleurotus cystidiosus* (50 mg/kg/body weight) significantly ($p < 0.05$) reduced fasting blood glucose levels.[123] The *Pleurotus citrinopileatus* polysaccharides prevent damage to the islets of Langerhans.[124] Oral administration of *Pleurotus tuber-regium* polysaccharides (20 mg/kg body weight/8 weeks) prevents obesity in diabetic rats by altering the composition of fatty acids and has hypoglycemic effects by increasing PPAR-α mRNA expression in the liver. The polysaccharides of this fungus seem to act as PPAR-α agonists and reduce triglycerides by increasing lipid metabolism.[6] They also reduced HbA1c levels in diabetic rats and inhibited lipid peroxidation in the liver.[6] *Pleurotus pulmonarius* extract up to 5000 mg/kg is not toxic to mice and can significantly reduce serum glucose. Consumption of this extract simultaneously with acarbose has a great antihyperglycemic effect.[125] Oral administration of *P. pulmonarius* (200 and 400 mg/kg) causes a significant ($p < 0.05$) reduction in blood sugar in diabetic Wistar albino rats after 4 weeks. This fungus controls the activity of the α-amylase and repairs the pancreas, liver, and kidney tissues.[67] Aqueous extract of *P. fossulatus* reduces blood glucose in diabetic albino Wistar rats by more than 50%. This extract regulates the function of liver enzymes and reduces the levels of creatinine, blood urea nitrogen, and uric acid.[126] The antidiabetic effect of *Pleurotus citrinopileatus* fruit bodies has also been reported.[1] Animal studies have also been performed on *Pleurotus eous* and *Pleurotus abalones*.[1]

9.2.12 *SCHIZOPHYLLUM COMMUNE*

Schizophyllum commune is an edible fungus used in traditional Chinese medicine to treat headaches, inflammation, obesity, rheumatism, and weakness.[56,127] (1→3)-β-D-glucan in this fungus binding to macrophage receptors and other cells causes the production of cytokines and strengthens the immune system.[128] Schizophyllan is a water-soluble glucan compound with various biological properties extracted from this fungus.[129] Studies show that the *S. commune* can inhibit the activity of the α-glucosidase enzyme by more than 90% and leads to a decrease in blood glucose levels.[56] 100 mg/kg of ethyl acetate extract of *S. commune* causes a significant reduction in blood glucose levels (56%) than acarbose (63%) in diabetic rats. One of the side effects of diabetes mellitus is weight loss due to increased fat and protein metabolism. The extract of this fungus causes the rats to gain weight after the end of the treatment period. The *S. commune* extract restores creatinine, blood urea nitrogen, and ion levels in the kidney. *S. commune* improves liver enzymes, including serum glutamic pyruvate transaminase (sGPT), serum glutamic oxalate transaminase (SGOT), and alkaline phosphatase (ALP).[56] Studies show that oxidative stress promotes diabetes and its complications. The extract of this fungus, which contains phenolic compounds and has antioxidant activity, modulates free radicals.[130,131] The *S. commune* polysaccharide with a molecular weight of 11 kDa has the highest antioxidant activity.[132] Chandrawanshi et al. observed that the hot water, methanol, and ethanol extract of this fungus have DPPH-free radical scavenging properties. The antioxidant properties of this fungus are higher than those of ascorbic acid. β-glucan of this fungus also lowers cholesterol and controls diabetes mellitus.[57,133] The use of *S. commune* (5 g/kg, 12 weeks) increases the goblet cell density and the thickness of the mucous layer. Lactobacillus populations also increase in mice with a low-fiber diet.[57] The major pathway for producing simple sugars such as glucose in humans is through the hydrolysis of α-1,4-glycosidic bonds in starch by α-amylase. Inhibition of this enzyme lowers plasma glucose levels after eating. In various studies, it has been observed that the extract of *S. commune* is an α-amylase inhibitor and can be used as an alternative to drugs used in the treatment of diabetes mellitus (IC50 =50.98 μg/ml).[134,135]

9.2.13 TREMELLA SPP.

Tremella is also known as jelly fungi and more than 100 species of this fungus are known. *Tremella fuciformis* and *Tremella aurantialba* are cultivated commercially for food and medicine. *T. aurantialba* is known as one of the immunostimulating fungi. This fungus increases the proliferation of mouse spleen lymphocytes.[136] *T. fuciformis* is rich in phenols, flavonoids, and dietary fiber with hypoglycemic, antioxidant, and hypolipidemic effects.[118,137] The aldolase reductase enzyme is involved in the formation and accumulation of sorbitol, which causes diabetic complications. *T. fuciformis* can inhibit the activity of this enzyme, improve insulin sensitivity, and regulate the insulin signaling pathway.[138,139] *T. fuciformis* polysaccharides, composed of mannose and galactose, help lower fasting blood glucose and improve glucose tolerance.[6] This fungus increased insulin sensitivity by regulating lipid metabolism.[1] Low molecular weight *Tremella aurantia* polysaccharides can be used to treat type 1 and type 2 diabetes by improving glucose metabolism and increasing insulin secretion in the body. Consuming this fungus (50 mg/kg) for 10 weeks prevents increased plasma glucose and TG in genetic type 2 diabetic KK-A^y mice.[140]

9.2.14 TRAMETES VERSICOLOR

Trametes versicolor is one of the most important medicinal fungi whose polysaccharides are commercially produced. Krestin is the most important secondary metabolite of this fungus, used as a supplement in many countries.[9,141] Another metabolite of this fungus is Tramesan, which has antioxidant and antimicrobial activity.[142] The compounds of this fungus can inhibit the α-glucosidase enzyme. Alvandi et al. (2020) observed that the growth and production of *T. versicolor* exopolysaccharides in a soy milk-based culture medium increased. Exopolysaccharides of this fungus can reduce blood sugar, TG, and cholesterol in diabetic rats by 50%, 89%, and 20%, respectively. In the acarbose-treated group, this reduction was 13.77%, 69%, and 9.5%, respectively.[9] 1500 mg/kg of methanolic extract of this fungus reduces serum blood glucose, TG, and ALT enzyme in male mice. Histopathological studies show inflammation, necrosis, and apoptosis in the liver of diabetic rats. *T. versicolor* extract improves liver tissue damage.[62] The aqueous extract of this fungus has more phenolic, flavonoid, and antioxidant activity than the alcoholic extract. Studies show that inhibiting free radicals plays an important role in treating many diseases, including type 2 diabetes.[143] The n-hexane extract of *T. versicolor* inhibits α-amylase activity.[91] This fungus (0.1 g/kg weight for 28 days) on the bone properties in diabetic Wistar rats was also studied. In addition to lowering blood sugar, *T. versicolor* increases proximal tibia volume, trabecular number, and femoral bone strength ($p < 0.01$).[63] Figure 9.1 shows the antidiabetic mechanism of fungal polysaccharides.

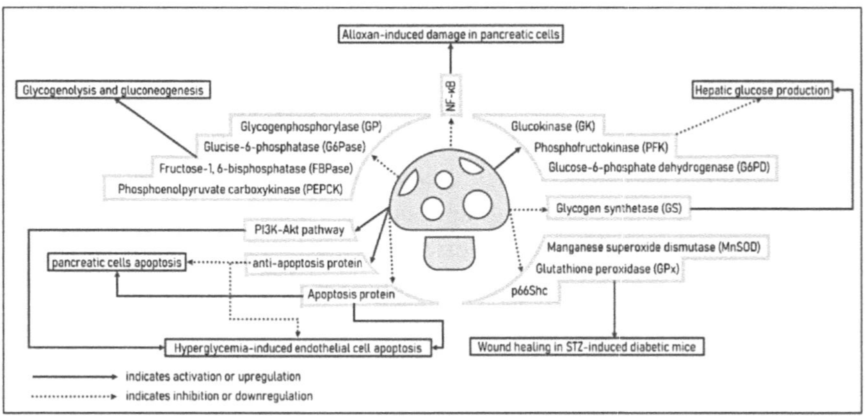

FIGURE 9.1 Schematic diagram of mushrooms polysaccharides antidiabetes properties.

9.2.15 OTHER FUNGI

Many fungi are used worldwide for their antidiabetic effect in traditional medicine, and studies on these fungi are still ongoing. In this section, we will look at some lesser-known fungi. *Coprinus comatus*, the shaggy ink cap, regulates the immune system, lowers blood sugar, lowers blood lipids, and has antitumor and antibacterial activities. The extracts of this fungus inhibit the activity of α-amylase and α-glucosidase.[103] Yu et al. investigated the antidiabetic effect of selenium-containing polysaccharides of this fungus. In addition to lowering blood glucose, these Se-polysaccharides significantly reduce MDA levels and increase the levels and activity of enzymatic antioxidants such as SOD, GSH-Px, and CAT, and nonenzymatic GSH in the liver and kidneys of all diabetic mice. These results confirm a close relationship between oxidative stress and the incidence of diabetes.[58] Oral administration of *Cerrena unicolor* (Bull.) Murrill, *Coprinus comatus* (O.F. Müll.) Pers. and *Lenzites betulina* (L.) Fr. polysaccharides (100 mg/kg body weight) for 7 days reduces blood sugar by 61.23%, 42.78%, and 40.08% in diabetic rats, respectively. Histopathological studies have shown that fungal polysaccharides cause enlargement of the Langerhans islets and angiogenesis in diabetic rats. The number of Langerhans islets cells was significantly increased in diabetic rats treated with *Cerrena unicolor* polysaccharide.[144] Studies show that streptozotocin-diabetic animals increase in red blood cell count (an antianemic effect) and fetal hemoglobin concentration. *Agaricus campetris* stimulates 2-deoxyglucose transfer, glucose oxidation, and glycogen increase in mice abdominal muscle.[145] Low and high molecular weight compounds in this fungus can induce insulin secretion.[1] Clinical studies show that consumption of *Agaricus sylvaticus* in 56 patients with colorectal cancer reduces fasting blood glucose, TG, and cholesterol.[1,146] *Catathelasma ventricosum* is used as food in southwestern China.[112] Se-containing polysaccharide of *C. ventricosum* has an antioxidant effect and antihyperglycemic.[147] 100 mg/kg/day polysaccharide of this fungus reduced the blood sugar of diabetic mice from 446.6 mg/dl to 228.6 mg/dl.[148] *Auricularia auricular* polysaccharides increase glucose uptake into HepG2 cells and decrease advanced glycation end products (AGEs).[112] *Ganoderma pfeifferi* has antioxidant activity and can repair pancreatic tissue in diabetic animals.[149] *Ganoderma applanatum* polysaccharides can lower plasma cholesterol, triglycerides, and plasma glucose levels.[47] *Sparassis crispa* β-glucans can heal the wounds of diabetic patients and increase the motility of macrophages and fibroblasts.[47] *Poria cocos* have been used alone or in combination with herbs to treat diabetes in traditional Chinese medicine. Triterpenes of this fungus lower glucose levels in db/db mice and increase insulin sensitivity.[150] Table 9.2 summarizes the clinical studies performed.

TABLE 9.2 Clinical Trials of Mushrooms for Antidiabetic Activity.

Mushroom	Clinical trial	Administration	Material	Result	Reference
A. bisporus	37 prediabetics	100 g for 16 daily weeks	Fruiting body	Increases antioxidant markers ORAS and anti-inflammatory hormones. It reduces oxidative stress factors, carboxymethyl lysine, and methylglyoxal in serum	[23]
Agaricus blazei	536 diabetic patients	1500 mg daily, 12 weeks	Powder extract of fruiting body	Lower HOMA IR index, increased plasma adiponectin concentration, improved insulin resistance	[29]
Cordyceps sinensis	20 diabetic patients	3 g/day	JinShuiBao capsule	Decrease in blood sugar levels	[48]
Ganoderma lucidum	71 diabetic patients	1800 mg three times daily, 12 weeks	Ganopoly (polysaccharide fractions extracted)	Reduce HbA1c and fasting blood glucose	[85]
Agaricus sylvaticus	56 patients with colorectal cancer	30 mg/kg/day, followed up for six months	Dietary supplementation	Reduces fasting blood glucose, TG, and cholesterol	[146]
Pleurotus ostreatus and *Pleurotus cystidiosus*	28 diabetic patients	50 mg/kg/body weight	Fruiting body powder	Decrease in blood sugar levels, increase glucokinase and insulin secretion	[123]

9.3 CONCLUSIONS AND FUTURE PROSPECTIVE

Diabetes mellitus is the fifth leading cause of death in the world and its prevalence is increasing dramatically worldwide. This disease is a defect in the secretion or function of insulin. The destructive effects of diabetes include advanced metabolic complications and lesions of various organs such as retinopathy, nephropathy, neuropathy, cardiovascular and cerebrovascular disease.[1,9] So far, various chemical drugs have been used to control diabetes, but the side effects of these chemical compounds have led researchers to look for natural compounds from plants and fungi.[9] Mushrooms have been used to treat diabetes in traditional medicine for thousands of years. Many in vitro, in vivo, and clinical studies have been performed on the antidiabetic effects of fungi. Medicinal fungi have hypoglycemic, antioxidant, and immune enhancement effects. These fungi protect liver and pancreas tissues by reducing cholesterol and triglycerides, improving fat metabolism and their enzymes function. The antioxidant activity of medicinal fungi reduces oxidative stress, increases the activity of antioxidant enzymes, and repairs the islets of Langerhans. They also have anti-inflammatory effects by regulating the production of cytokines.[1,6,11,47,86,107] Numerous studies have been performed on the physicochemical conditions of fungal culture and the optimal conditions for the growth and production of metabolites of many fungi have been identified.[27] Fungal cultivation in solid-bed bioreactors is also widespread in some countries, especially Brazil.[151] The study of using different elicitors on the growth and production of different metabolites is also very popular. It has been observed that physical (ultrasound), chemical (rifampin) elicitors and microbial volatile can affect the growth and production of the *G. lucidum* metabolite.[70,152,153] The effect of adding elements such as selenium and zinc to the culture medium of fungi such as *H. erinaceus*, *T. versicolor*, and *F. fomentarius* has also been investigated.[154–156] Some medicinal fungi such as *G. lucidum*, *C. sinensis*, *C. militaris*, and *A. blazei* are commercially produced. Fungal supplements include mycelium, polysaccharides, and other fungal metabolites. Some of these antidiabetic capsules also contain two or more fungi.[1] One of the challenges of using medicinal fungi is the low solubility and stability of their polysaccharides. Therefore, the use of nanotechnology and drug delivery systems can be a good solution to this problem. The use of nanosystems based on liposomes and polymers, in addition to increasing the solubility and stability of fungal metabolites, allows them to target specific organs (such as the liver or pancreas).[157,158] The loading of fungal polysaccharides in nanocarriers has been studied. Li et al.[159] observed that loading *G. lucidum* polysaccharides into chitosan nanoparticles increased the antiproliferative activity against cancer cells. Our recent study loaded *T. versicolor* polysaccharides into solid lipid nanoparticles (SLNs) and investigated its antidiabetic effect (our study, unpublished). Studies in this field are not yet complete and it is necessary to load different nanocarriers with fungal polysaccharides and investigate its antidiabetic effects both in vitro and in vivo. Medicinal fungi can be used as dietary supplements and medications in the treatment of diabetes, and their combination with nanodrug delivery systems can make a huge difference in the prevention and treatment of diabetes.

KEYWORDS

- **antidiabetic**
- **mushrooms**
- **clinical trials**
- **type 1 diabetes**
- **type 2 diabetes**

REFERENCES

1. De Silva, D. D.; Rapior, S.; Hyde, K. D.; Bahkali, A. H. Medicinal Mushrooms in Prevention and Control of Diabetes Mellitus. *Fungal Divers.* **2012,** *56* (1), 1–29.
2. Jia, J.; Zhang, X.; Hu, Y.-S.; Wu, Y.; Wang, Q.-Z.; Li, N.-N.; Guo, Q.-C.; Dong, X.-C. Evaluation of in Vivo Antioxidant Activities of *Ganoderma lucidum* Polysaccharides in STZ-diabetic Rats. *Food Chem.* **2009,** *115* (1), 32–36.
3. Prabu, M.; Kumuthakalavalli, R. Antidiabetic Potential of the Oyster Mushroom *Pleurotus florida* (Mont.) Singer. *Int. J. Curr. Pharm. Res.* **2017,** *9* (4), 51–54.
4. Veiseh, O.; Tang, B. C.; Whitehead, K. A.; Anderson, D. G.; Langer, R. Managing Diabetes with Nanomedicine: Challenges and Opportunities. *Nat. Rev. Drug Discov.* **2015,** *14* (1), 45–57.
5. Chaudhury, A.; Duvoor, C.; Reddy Dendi, V. S.; Kraleti, S.; Chada, A.; Ravilla, R.; Marco, A.; Shekhawat, N. S.; Montales, M. T.; Kuriakose, K. Clinical Review of

Antidiabetic Drugs: Implications for Type 2 Diabetes Mellitus Management. *Front. Endocrinol.* **2017,** *8*, 6.
6. Friedman, M. Mushroom Polysaccharides: Chemistry and Antiobesity, Antidiabetes, Anticancer, and Antibiotic Properties in Cells, Rodents, and Humans. *Foods* **2016,** *5* (4), 80.
7. Yan, J.-K.; Pei, J.-J.; Ma, H.-L.; Wang, Z.-B.; Liu, Y.-S. Advances in Antitumor Polysaccharides from *Phellinus sensu* Lato: Production, Isolation, Structure, Antitumor Activity, and Mechanisms. *Crit. Rev. Food Sci.* **2017,** *57* (6), 1256–1269.
8. Huang, C.-H.; Lin, W.-K.; Chang, S. H.; Tsai, G.-J. Evaluation of the Hypoglycaemic and Antioxidant Effects of Submerged *Ganoderma lucidum* Cultures in Type 2 Diabetic Rats. *Mycology* **2020,** *12* (2), 82–93.
9. Alvandi, H.; Ghahremani, M.; Hatamian-Zarmi, A.; Hosseinzadeh, B. E.; Mokhtari-Hosseini, Z. B.; Farjam, S. N. J. Optimization of Soy-based Media for the Production of Biologically Active Exopolysaccharides by Medicinal Mushroom *Trametes versicolor*. *Appl. Food Biotechnol.* **2020,** *7* (4), 251–261.
10. Li, F.; Zhang, Y.; Zhong, Z. Antihyperglycemic Effect of *Ganoderma lucidum* Polysaccharides on Streptozotocin-induced Diabetic Mice. *Int. J. Mol. Sci.* **2011,** *12* (9), 6135–6145.
11. Gulati, V.; Singh, M. D.; Gulati, P. Role of Mushrooms in Gestational Diabetes Mellitus. *AIMS Med. Sci.* **2019,** *6* (1), 49–66.
12. Atila, F.; Owaid, M. N.; Shariati, M. A. The Nutritional and Medical Benefits of *Agaricus bisporus*: A Review. *J. Microbiol., Biotechnol. Food Sci.* **2021,** *2021*, 281–286.
13. Jeong, S. C.; Jeong, Y. T.; Yang, B. K.; Islam, R.; Koyyalamudi, S. R.; Pang, G.; Cho, K. Y.; Song, C. H. White Button Mushroom (*Agaricus bisporus*) Lowers Blood Glucose and Cholesterol Levels in Diabetic and Hypercholesterolemic Rats. *Nutr. Res. Rev.* **2010,** *30* (1), 49–56.
14. Mircea, C.; Cioancă, O.; Bild, V.; Iancu, C.; Stan, C.; Hăncianu, M. In Vivo Antioxidant Properties of Some Mushroom Extracts in Experimentally Induced Diabetes. *Farm* **2018,** *66* (2), 257–261.
15. Reis, F. S.; Martins, A.; Barros, L.; Ferreira, I. C. Antioxidant Properties and Phenolic Profile of the Most Widely Appreciated Cultivated Mushrooms: A Comparative Study between in Vivo and in Vitro Samples. *Food Chem. Toxicol.* **2012,** *50* (5), 1201–1207.
16. Holy, B.; Ngoye, B. O. Clinical Relevance of Superoxide Dismutase and Glutathione Peroxidase Levels in Management of Diabetes Type 2. *Int. J. Contemp. Med. Res.* **2016,** *3* (5), 1380–1382.
17. Liu, J.; Jia, L.; Kan, J.; Jin, C.-H. In Vitro and in Vivo Antioxidant Activity of Ethanolic Extract of White Button Mushroom (*Agaricus bisporus*). *Food Chem. Toxicol.* **2013,** *51*, 310–316.
18. Abou Zaid, O. A.; Sonbaty, S. E.; Neama, M. Anti-diabetic Activity of *Agaricus bisporus*: A Biochemical and Pathological Study. *Int. J. Pharm. Sci. Res.* **2017,** *7* (2), 1740–1745.
19. Flatt, P. R.; Bailey, C. J. Role of Dietary Factors in the Hyperinsulinemia of Genetically Obese Hyperglycemic (ob/ob) Mice. *Nutr. J.* **1982,** *112* (12), 2212–2216.

20. Vishvakarma, R.; Mishra, A. Effect of Protease Inhibitor from *Agaricus bisporus* on Glucose Uptake and Oxidative Stress in 3T3-L1 Adipocytes. *Asian Pac. J. Trop. Biomed.* **2020,** *10* (3), 136–146.
21. Ekowati, N.; Yuniati, N. I.; Hernayanti, H.; Ratnaningtyas, N. I. Antidiabetic Potentials of Button Mushroom (*Agaricus bisporus*) on Alloxan-induced Diabetic Rats. *Biosaintif.: J. Biol. Biol. Educ.* **2018,** *10* (3), 655–662.
22. Brahmachari, G. Bio-flavonoids with Promising Antidiabetic Potentials: A Critical Survey. *Signpost* **2011,** *661* (2), 187–212.
23. Calvo, M. S.; Mehrotra, A.; Beelman, R. B.; Nadkarni, G.; Wang, L.; Cai, W.; Goh, B. C.; Kalaras, M. D.; Uribarri, J. A Retrospective Study in Adults with Metabolic Syndrome: Diabetic Risk Factor Response to Daily Consumption of *Agaricus bisporus* (White Button Mushrooms). *Plant Foods Hum. Nutr.* **2016,** *71* (3), 245–251.
24. Ali, M. M.; Baig, M. T.; Jabeen, A.; Aslam, M.; Shahid, U. Therapeutic Value of Medicinal Mushroom *Agaricus blazei* Murill. *Pak. J. Med. Dent.* **2021,** *10*, 83–89.
25. Firenzuoli, F.; Gori, L.; Lombardo, G. The Medicinal Mushroom *Agaricus blazei* Murrill: Review of Literature and Pharmaco-toxicological Problems. *Evid.-Based Complement. Alternat. Med.* **2008,** *5* (1), 3–15.
26. Ellertsen, L. K.; Hetland, G. An Extract of the Medicinal Mushroom *Agaricus blazei* Murill Can Protect against Allergy. *Clin. Mol. Allergy* **2009,** *7* (1), 1–10.
27. Alvandi, H.; Hatamian-Zarmi, A.; Ebrahimi Hosseinzadeh, B.; Mokhtari-Hosseini, Z.-B.; Aghajani, H. Effect of Production, Extraction and Purification methods on Anti-cancer Property of Fungal Polysaccharides. *Dev. Biol.* **2020,** *12* (1), 27–42.
28. Wei, Q.; Zhan, Y.; Chen, B.; Xie, B.; Fang, T.; Ravishankar, S.; Jiang, Y. Assessment of Antioxidant and Antidiabetic Properties of *Agaricus blazei* Murill Extracts. *Food. Sci. Nutr.* **2020,** *8* (1), 332–339.
29. Hsu, C.-H.; Liao, Y.-L.; Lin, S.-C.; Hwang, K.-C.; Chou, P. The Mushroom *Agaricus blazei* Murill in Combination with Metformin and Gliclazide Improves Insulin Resistance in Type 2 Diabetes: A Randomized, Double-blinded, and Placebo-controlled Clinical Trial. *J. Altern. Complement. Med.* **2007,** *13* (1), 97–102.
30. Misgiati, M., Ed. The Effect of *Agaricus blazei* Murill on Haematological Parameter, Random Blood Sugar, Total Cholesterol, and Uric Acid of Wistar Rats (Sprague Dawley). *J. Sci. Res. Stud.* **2015,** *2* (2), 56–62.
31. Vitak, T.; Yurkiv, B.; Wasser, S.; Nevo, E.; Sybirna, N. Effect of Medicinal Mushrooms on Blood Cells under Conditions of Diabetes Mellitus. *World J. Diabetes* **2017,** *8* (5), 187.
32. Vitak, T. Y.; Wasser, S. P.; Nevo, E. D.; Sybirna, N. O. The Effect of the Medicinal Mushrooms *Agaricus brasiliensis* and *Ganoderma lucidum* (Higher Basidiomycetes) on the Erythron System in Normal and Streptozotocin-induced Diabetic Rats. *Int. J. Med. Mushrooms* **2015,** *17* (3), 277–286.
33. Vitak, T. Y.; Wasser, S. P.; Nevo, E. D.; Sybirna, N. O. Structural changes of erythrocyte surface glycoconjugates after treatment with medicinal mushrooms. *Int. J. Med. Mushrooms* **2015,** *17* (9), 867–878.
34. Kim, D. J.; Kang, Y. H.; Kim, K. K.; Kim, T. W.; Park, J. B.; Choe, M. Increased Glucose Metabolism and Alpha-glucosidase Inhibition in *Cordyceps militaris* Water Extract-treated HepG2 Cells. *Nutr. Res. Pract.* **2017,** *11* (3), 180.

35. Jo, W.-S.; Nam, B.-H.; Oh, S.-J.; Choi, Y.-J.; Kang, E.-Y.; Hong, S.-H.; Lee, S.-H.; Jeong, M.-H. Hepatic Protective Effect and Single-dose Toxicity Study of Water Extract of *Cordyceps militaris* Grown upon *Protaetia dreujtarsis*. *Korean J. Food Sci. Technol.* **2008,** *40* (1), 106–110.
36. Kim, H.-S.; Roh, Y.-J.; Choe, M. *Cordyceps militaris* Increases Hepatic Glucokinase Activities. *J. Korean Soc. Food Sci. Nutr.* **2005,** *34* (2), 158–161.
37. Kim, D.-H.; Yang, B.-K.; Jeong, S.-C.; Hur, N.-J.; Surajit, D.; Yun, J.-W.; Choi, J.-W.; Lee, Y.-S.; Song, C.-H. A Preliminary Study on the Hypoglycemic Effect of the Exo-polymers Produced by Five Different Medicinal Mushrooms. *J. Microbiol Biotechnol.* **2001,** *11* (1), 167–171.
38. Dong, Y.; Jing, T.; Meng, Q.; Liu, C.; Hu, S.; Ma, Y.; Liu, Y.; Lu, J.; Cheng, Y.; Wang, D. Studies on the Antidiabetic Activities of *Cordyceps militaris* Extract in Diet-streptozotocin-induced Diabetic Sprague-Dawley Rats. *Biomed. Res. Int.* **2014,** *2014*, 160980.
39. Patel, K.; Ingalhalli, R. *Cordyceps militaris* (L.: Fr.) Link—An Important Medicinal Mushroom. *J. Pharmacogn. Phytochem.* **2013,** *2* (1), 315–319.
40. Yun, Y.-H.; Han, S.-H.; Lee, S.-J.; Ko, S.-K.; Lee, C.-K.; Ha, N.-J.; Kim, K.-J. Anti-diabetic Effects of CCCA, CMESS, and Cordycepin from *Cordyceps militaris* and the Immune Responses in Streptozotocin-induced Diabetic Mice. *Nat. Prod. Sci.* **2003,** *9* (4), 291–298.
41. Ashraf, S. A.; Elkhalifa, A. E. O.; Siddiqui, A. J.; Patel, M.; Awadelkareem, A. M.; Snoussi, M.; Ashraf, M. S.; Adnan, M.; Hadi, S. Cordycepin for Health and Wellbeing: A Potent Bioactive Metabolite of an Entomopathogenic Cordyceps Medicinal Fungus and Its Nutraceutical and Therapeutic Potential. *Molecules* **2020,** *25* (12), 2735.
42. Shin, S.; Lee, S.; Kwon, J.; Moon, S.; Lee, S.; Lee, C.-K.; Cho, K.; Ha, N.-J.; Kim, K. Cordycepin Suppresses Expression of Diabetes Regulating Genes by Inhibition of Lipopolysaccharide-Induced Inflammation in Macrophages. *Immune Netw.* **2009,** *9* (3), 98.
43. Cao, T.; Xu, R.; Xu, Y.; Liu, Y.; Qi, D.; Wan, Q. The Protective Effect of Cordycepin on Diabetic Nephropathy through Autophagy Induction in Vivo and in Vitro. *Int. Urol. Nephrol.* **2019,** *51* (10), 1883–1892.
44. Liu, C.; Song, J.; Teng, M.; Zheng, X.; Li, X.; Tian, Y.; Pan, M.; Li, Y.; Lee, R. J.; Wang, D. Antidiabetic and Antinephritic Activities of Aqueous Extract of *Cordyceps militaris* Fruit Body in Diet-streptozotocin-induced Diabetic Sprague Dawley Rats. *Oxid. Med. Cell Longev.* **2016,** *2016*, 9685257.
45. Zhang, Q.; Olatunji, O. J.; Chen, H.; Tola, A. J.; Oluwaniyi, O. O. Evaluation of the Anti-diabetic Activity of Polysaccharide from *Cordyceps cicadae* in Experimental Diabetic Rats. *Chem. Biodivers.* **2018,** *15* (8), e1800219.
46. Liu, R.-M.; Dai, R.; Luo, Y.; Xiao, J.-H. Glucose-lowering and Hypolipidemic Activities of Polysaccharides from *Cordyceps taii* in Streptozotocin-induced Diabetic Mice. *BMC Complement. Altern. Med.* **2019,** *19* (1), 1–10.
47. Dubey, S. K.; Chaturvedi, V. K.; Mishra, D.; Bajpeyee, A.; Tiwari, A.; Singh, M. Role of Edible Mushroom as a Potent Therapeutics for the Diabetes and Obesity. *3 Biotech* **2019,** *9* (12), 1–12.
48. Guo, Q.; Zhang, C. Clinical Observations of Adjunctive Treatment of 20 Diabetic Patients with JinShuiBao Capsule. *J. Admin. Trad. Chin. Med* **1995,** *5*, 22.

49. Kan, W.-C.; Wang, H.-Y.; Chien, C.-C.; Li, S.-L.; Chen, Y.-C.; Chang, L.-H.; Cheng, C.-H.; Tsai, W.-C.; Hwang, J.-C.; Su, S.-B. Effects of Extract from Solid-state Fermented *Cordyceps sinensis* on Type 2 Diabetes Mellitus. *Evid.-Based Complement. Alternat. Med.* **2012,** *2012*, 743107.
50. Alvandi, H.; Hatamian-Zarmi, A.; Ebrahimi Hosseinzadeh, B.; Mokhtari-Hosseini, Z.-B. Optimization of Production Conditions for Bioactive Polysaccharides from *Fomes fomentarius* and Investigation of Antibacterial and Antitumor Activities. *Iran. J. Microbiol.* **2020,** *14* (6), 596–611.
51. Sairi, A. M.; Ismail, S. I.; Sukor, A.; Rashid, N.; Saad, N.; Jamian, S.; Abdullah, S. Cytotoxicity and Anticancer Activity of *Donkioporiella mellea* on MRC5 (Normal Human Lung) and A549 (Human Lung Carcinoma) Cells Lines. *Evid.-Based Complement. Alternat. Med.* **2020,** *2020*. https://doi.org/10.1155/2020/7415672
52. Pelcaru, C. F.; Ene, M.; Petrache, A.-M.; Neguţ, D. C. Low Doses of Gamma Irradiation Stimulate Synthesis of Bioactive Compounds with Antioxidant Activity in *Fomes fomentarius* Living Mycelium. *Appl. Sci.* **2021,** *11* (9), 4236.
53. Elkhateeb, W.; Elnahas, M.; Paul, W.; Daba, T. *Fomes fomentarius* and *Polyporus squamosus* Models of Marvel Medicinal Mushrooms. *Biomed. Res. Rev.* **2020,** *3*, 119.
54. Maljurić, N.; Golubović, J.; Ravnikar, M.; Žigon, D.; Štrukelj, B.; Otašević, B. Isolation and Determination of Fomentariol: Novel Potential Antidiabetic Drug from Fungal Material. *J. Anal. Methods Chem.* **2018,** *2018*. https://doi.org/10.1155/2018/2434691
55. Seo, D.-W.; Yi, Y.-J.; Lee, M.-S.; Yun, B.-S.; Lee, S.-M. Differential Modulation of Lipopolysaccharide-induced Inflammatory Cytokine Production by and Antioxidant Activity of Fomentariol in RAW264.7 Cells. *Mycobiology* **2015,** *43* (4), 450–457.
56. Sharma, A.; Kaur, R.; Kaur, J.; Garg, S.; Bhatti, R.; Kaur, A. An Endophytic *Schizophyllum commune* Fr. Exhibits in-Vitro and in-Vivo Antidiabetic Activity in Streptozotocin Induced Diabetic Rats. *AMB Express* **2021,** *11* (1), 1–11.
57. Muthuramalingam, K.; Singh, V.; Choi, C.; Choi, S. I.; Park, S.; Kim, Y. M.; Unno, T.; Cho, M. Effect of Mushroom (*Schizophyllum* Spp.) Derived β-Glucan on Low-fiber Diet Induced Gut Dysbiosis. *J. Appl. Biol. Chem.* **2019,** *62* (2), 211–217.
58. Yu, J.; Cui, P.-J.; Zeng, W.-L.; Xie, X.-L.; Liang, W.-J.; Lin, G.-B.; Zeng, L. Protective Effect of Selenium-polysaccharides from the Mycelia of *Coprinus comatus* on Alloxan-induced Oxidative Stress in Mice. *Food Chem.* **2009,** *117* (1), 42–47.
59. Liang, B.; Guo, Z.; Xie, F.; Zhao, A. Antihyperglycemic and Antihyperlipidemic Activities of Aqueous Extract of *Hericium erinaceus* in Experimental Diabetic Rats. *BMC Complement. Altern. Med.* **2013,** *13* (1), 1–7.
60. Lu, X.; Chen, H.; Dong, P.; Fu, L.; Zhang, X. Phytochemical Characteristics and Hypoglycaemic Activity of Fraction from Mushroom *Inonotus obliquus*. *J. Sci. Food Agric.* **2010,** *90* (2), 276–280.
61. Wang, J.; Wang, C.; Li, S.; Li, W.; Yuan, G.; Pan, Y.; Chen, H. Anti-diabetic Effects of *Inonotus obliquus* Polysaccharides in Streptozotocin-induced Type 2 Diabetic Mice and Potential Mechanism Via PI3K-Akt Signal Pathway. *Biomed. Pharmacother.* **2017,** *95*, 1669–1677.
62. Shokrzadeh, M.; Azdo, S.; Habibi, E. Anti-diabetic Effect of Methanol Extract of *Trametes versicolor* on Male Mice. *J. Maz. Univ. Med. Sci.* **2017,** *26* (145), 165–175.

63. Chen, C.-H.; Kang, L.; Lo, H.-C.; Hsu, T.-H.; Lin, F.-Y.; Lin, Y.-S.; Wang, Z.-J.; Chen, S.-T.; Shen, C.-L. Polysaccharides of *Trametes versicolor* Improve Bone Properties in Diabetic Rats. *J. Agric. Food Chem.* **2015,** *63* (42), 9232–9238.
64. Afiati, F.; Firza, S. F.; Kusmiati; Aliya, L. S., Eds. The Effectiveness β-glucan of Shiitake Mushrooms and *Saccharomyces cerevisiae* as Antidiabetic and Antioxidant in Mice Sprague Dawley Induced Alloxan. In *AIP Conference Proceedings*; AIP Publishing LLC, 2019.
65. Yang, H. J.; Kim, M. J.; Kwon, D. Y.; Kim, D. S.; Zhang, T.; Ha, C.; Park, S. Combination of Aronia, Red Ginseng, Shiitake Mushroom and Nattokinase Potentiated Insulin Secretion and Reduced Insulin Resistance with Improving Gut Microbiome Dysbiosis in Insulin Deficient Type 2 Diabetic Rats. *Nutrients* **2018,** *10* (7), 948.
66. Hata, K. In Vitro and in Vivo Antidiabetic Effects of the Ethanol Extract from *Lentinula edodes* (Shiitake). *J. Funct. Foods* **2021**. doi: 10.17470/NF-016-1007-4.
67. Balaji, P.; Madhanraj, R.; Rameshkumar, K.; Veeramanikandan, V.; Eyini, M.; Arun, A.; Thulasinathan, B.; Al Farraj, D.; Elshikh, M.; Alokda, A. Evaluation of Antidiabetic Activity of *Pleurotus pulmonarius* against Streptozotocin-nicotinamide Induced Diabetic Wistar Albino Rats. *Saudi J. Biol. Sci.* **2020,** *27* (3), 913–924.
68. Omale, S.; Aguiyi, J.; Bukar, B.; Ede, S.; Amagon, K.; Amagon, L.; Usman, O.; Chinello, V.; Oshibanjo, D. Fruiting Body of *Pleurotus ostreatus* Reduces Serum Glucose and Modifies Oxidative Stress in Type 2 Diabetic: *Drosophila melanogaster* (Fruit-Fly). *Adv. Pharmacol. Pharmacy* **2020,** *8* (3), 41–50.
69. Heydarian, M.; Hatamian-Zarmi, A.; Amoabediny, G.; Ebrahimi-Hosseinzadeh, B.; Alvandi, H.; Doryab, A.; Salehi, A. Growth Kinetics and Ganoderic Acid Production from *Ganoderma lucidum* GIRAN17: A Real-time Monitoring Platform. *Iran. J. Microbiol.* **2021,** *15* (1), 67–84.
70. Kalantari-Dehaghi, S.; Hatamian-Zarmi, A.; Ebrahimi-Hosseinzadeh, B.; Mokhtari-Hosseini, Z.-B.; Nojoki, F.; Hamedi, J.; Hosseinkhani, S. Effects of Microbial Volatile Organic Compounds on *Ganoderma lucidum* Growth and Ganoderic Acids Production in Co-V-Cultures (Volatile Co-cultures). *Prep. Biochem. Biotechnol.* **2019,** *49* (3), 286–297.
71. Bach, E. E.; Hi, E. M. B.; Martins, A. M. C.; Nascimento, P. A.; Wadt, N. S. Y. Hypoglicemic and Hypolipedimic Effects of *Ganoderma lucidum* in Streptozotocin-induced Diabetic Rats. *J. Med.* **2018,** *5* (3), 78.
72. Ma, H.-T.; Hsieh, J.-F.; Chen, S.-T. Anti-diabetic Effects of *Ganoderma lucidum*. *Phytochemistry* **2015,** *114*, 109–113.
73. Xiao, C.; Wu, Q.-P.; Cai, W.; Tan, J.-B.; Yang, X.-B.; Zhang, J.-M. Hypoglycemic Effects of *Ganoderma lucidum* Polysaccharides in Type 2 Diabetic Mice. *Arch. Pharm. Res.* **2012,** *35* (10), 1793–1801.
74. Hikino, H.; Ishiyama, M.; Suzuki, Y.; Konno, C. Mechanisms of Hypoglycemic Activity of Ganoderan B: A Glycan of *Ganoderma lucidum* Fruit Bodies. *Planta Med.* **1989,** *55* (05), 423–428.
75. Chen, J.; Yang, H.; Pei, R.; Wang, L. *Ganoderma lucidum* Polysaccharides on Hepatic Ischemia–Reperfusion Injury. *J. Pract. Med.* **2010,** *28* (04), 700–701.

76. Zalba, G.; José, G. S.; Moreno, M. U.; Fortuño, M. A.; Fortuño, A.; Beaumont, F. J.; Díez, J. Oxidative Stress in Arterial Hypertension: Role of NAD(P)H Oxidase. *Hypertension* **2001,** *38* (6), 1395–1399.
77. Zeng, P.; Guo, Z.; Zeng, X.; Hao, C.; Zhang, Y.; Zhang, M.; Liu, Y.; Li, H.; Li, J.; Zhang, L. Chemical, Biochemical, Preclinical and Clinical Studies of *Ganoderma lucidum* Polysaccharide as an Approved Drug for Treating Myopathy and Other Diseases in China. *J. Cell Mol. Med.* **2018,** *22* (7), 3278–3297.
78. Seto, S.; Lam, T.; Tam, H.; Au, A.; Chan, S. W.; Wu, J.; Yu, P.; Leung, G.; Ngai, S.; Yeung, J. H. Novel Hypoglycemic Effects of *Ganoderma lucidum* Water-extract in Obese/Diabetic (+db/+db) Mice. *Phytomedicine* **2009,** *16* (5), 426–436.
79. Jung, K. H.; Ha, E.; Kim, M.-J.; Uhm, Y. K.; Kim, H. K.; Hong, S.-J.; Chung, J.-H.; Yim, S.-V. *Ganoderma lucidum* Extract Stimulates Glucose Uptake in L6 Rat Skeletal Muscle Cells. *Acta Biochim. Pol.* **2006,** *53* (3), 597–601.
80. Huang, C.-H.; Lin, W.-K.; Chang, S. H.; Tsai, G.-J. *Ganoderma lucidum* Culture Supplement Ameliorates Dyslipidemia and Reduces Visceral Fat Accumulation in Type 2 Diabetic Rats. *Mycology* **2021,** *12* (2), 94–104.
81. Teng, B.-S.; Wang, C.-D.; Zhang, D.; Wu, J.; Pan, D.; Pan, L.; Yang, H.; Zhou, P. Hypoglycemic Effect and Mechanism of a Proteoglycan from *Ganoderma lucidum* on Streptozotocin-induced Type 2 Diabetic Rats. *Eur. Rev. Med. Pharmacol. Sci.* **2012,** *16* (2), 166–175.
82. Pan, D.; Zhang, D.; Wu, J.; Chen, C.; Xu, Z.; Yang, H.; Zhou, P. Antidiabetic, Antihyperlipidemic and Antioxidant Activities of a Novel Proteoglycan from *Ganoderma lucidum* Fruiting Bodies on db/db Mice and the Possible Mechanism. *PLoS ONE* **2013,** *8* (7), e68332.
83. Prihastuti, C. C. The Lingzhi Mushroom (*Ganoderma lucidum*) Extract Reduce the Number of Lymphocyte in Diabetics Rats with Periodontitis: In Vivo Experimental on Sprague Dawley Rats. **2021**. In *Proceedings of the 1st Jenderal Soedirman International Medical Conference in conjunction with the 5th Annual Scientific Meeting (Temilnas) Consortium of Biomedical Science Indonesia (JIMC 2020)*; pp 254–259.
84. Zhang, H.-N.; Lin, Z.-B. Hypoglycemic Effect of *Ganoderma lucidum* Polysaccharides. *Acta Pharmacol. Sin.* **2004,** *25* (2), 191–195.
85. Gao, Y.; Lan, J.; Dai, X.; Ye, J.; Zhou, S. A Phase I/II study of Ling Zhi Mushroom *Ganoderma lucidum* (W. Curt.: Fr.) Lloyd (Aphyllophoromycetideae) Extract in Patients with Type II Diabetes Mellitus. *Int. J. Med. Mushrooms* **2004,** *6* (1). doi: 10.1615/IntJMedMushr.v6.i1.30.
86. Martel, J.; Ojcius, D. M.; Chang, C.-J.; Lin, C.-S.; Lu, C.-C.; Ko, Y.-F.; Tseng, S.-F.; Lai, H.-C.; Young, J. D. Anti-obesogenic and Antidiabetic Effects of Plants and Mushrooms. *Nat. Rev. Endocrinol.* **2017,** *13* (3), 149–160.
87. Canfora, E. E.; Jocken, J. W.; Blaak, E. E. Short-chain Fatty Acids in Control of Body Weight and Insulin Sensitivity. *Nat. Rev. Endocrinol.* **2015,** *11* (10), 577.
88. Cheng, P.-G.; Phan, C.-W.; Sabaratnam, V.; Abdullah, N.; Abdulla, M. A.; Kuppusamy, U. R. Polysaccharides-rich Extract of *Ganoderma lucidum* (MA Curtis: Fr.) P. Karst Accelerates Wound Healing in Streptozotocin-induced Diabetic Rats. *Evid.-Based Complement. Alternat. Med.* **2013,** *2013*.

89. Chen, Y.; Liu, D.; Wang, D.; Lai, S.; Zhong, R.; Liu, Y.; Yang, C.; Liu, B.; Sarker, M. R.; Zhao, C. Hypoglycemic Activity and Gut Microbiota Regulation of a Novel Polysaccharide from *Grifola frondosa* in Type 2 Diabetic Mice. *Food Chem. Toxicol.* **2019,** *126*, 295–302.
90. Li, Q.; Zhang, F.; Chen, G.; Chen, Y.; Zhang, W.; Mao, G.; Zhao, T.; Zhang, M.; Yang, L.; Wu, X. Purification, Characterization and Immunomodulatory Activity of a Novel Polysaccharide from *Grifola frondosa*. *Int. J. Biol. Macromol.* **2018,** *111*, 1293–1303.
91. Su, C.-H.; Lai, M.-N.; Ng, L.-T. Inhibitory Effects of Medicinal Mushrooms on α-Amylase and α-Glucosidase–Enzymes Related to Hyperglycemia. *Food Funct.* **2013,** *4* (4), 644–649.
92. Guo, W.-L.; Deng, J.-C.; Pan, Y.-Y.; Xu, J.-X.; Hong, J.-L.; Shi, F.-F.; Liu, G.-L.; Qian, M.; Bai, W.-D.; Zhang, W. Hypoglycemic and Hypolipidemic Activities of *Grifola frondosa* Polysaccharides and Their Relationships with the Modulation of Intestinal Microflora in Diabetic Mice Induced by High-fat Diet and Streptozotocin. *Int. J. Biol. Macromol.* **2020,** *153*, 1231–1240.
93. Larsen, N.; Vogensen, F. K.; Van Den Berg, F. W.; Nielsen, D. S.; Andreasen, A. S.; Pedersen, B. K.; Al-Soud, W. A.; Sørensen, S. J.; Hansen, L. H.; Jakobsen, M. Gut Microbiota in Human Adults with Type 2 Diabetes Differs from Non-diabetic Adults. *PLoS ONE* **2010,** *5* (2), e9085.
94. Makiura, N.; Ojima, M.; Kou, Y.; Furuta, N.; Okahashi, N.; Shizukuishi, S.; Amano, A. Relationship of *Porphyromonas gingivalis* with Glycemic Level in Patients with Type 2 Diabetes Following Periodontal Treatment. *Oral Microbiol. Immunol.* **2008,** *23* (4), 348–351.
95. Kou, L.; Du, M.; Liu, P.; Zhang, B.; Zhang, Y.; Yang, P.; Shang, M.; Wang, X. Anti-diabetic and Anti-nephritic Activities of *Grifola frondosa* Mycelium Polysaccharides in Diet-streptozotocin-induced Diabetic Rats Via Modulation on Oxidative Stress. *Appl. Biochem. Biotechnol.* **2019,** *187* (1), 310–322.
96. Thongbai, B.; Rapior, S.; Hyde, K. D.; Wittstein, K.; Stadler, M. *Hericium erinaceus*, an Amazing Medicinal Mushroom. *Mycol. Prog.* **2015,** *14* (10), 1–23.
97. Wang, J. C.; Hu, S. H.; Wang, J. T.; Chen, K. S.; Chia, Y. C. Hypoglycemic Effect of Extract of *Hericium erinaceus*. *J. Sci. Food Agric.* **2005,** *85* (4), 641–646.
98. Yang, B.-K.; Park, J.-B.; Song, C.-H. Hypolipidemic Effect of an Exo-biopolymer Produced from a Submerged Mycelial Culture of *Hericium erinaceus*. *Biosci. Biotechnol. Biochem.* **2003,** *67* (6), 1292–1298.
99. Cai, W.-D.; Ding, Z.-C.; Wang, Y.-Y.; Yang, Y.; Zhang, H.-N.; Yan, J.-K. Hypoglycemic Benefit and Potential Mechanism of a Polysaccharide from *Hericium erinaceus* in Streptozotoxin-induced Diabetic Rats. *Process Biochem.* **2020,** *88*, 180–188.
100. Cui, Y.; Kim, D.-S.; Park, K.-C. Antioxidant Effect of *Inonotus obliquus*. *J. Ethnopharmacol.* **2005,** *96* (1–2), 79–85.
101. Xu, X.; Wu, Y.; Chen, H. Comparative Antioxidative Characteristics of Polysaccharide-enriched Extracts from Natural Sclerotia and Cultured Mycelia in Submerged Fermentation of *Inonotus obliquus*. *Food Chem.* **2011,** *127* (1), 74–79.
102. Zhang, J.-J.; Li, Y.; Zhou, T.; Xu, D.-P.; Zhang, P.; Li, S.; Li, H.-B. Bioactivities and Health Benefits of Mushrooms Mainly from China. *Molecules* **2016,** *21* (7), 938.

103. Stojkovic, D.; Smiljkovic, M.; Ciric, A.; Glamoclija, J.; Van Griensven, L.; Ferreira, I. C.; Sokovic, M. An Insight into Antidiabetic Properties of Six Medicinal and Edible Mushrooms: Inhibition of α-Amylase and α-Glucosidase Linked to Type-2 Diabetes. *S. Afr. J. Bot.* **2019,** *120*, 100–103.
104. Ying, Y.-M.; Zhang, L.-Y.; Zhang, X.; Bai, H.-B.; Liang, D.-E.; Ma, L.-F.; Shan, W.-G.; Zhan, Z.-J. Terpenoids with Alpha-glucosidase Inhibitory Activity from the Submerged Culture of *Inonotus obliquus*. *Phytochemistry* **2014,** *108*, 171–176.
105. Chen, H.; Lu, X.; Qu, Z.; Wang, Z.; Zhang, L. Glycosidase Inhibitory Activity and Antioxidant Properties of a Polysaccharide from the Mushroom *Inonotus obliquus*. *J. Food Biochem.* **2010,** *34*, 178–191.
106. Sun, J.-E.; Ao, Z.-H.; Lu, Z.-M.; Xu, H.-Y.; Zhang, X.-M.; Dou, W.-F.; Xu, Z.-H. Antihyperglycemic and Antilipidperoxidative Effects of Dry Matter of Culture Broth of *Inonotus obliquus* in Submerged Culture on Normal and Alloxan-diabetes Mice. *J. Ethnopharmacol.* **2008,** *118* (1), 7–13.
107. Jiang, X.; Meng, W.; Li, L.; Meng, Z.; Wang, D. Adjuvant Therapy with Mushroom Polysaccharides for Diabetic Complications. *Front. Pharmacol.* **2020,** *11*, 168.
108. Sheng, K.; Wang, C.; Chen, B.; Kang, M.; Wang, M.; Liu, K.; Wang, M. Recent Advances in Polysaccharides from *Lentinus edodes* (Berk.): Isolation, Structures and Bioactivities. *Food Chem.* **2021,** *358*, 129883.
109. Nisar, J.; Mustafa, I.; Anwar, H.; Sohail, M. U.; Hussain, G.; Ullah, M. I.; Faisal, M. N.; Bukhari, S. A.; Basit, A. Shiitake Culinary-medicinal Mushroom, *Lentinus edodes* (Agaricomycetes): A Species with Antioxidant, Immunomodulatory, and Hepatoprotective Activities in Hypercholesterolemic Rats. *Int. J. Med. Mushrooms* **2017,** *19* (11), 981–990.
110. Handayani, D.; Chen, J.; Meyer, B. J.; Huang, X.-F. Dietary Shiitake Mushroom (*Lentinus edodes*) Prevents Fat Deposition and Lowers Triglyceride in Rats Fed a High-fat Diet. *J. Obes.* **2011,** *2011*, 258051.
111. Laurino, L. F.; Viroel, F. J.; Pickler, T. B.; Gerenutti, M. Functional Foods in Gestational Diabetes: Evaluation of the Oral Glucose Tolerance Test (OGTT) in Pregnant Rats Treated with Mushrooms. *Reprod. Toxicol.* **2017,** *72*, 36.
112. Khursheed, R.; Singh, S. K.; Wadhwa, S.; Gulati, M.; Awasthi, A. Therapeutic Potential of Mushrooms in Diabetes Mellitus: Role of Polysaccharides. *Int. J. Biol. Macromol.* **2020**, *164*, 1194–1205.
113. Feng, H.; Zhang, S.; Wan, J. M.-F.; Gui, L.; Ruan, M.; Li, N.; Zhang, H.; Liu, Z.; Wang, H. Polysaccharides Extracted from *Phellinus linteus* Ameliorate High-fat High-fructose Diet Induced Insulin Resistance in Mice. *Carbohydr. Polym.* **2018,** *200*, 144–153.
114. Kim, H. M.; Kang, J. S.; Kim, J. Y.; Park, S.-K.; Kim, H. S.; Lee, Y. J.; Yun, J.; Hong, J. T.; Kim, Y.; Han, S.-B. Evaluation of Antidiabetic Activity of Polysaccharide Isolated from *Phellinus linteus* in Non-obese Diabetic Mouse. *Int. Immunopharmacol.* **2010,** *10* (1), 72–78.
115. Yang, K.; Zhang, S.; Ying, Y.; Li, Y.; Cai, M.; Guan, R.; Hu, J.; Sun, P. Cultivated Fruit Body of *Phellinus baumii*: A Potentially Sustainable Antidiabetic Resource. *ACS Omega* **2020,** *5* (15), 8596–8604.
116. Yang, K.; Zhang, S.; Geng, Y.; Tian, B.; Cai, M.; Guan, R.; Li, Y.; Ye, B.; Sun, P. Anti-Inflammatory Properties in Vitro and Hypoglycaemic Effects of Phenolics from

Cultivated Fruit Body of *Phellinus baumii* in Type 2 Diabetic Mice. *Molecules* **2021,** *26* (8), 2285.
117. Cho, J.-H.; Park, H.-S.; Han, J.-G.; Lee, K.-H.; Jhune, C.-S. Anti-diabetic Efficacy of the Alcoholic Extracts in *Ganoderma* sp. and *Phellinus Baumi*. *J. Mushrooms* **2015,** *13* (4), 326–329.
118. Elkhateeb, W. A.; Daba, G. M. Mycotherapy of the Good and the Tasty Medicinal Mushrooms *Lentinus*, *Pleurotus*, and *Tremella*. *J. Pharm. Sci. Res.* **2021,** *4* (3). https://doi.org/10.31579/2693-7247/029
119. Li, J.-P.; Lei, Y.-l.; Zhan, H. The Effects of the King Oyster Mushroom *Pleurotus eryngii* (Higher Basidiomycetes) on Glycemic Control in Alloxan-induced Diabetic Mice. *Int. J. Med. Mushrooms* **2014,** *16* (3), 219–225.
120. Chen, R.-R.; Liu, Z.-K.; Liu, F.; Ng, T. B. Antihyperglycaemic Mechanisms of an Aceteoside Polymer from Rose Flowers and a Polysaccharide–Protein Complex from Abalone Mushroom. *Nat. Prod. Res.* **2015,** *29* (6), 558–561.
121. Jayakumar, T.; Thomas, P. A.; Isai, M.; Geraldine, P. An Extract of the Oyster Mushroom, *Pleurotus ostreatus*, Increases Catalase Gene Expression and Reduces Protein Oxidation during Aging in Rats. *Zhong xi yi jie he xue bao= J. Chin. Integr. Med.* **2010,** *8* (8), 774–780.
122. Xiong, M.; Huang, Y.; Liu, Y.; Huang, M.; Song, G.; Ming, Q.; Ma, X.; Yang, J.; Deng, S.; Wen, Y. Antidiabetic Activity of Ergosterol from *Pleurotus ostreatus* in KK-Ay Mice with Spontaneous Type 2 Diabetes Mellitus. *Mol. Nutr. Food Res.* **2018,** *62* (3), 1700444.
123. Jayasuriya, W. B. N.; Wanigatunge, C. A.; Fernando, G. H.; Abeytunga, D. T. U.; Suresh, T. S. Hypoglycaemic Activity of Culinary *Pleurotus ostreatus* and *P. cystidiosus* Mushrooms in Healthy Volunteers and Type 2 Diabetic Patients on Diet Control and the Possible Mechanisms of Action. *Phytother. Res.* **2015,** *29* (2), 303–309.
124. Hu, S. H.; Liang, Z. C.; Chia, Y. C.; Lien, J. L.; Chen, K S.; Lee, M. Y.; Wang, J. C. Antihyperlipidemic and Antioxidant Effects of Extracts from *Pleurotus citrinopileatus*. *J. Agric. Food Chem.* **2006,** *54* (6), 2103–2110.
125. Badole, S. L.; Bodhankar, S. L. Interaction of Aqueous Extract of *Pleurotus pulmonarius* (Fr.) Quel-champ. with Acarbose in Alloxan Induced Diabetic Mice. *Interaction* **2007,** *5* (3), 157–166.
126. Dubey, S.; Yadav, C.; Bajpeyee, A.; Singh, M. P. Effect of *Pleurotus fossulatus* Aqueous Extract on Biochemical Properties of Liver and Kidney in Streptozotocin-induced Diabetic Rat. *Diabetes Metab. Syndr. Obes.: Targets Ther.* **2020,** *13*, 3035.
127. Kamalebo, H. M.; Malale, H. N. S. W.; Ndabaga, C. M.; Degreef, J.; De Kesel, A. Uses and Importance of Wild Fungi: Traditional Knowledge from the Tshopo Province in the Democratic Republic of the Congo. *J. Ethnobiol. Ethnomed.* **2018,** *14* (1), 1–12.
128. Hobbs, C. The Chemistry, Nutritional Value, Immunopharmacology, and Safety of the Traditional Food of Medicinal Split-gill Fugus *Schizophyllum commune* Fr.:Fr. (Schizophyllaceae). A Literature Review. *Int. J. Med. Mushrooms* **2005,** *7* (1–2), 127–140.
129. Hao, L.-M.; Xing, X.-H.; Li, Z.; Zhang, J.-C.; Sun, J.-X.; Jia, S.-R.; Qiao, C.-S.; Wu, T. Optimization of Effect Factors for Mycelial Growth and Exopolysaccharide

Production by *Schizophyllum commune*. *Appl. Biochem. Biotechnol.* **2010,** *160* (2), 621–631.
130. Tiwari, B. K.; Pandey, K. B.; Abidi, A.; Rizvi, S. I. Markers of Oxidative Stress during Diabetes Mellitus. *J. Biomark.* **2013,** *2013*. https://doi.org/10.1155/2013/378790
131. Wanna, C.; Sudhadham, M. The Effect of Coconut Water and Boiling on Antioxidant Activity and Total Phenolic Contents in *Schizophyllum commune* Fr. *Pharmacogn. Mag.* **2018,** *10* (5), 925–931.
132. Chen, Z.; Yin, C.; Fan, X.; Ma, K.; Yao, F.; Zhou, R.; Shi, D.; Cheng, W.; Gao, H. Characterization of Physicochemical and Biological Properties of *Schizophyllum commune* Polysaccharide Extracted with Different Methods. *Int. J. Biol. Macromol.* **2020,** *156*, 1425–1434.
133. Chandrawanshi, N. K.; Tandia, D. K.; Jadhav, S. Nutraceutical Properties Evaluation of *Schizophyllum commune*. *Indian J. Sci. Res.* **2017,** *13* (2), 57–62.
134. Kumar, A.; Dandapat, S.; Kumar, M.; Sinha, M. Anti-inflammatory and Amylase Inhibitory Properties of Indian Edible Macrofungi *Dacryopinax spathularia* (Schwein) and *Schizophyllum commune* (Fries). *Bioscan* **2018,** *13* (2), 715–718.
135. Chandrawanshi, N. K.; Tandia, D. K.; Jadhav, S. Determination of Anti-diabetic Property of Organic and Nonorganic Solvent Extracts of *Schizophyllum commune*. *NewBioWorld* **2019,** *1* (1), 5–8.
136. Du, X.-J.; Zhang, J.-S.; Yang, Y.; Tang, Q.-J.; Jia, W.; Pan, Y.-J. Purification, Chemical Modification and Immunostimulating Activity of Polysaccharides from *Tremella aurantialba* Fruit Bodies. *J. Zhejiang Univ. Sci. B* **2010,** *11* (6), 437–442.
137. Wu, Y.-J.; Wei, Z.-X.; Zhang, F.-M.; Linhardt, R. J.; Sun, P.-L.; Zhang, A.-Q. Structure, Bioactivities and Applications of the Polysaccharides from *Tremella fuciformis* Mushroom: A Review. *Int. J. Biol. Macromol.* **2019,** *121*, 1005–1010.
138. Wu, T.; Xu, B. B. Antidiabetic and Antioxidant Activities of Eight Medicinal Mushroom Species from China. *Int. J. Med. Mushrooms* **2015,** *17* (2), 129–140.
139. Yoon, Y.-C.; Kim, B.-H.; Kim, J.-G.; Lee, J.-H.; Park, Y.; Park, H.-S.; Hwang, H.-S.; Kwon, G.-S.; Lee, J.-B. Anti-obesity and Anti-diabetic Effects of the Fermented Ethanol Extracts from White Jelly Fungus (*Tremella fuciformis* Berk) with *Lactobacillus rhamnosus* BHN-LAB 76. *Microbiol. Biotechnol. Lett.* **2019,** *47* (3), 323–331.
140. Lo, H.-C.; Wasser, S. P. Medicinal Mushrooms for Glycemic Control in Diabetes Mellitus: History, Current Status, Future Perspectives, and Unsolved Problems. *Int. J. Med. Mushrooms* **2011,** *13* (5), 401–426.
141. Price, L. A.; Wenner, C. A.; Sloper, D. T.; Slaton, J. W.; Novack, J. P. Role for Toll-like Receptor 4 in TNF-alpha Secretion by Murine Macrophages in Response to Polysaccharide Krestin, a *Trametes versicolor* Mushroom Extract. *Fitoterapia* **2010,** *81* (7), 914–919.
142. Scarpari, M.; Reverberi, M.; Parroni, A.; Scala, V.; Fanelli, C.; Pietricola, C.; Zjalic, S.; Maresca, V.; Tafuri, A.; Ricciardi, M. R. Tramesan, a Novel Polysaccharide from *Trametes versicolor*. Structural Characterization and Biological Effects. *PLoS ONE* **2017,** *12* (8), e0171412.
143. Puia, I. C.; Aida, P.; Chedea, V. S.; Leopold, N.; Bocsan, I. C.; Buzoianu, A. D. Characterization of *Trametes versicolor*: Medicinal Mushroom with Important Health Benefits. *Nat. Bot. Hortic. Agrobot. Cluj Napoca* **2018,** *46* (2), 343–349.

144. Yamac, M.; Zeytinoglu, M.; Kanbak, G.; Bayramoglu, G.; Senturk, H. Hypoglycemic Effect of Crude Exopolysaccharides Produced by *Cerrena unicolor*, *Coprinus comatus*, and *Lenzites betulina* Isolates in Streptozotocin-induced Diabetic Rats. *Pharm. Biol.* **2009,** *47* (2), 168–174.
145. Gray, A.; Flatt, P. Insulin-releasing and Insulin-like Activity of *Agaricus campestris* (Mushroom). *J. Endocrinol.* **1998,** *157* (2), 259–266.
146. Fortes, R. C.; Recôva, V.; Melo, A.; Novaes, M. Effects of Dietary Supplementation with Medicinal Fungus in Fasting Glycemia Levels of Patients with Colorectal Cancer: A Randomized, Double-blind, Placebo-controlled Clinical Study. *Nutr. Hosp.* **2008,** *23* (6), 591–598.
147. Liu, Y.; Sun, J.; Rao, S.; Su, Y.; Li, J.; Li, C.; Xu, S.; Yang, Y. Antidiabetic Activity of Mycelia Selenium-polysaccharide from *Catathelasma ventricosum* in STZ-induced Diabetic Mice. *Food Chem. Toxicol.* **2013,** *62*, 285–291.
148. Liu, Y.; Chen, D.; You, Y.; Zeng, S.; Hu, Y.; Duan, X.; Liu, A.; Chen, H.; Hu, X.; Chen, S. Structural Characterization and Antidiabetic Activity of a Glucopyranose-rich Heteropolysaccharide from *Catathelasma ventricosum*. *Carbohydr. Polym.* **2016,** *149*, 399–407.
149. Rašeta, M.; Popović, M.; Čapo, I.; Stilinović, N.; Vukmirović, S.; Milošević, B.; Karaman, M. Antidiabetic Effect of Two Different *Ganoderma* Species Tested in Alloxan Diabetic Rats. *RSC Adv.* **2020,** *10* (17), 10382–10393.
150. Li, T.-H.; Hou, C.-C.; Chang, C. L.-T.; Yang, W.-C. Anti-hyperglycemic Properties of Crude Extract and Triterpenes from *Poria cocos*. *Evid.-Based Complement. Alternat. Med.* **2010,** *2011*. https://doi.org/10.1155/2011/128402
151. Soccol, C. R.; Vandenberghe, L. P. Overview of Applied Solid-state Fermentation in Brazil. *Biochem. Eng. J.* **2003,** *13* (2–3), 205–218.
152. Nojoki, F.; Hatamian-Zarmi, A.; Hosseinzadeh, B. E.; Mir-derikvand, M. Investigation and Optimization Effects of Ultrasound Waves to Produce Ganoderic Acid, Anti-cancer Mushrooms Metabolite. *Iran. J. Microbiol.* **2017,** *11* (1), 58–66.
153. Nojoki, F.; Hatamian-Zarmi, A.; Mir-Drikvand, M.; Ebrahimi-Hosseinzadeh, B.; Mokhtari-Hosseini, Z.-B.; Kalantari-Dehaghi, S.; Esmaeilifar, M. Impact of Rifampin Induction on the Fermentation Production of Ganoderic Acids by Medicinal Mushroom *Ganoderma lucidum*. *Appl. Food Biotechnol.* **2016,** *3* (2), 91–98.
154. Malinowska, E.; Krzyczkowski, W.; Herold, F.; Łapienis, G.; Ślusarczyk, J.; Suchocki, P.; Kuraś, M.; Turło, J. Biosynthesis of Selenium-containing Polysaccharides with Antioxidant Activity in Liquid Culture of *Hericium erinaceum*. *Enzyme Microb. Technol.* **2009,** *44* (5), 334–343.
155. Miletić, D.; Turło, J.; Podsadni, P.; Pantić, M.; Nedović, V.; Lević, S.; Nikšić, M. Selenium-enriched *Coriolus versicolor* Mushroom Biomass: Potential Novel Food Supplement with Improved Selenium Bioavailability. *J. Sci. Food Agric.* **2019,** *99* (11), 5122–5130.
156. Alvandi, H.; Hatamian-Zarmi, A.; Hoseinzadeh, B. E.; Mokhtari-Hosseini, Z. B.; Langer, E.; Aghajani, H. Improving the Biological Properties of *Fomes fomentarius* MG835861 Exopolysaccharide by Bioincorporating Selenium into Its Structure. *Carbohydr. Polym. Technol. Appl.* **2021,** 100159. doi: 10.1016/j.carpta.2021.100159.

157. Xu, Y.; Zhang, L.; Chen, G.; Chen, P., Eds. Thinking on the Application of Nanotechnology in the Mechanism Research on the Traditional Chinese Medicine Diagnosis and Treatment of Diabetes Mellitus. *J. Phys.: Conf. Ser.* **2011,** *276,* 012050.
158. Hu, T.; Jiang, J.-G. Application of Nanotechnology in Traditional Chinese Medicine. *Curr. Nanosci.* **2012,** *8* (3), 474–484.
159. Li, N.; Hu, Y. L.; He, C. X.; Hu, C. J.; Zhou, J.; Tang, G. P.; Gao, J. Q. Preparation, Characterisation and Anti-tumour Activity of *Ganoderma lucidum* Polysaccharide Nanoparticles. *J. Pharm. Pharmacol.* **2010,** *62* (1), 139–144.

CHAPTER 10

Antidiabetic Mushrooms: Market Products, Safety, and Challenges

HARWINDER K.[1], MRIDU[2*], AND AMITA[3]

[1]Department of Botany, Akal University, Talwandi Sabo Bathinda 151302, Punjab, India

[2]Department of Biotechnology, Dyal Singh College, Karnal 132001, Haryana, India

[3]Depertment of Botany, Punjabi University, Patiala 147002, Punjab, India

**Corresponding author. E-mail: mriduphd@gmail.com*

ABSTRACT

Mushrooms have been known for their multifarious benefits in the biosphere since times immemorial. Besides the ecological services, they provide in the overall growth and replenishment of the ecosystem, many of these are in use as a source of food and medicine. The traditional ways of using mushrooms by people, all around the world, are a treasure for humankind which needs to be documented faithfully. Mushrooms are quite rich in nutritional and bioactive components, which accounts for a broad spectrum of their application in therapeutics as antioxidants, anti-bacterial, antifungal, immunostimulatory, and a lot more such properties. Mushrooms are such a magical wonder that making them a regular part of diet can prevent or delay the onset of many life-threatening diseases such as atherosclerosis, hypertension, hypercholesterolemia, diabetes, AIDS,

Therapeutic Mushrooms for Diabetes Mellitus: Current Evidences and Future Scope. Uzma Azeem, Khalid Rehman Hakeem, (Eds.)

and cancer. In this article, the information available on mushrooms as a source of antidiabetic products, their safety aspects and challenges have been reviewed. Diabetes mellitus is a serious metabolic disorder and very common among the people of all age groups nowadays and the long-term use of drugs that are taken for the treatment of this disorder affects various organs adversely. In such cases, mushrooms serve as one of the wonderful gifts of nature with antidiabetic properties due to the presence of certain specific biochemicals such as enzymes, polysaccharides, glucoproteins, alkaloids, lipopolysaccharides, phenols, sterols, and terpenoids, which target various metabolic pathways and help in reducing the blood glucose level and managing insulin concentrations. Some such mushroom species with antidiabetic potential are *Hericium erinaceus* (Bull.) Pers., *Inonotus obliquus* (Ach. ex Pers.) Pilát, *Ganoderma lucidum* (Curtis) P. Karst, *Pleurotus ostreatus* (Jacq.) P. Kumm., *Cordyceps militaris* (L.) Link, *Agaricus blazei* Murrill, *Grifola frondosa* (Dicks.) Gray, etc. Nowadays, various brands have started manufacturing and marketing the antidiabetic products in the form of extracts, powder, tablets, and capsules from such medicinal mushroom species. Even the consumption of dried fruit bodies of such mushrooms is recommended for consumption as dietary supplements. The presently available major antidiabetic products manufactured under different brands, their safety concerns, as well as challenges associated with such products have been documented in the ongoing account.

10.1 INTRODUCTION

As per the latest global report (2019) of World Health Organization, approximately 4.22 million people are suffering from diabetes; nearly 3.7 million people are reported to have died due to diabetes and high blood glucose level. As many as 1.5 million deaths are exclusively attributed to diabetes, which is reported to be the eighth major cause of fatality. If remain uncontrolled for a long time diabetes is reported to cause serious damage to various organs of the human body leading to heart attacks and strokes, kidney failure, blindness, etc. Besides this, even in case of Covid-19 and Coronavirus 2 (SARS-CoV-2) infections, severe consequences have been observed in the patients suffering from diabetes. During the present times, diabetic patients are being admitted to the hospitals at higher rates and they are at higher risks of severe pneumonia and mortality as compared to the nondiabetic patients.[1] Even the diabetic patients suffering from Covid-19 and Coronavirus 2 (SARS-CoV-2) infections are found to be more prone to mucormycosis.[2] Maintaining blood glucose level, thus, is necessary for a healthy and safe life. World Health Organization has suggested that a simple lifestyle is the best way to prevent or delay the onset of the most common type of diabetes, i.e., type 2 diabetes. A simple lifestyle includes maintaining healthy body weight, doing physical activity regularly, avoiding use of tobacco, and most importantly having a healthy diet, which must include those foods in the diet, which are low in sugar and fat content and rich in vitamins, minerals, and fibers. There are many such natural food items including mushrooms, which are highly nutritious and associated with a number of health benefits since these contain some additional ingredients designed to improve health because of which mushrooms are classified under the category of functional foods. Edible mushrooms fall in the category of "Super Food" because of the presence of nutritional and nutraceutical important constituents in them.[3,4] In them, there are present number of amino acids, vitamins, minerals,[5–7] and secondary metabolites, which accounts for their antioxidant, anticancer, antiallergic, anti-inflammatory, antidiabetic, antiviral, antibacterial, antiparasitic, antifungal, anticholesterolemic, and immunomodulatory properties.[8–12] Also, the number of enzymes such as laccase and peroxidase; polysaccharides such as β-D-glucans; glucoproteins, lectins, proteins, alkaloids, phenols, sterols, terpenoids, lipopolysaccharides, etc. are a part and parcel of mushroom composition. These biochemical constituents have been reported to target different metabolic pathways that help to reduce the blood glucose level and maintain insulin concentration.[13,14] Number of mushrooms that have been investigated for their antidiabetic potential include *Ganoderma lucidum* (Curtis) P. Karst., *Pleurotus florida* Singer, *Pleurotus ostreatus* (Jacq.) P. Kumm., *Astraeus hygrometricus* (Pers.) Morgan, *Agaricus sylvaticus* Sacc., *A. blazei* Murrill, *Agaricus bisporus* Murrill, *Agaricus campestris* L., *Agaricus subrufescens* Peck, *Auricularia auricula-judae*, *Coprinus comatus* (O.F. Mull.) Pers., *Cordyceps militaris* (L.) Link, *Cordyceps sinensis* (Berk) Sacc., *Grifola frondosa* (Dicks.) Gray, *Hericium erinaceus* (Bull.) Pers., *Inonotus obliquus* (Ach. ex Pers.) Pilat, *Lentinula edodes* (Berk.) Pegler, *Phellinus* spp., *Tremella mesenterica* Retz., *Tremella fuciformis* Berk., *Wolfiporia extensa* (Peck.) Ginns, etc.[15–17] Information about their specific bioactive components and the antidiabetic mode of action of each such component is given in Table 10.1.

During the past few years some companies have started preparing dietary supplements using extracts or powder of such nutritionally and nutraceutically important mushrooms in the form of tablets, capsules, powder, liquid, etc. at commercial scale.[18] This unique initiative has helped in extending the benefits of this magical gift of nature to the common consumers. Even dried fruit bodies of these mushrooms are being sold commercially. This communication is an attempt to provide the available information about various antidiabetic market products prepared from different mushrooms at one place.

10.2 ANTIDIABETIC MARKET PRODUCTS OF MUSHROOMS

Commercialization of mushroom products has opened the doors for easy prophylactics in case of various diseases. People in any part of the world can benefit from these mushrooms through these products even where they do not grow naturally. Like for the people living in urban areas or the areas with extreme climatic conditions, the wild mushrooms are almost inaccessible. Most of these products are available for online shopping through the manufacturer's website of various online shopping sites. Besides this, these platforms also provide the facility of shipping to different parts of the world. Secondly, the various extraction processes give out the concentrated amount of desired bioactive components such as polysaccharides, which can be more effective for a specific purpose as compared to the use of fresh mushrooms as a whole. Therefore, bringing out the products made from mushrooms bears a great potential for their better utilization.

10.2.1 AGARICUS BLAZEI MURRILL AS A SOURCE OF ANTIDIABETIC PRODUCTS

A. blazei is traditionally used in folk medicine for the treatment of various chronic metabolic diseases such as cancer, chronic hepatitis, arteriosclerosis, hyperlipidemia, and diabetes.[31] There are a number of reports demonstrating that this species has a good immunomodulating and antioxidative potential.[20] It is reported to inhibit α-glucosidase enzyme,[32,33] which provides an effective solution to control blood glucose level in persons suffering from type 2 diabetes. Metformin, a commonly

TABLE 10.1 Bioactive Components of Some Mushroom Species and Their Antidiabetic Mode of Action.

S. No.	Name of the species	Bioactive component	Mode of action	References
1.	*Hericium erinaceus* (Bull.) Pers.	Polysaccharides	Reduce blood glucose level (BGL), increase insulin level, reduce lipid levels, and enhance the actions of catalase (CAT), superoxide dismutase (SOD), glutathione peroxidase (GSH-Px), and glutathione (GSH)	[19–21]
2.	*Phellinus linteus* (Berk. & M.A. Curtis) Teng	Polysaccharides, hispidin	Decrease fasting blood glucose and improve glucose intolerance by altering metabolism of hepatic phospholipids and rescuing insulin signaling transduction via FOXO signaling pathway Hispidin prevents β-cells from deterioration due to increased ROS in case of diabetes mellitus	[15,22,23]
3.	*Agaricus subrufescens* Peck	Minerals (potassium, calcium, and zinc) and beta-glucans	Reduce BGL, oxidative stress, and HbA1c	[13]
4.	*Lentinula edodes* (Berk.) Pegler	Ergosterol and glycogen-like polysaccharides	Increase plasma insulin and reduce BGL	[13]
5.	*Auricularia auricula-judae* (Bull.) Quél.	Polysaccharides	Increase glucose absorption of HepG2 cells and reduce advanced glycation end products	[24]
6.	*Catathelasma ventricosum* (Peck) Singer	*C. ventricosum* polysaccharides (CVPs)	Reduce BGL; prevent injuries due to increased BGL in liver, kidney, and pancreas	[25,26]
7.	*Pleurotus florida* Singer	Polysaccharides	Reduce blood glucose level	[27]
8.	*Agaricus bisporus* (J.E. Lange) Imbach	Polysaccharides, polyphenols, ergothioneine, lectins	Increase the insulin and glucagon secretion from islets cells, enhance uptake of glucose	[28]
9.	*Agaricus brasiliensis* Fr.	Polysaccharides, α-glucan, and β-glucan	Increase in plasma insulin, decrease in glucagon, increase in insulin sensitivity, scavenge-free radicals, and lipid peroxidation	[29]
10.	*Ganoderma lucidum* (Curtis) P. Karst	Polysaccharides	Increased nonenzymatic and enzymatic antioxidants and serum insulin levels, and reduced lipid peroxidation and blood glucose levels	[18,30]

used drug for the management of blood sugar levels, works on the similar mechanism.[33] The extracts of *A. blazei* have also been reported to inhibit α-glucosidase enzyme that is why various brands are cultivating this mushroom and manufacturing dietary supplements in various forms to be sold in the market. Details about some such products are given below.

10.2.1.1 SUPER ROYAL AGARICUS

This product is a dietary supplement manufactured by Mushroom Wisdom, Inc., New Jersey. It is available in the form of tablets, which are made up of concentrated hot water extract of fruiting body of *Agaricus blazei.* and some other ingredients like Vitamin C, Microcrystalline Cellulose, Croscarmellose Sodium, Dicalcium Phosphate, Calcium Stearate, Silicon Dioxide, Hydroxypropyl Methylcellulose, and Glycerin. The manufacturer advises to take one tablet once a day or two tablets twice a day to maintain a healthy blood sugar level (Fig. 10.1a).

Price: $34.95 per pack of 120 tablets.

Certifications: The manufacturer has declared that the product has been manufactured under certified cGMP facility.

10.2.1.2 SUPERFOOD SCIENCE AGARICUS BIO® WELLNESS POWDER CAPSULES AND SUPERFOOD SCIENCE AGARICUS BIO® SUPER LIQUID

These products are manufactured by Atlas World USA, Inc. As per the information available on the manufacturer's website, these products are made of 100% USDA-certified organic *Agaricus blazei* mushroom. The manufacturer has converted the extract of the fruit body of *Agaricus blazei* into two forms that are powder capsules and liquid. SuperFood Science Agaricus Bio® Super Liquid is in a liquid tincture form, which is highly absorbable and especially useful for those who have weak digestive system and cannot digest the powdered form well. Another product Atlas Agaricus Ekismate® is manufactured by a unique extraction method (MSPS extraction) which supports the immune system even in serious conditions 16 times more than the liquid made from a general extraction process. The company claims that these products help in maintaining healthy blood sugar and cholesterol levels as well as promote antioxidant activity, regulation of abnormal cell growth, and support a strong immune system. Each powder capsule contains 600 mg of *A. blazei* powder and each liquid drop contains 25 mg of *A. blazei* fruit body extract. The doses of these products vary according to the purpose of consumption. For a healthy blood sugar level, it is recommended to start with 1 ml of SuperFood Science Agaricus Bio® Super Liquid per day, 2–5 drops of Atlas Agaricus Ekismate® per day, or 1 capsule per day (Fig. 10.1b and c).

Price: SuperFood Science Agaricus Bio® Wellness powder capsules—$33.19 per pack of 60 capsules.

SuperFood Science Agaricus Bio® Super Liquid—$28.95 per pack of 30 ml.

Certifications and warnings: The manufacturer claims that these products are manufactured from 100% USDA-certified organic *Agaricus blazei* mushroom. The company also warns that pregnant or breastfeeding women should consult with health professionals before using these products and those who are hypersensitive to mushrooms or bamboo should not use them.

10.2.1.3 ATLAS AGARICUS EKISMATE®

Another product Atlas Agaricus Ekismate® is manufactured by a unique extraction method (MSPS extraction) which is reported to support the immune system even in serious conditions 16 times more than the liquid made from a general extraction process. The company claims that these products help in maintaining healthy blood sugar and cholesterol levels as well as promote antioxidant activity, regulation of abnormal cell growth and support a strong immune system. Each powder capsule contains 600 mg of *A. blazei* powder and each liquid drop contains 25 mg of *A. blazei* fruit body extract. The doses of these products vary according to the purpose of consumption. For a healthy blood sugar level, it is recommended to start with 1 ml of SuperFood Science Agaricus Bio® Super Liquid per day, 2–5 drops of Atlas Agaricus Ekismate® per day, or 1 capsule per day (Fig. 10.1d).

Price: $75.00 per pack of 10 g.

Certifications and warnings: The manufacturer claims that these products are manufactured from 100% USDA-certified organic *Agaricus blazei* mushroom. The company also warns that pregnant or breastfeeding women should consult with health professionals before using these products and those who are hypersensitive to mushrooms or bamboo should not use them.

10.2.1.4 OTHER PRODUCTS OF A. BLAZEI

Urban Platter *Agaricus blazei* Murill (ABM) Mushroom Extract Powder, Swanson Superior Herbs—*Agaricus blazei* Mushroom Extract, DXN *Agaricus blazei* Murill capsules are some other commercially available products prepared from *A. blazei.*

10.2.2 GRIFOLA FRONDOSA (DICKS.) GRAY AS A SOURCE OF ANTIDIABETIC PRODUCTS

Grifola frondosa, commonly known as Maitake, is a widely consumed mushroom for its high nutritional and medicinal values.[18] It is recognized as highly priced traditional medicinal mushrooms in the materia medica of China and Japan.[36,37] This species has been reported to contain a good amount of various chemical constituents such as flavonoids, alkaloids, steroids, coumarins, terpene lactones, triterpenes, and organic acids.[38] But from the pharmacological point of view, polysaccharides are reported to be the main components of interest. *G. frondosa* is distinctly rich in water-soluble polysaccharides on dry weight basis and among them, 13.2% are (1 → 3, 1 → 6) β-D-glucans. It also contains a good level of β-D-glucans.[39] As per the available information in literature, therapeutically more than 40 polysaccharides and a large number of pharmaceutically important fractions have been obtained from this species. Some of these fractions include MD-fraction, SX-fraction, SZ-fraction, and Grifolians.[40–42] These fractions vary in their glucan/protein ratio. Polysaccharides of *G. frondosa* have promising antidiabetic potential as well as other bioactivities.[43] Therefore, this mushroom is being utilized commercially to develop various healthcare products, some of them are discussed here.

10.2.2.1 SX-FRACTION®

This product contains tablets prepared using 750 mg fruiting body powder of *Grifola frondosa*, fruiting body and extract concentrate of a glycoprotein along with the other basic components such as microcrystalline cellulose, dicalcium phosphate, etc. The manufacturer Mushroom Wisdom, Inc. New Jersey has patented the active constituent and extraction process of the product. It has been directed by the company to consume 3 tablets of this product daily as a dietary supplement. As claimed by the manufacturer, SX-Fraction® supports healthy blood sugar and insulin function as well as supports cardiovascular health maintenance (Fig. 10.1e).

Price: $129.95 per pack of 270 tablets.

Certifications: The product has been manufactured in a certified cGMP facility.

10.2.2.2 SUPER MAITAKE

Mushroom Wisdom, Inc. manufactures this product from the fruiting body powder of *Grifola frondosa* and Vitamin C along with other basic ingredients of tablet formulations. The company claims that this product helps in maintaining a healthy immune system, liver, blood sugar, and blood pressure. 3–4 tablets are recommended to be taken per day as a dietary supplement (Fig. 10.1f).

Price: $19.95 per pack of 90 tablets.

Certifications and warnings: The product has been manufactured in cGMP facility. The manufacturer also warns of its reproductive harm.

10.2.2.3 MAITAKE EXTRACT

This product is made up of triple extracted USDA-certified organic mushroom mycelium and fruit bodies of Maitake (*Grifola frondosa*). It is manufactured by Host Defense Mushroom™. According to the information available at the manufacturer's website, this product promotes a healthy glycemic balance by supporting normal blood sugar metabolism. It is rich in 1–3, 1–4, and 1–6 β-glucans, well known for promoting immune health, and also supports cellular health. It is suggested to take 1 ml twice a day as a dietary supplement (Fig. 10.1g).

Price: $19.95 per pack of 60 ml.

Certifications and warnings: The Company has mentioned that USDA-certified organic mushroom has been used in the manufacturing of this product. In case of pregnancy, healthcare advisors should be consulted before use and the product should be kept away from the reach of children.

10.2.2.4 MAITAKE ORGANIC MUSHROOM POWDER

A California-based company Om Mushroom Superfood® is the manufacturer of this product. It is a dietary supplement made in the form of powder blend of mycelial biomass and primordia of *Grifola frondosa.* This product supports healthy blood sugar levels and helps in controlling body weight. This powder can be consumed in various forms like by adding 1 tablespoon (2g) to smoothies, coffee, etc. For optimal support, it is suggested to take 4 g of this powder per day (Fig. 10.1h).

Price: $24.99 per pack of 100 g.

Certifications: This product is USDA Organic certified and Non GMO project verified.

10.2.2.5 OTHER PRODUCTS OF G. FRONDOSA

Urban platter Maitake mushroom extract powder, planetary herbals full spectrum Maitake, bluebonnet nutrition Maitake gold mushroom extract, NFH Maitake SAP hot water extract, etc. are some other products from Maitake mushroom.

10.2.3 CORDYCEPS MILITARIS (L.) LINK AS A SOURCE OF ANTIDIABETIC PRODUCTS

Cordyceps militaris is a cherished mushroom used traditionally by the populace in various regions in the world. It is also a source of livelihood as it is sold at very high rates due to the medicinal qualities it retains.[42] There are several reports documenting hypoglycemic activities of this species.[43,44]

It has been demonstrated that polysaccharides present in *C. militaris* are reported to reduce lipid peroxidation, blood glucose level, and lipid levels, enhance antioxidant enzyme actions, improve insulin resistance, and reduce fasting blood glucose, etc.[43,45,46] In another study by Ref. [47] it was shown that exopolysaccharides from *C. militaris* result in improved weight loss and glucose tolerance, reduced plasma glucose concentration, protect immune organs, and repair dyslipidemia to relieve diabetes in STZ-induced diabetic mice. Therefore, taking into consideration the antidiabetic properties of *C. militaris*, various products have been launched in the market by some brands, some of which are discussed below.

10.2.3.1 ROOTED ACTIVE NATURALS CORDYCEPS MILITARIS

This product contains pure dried fruit bodies of *Cordyceps militaris* manufactured by Manger Health Dynamics Pvt. Ltd., Faridabad, India. It provides blood sugar support along with many other health benefits and can be consumed in various ways like as a tea, by adding 5–7 strands of it in boiling water or by adding in coffee, warm milk, soups, or juices. Besides this, the strands of this dried fruit body can also be chewed (Fig. 10.1i).

Price: ₹1530 per pack of 15 g.

Certifications and warnings: The manufacturer claims that their product is lab tested for no toxins or fillers. There is a warning of using this product after consulting a physician if pregnant, nursing mother, or with any other medical condition.

10.2.3.2 VN ORGANICS LIFELINE CAPSULES AND CORDYCEPS LIFELINE TEA

These products are made up of *Cordyceps militaris* cultivated on organic rice in India and manufactured by VN Organics Pvt. Ltd., Madhya Pradesh, India. Each *Cordyceps* Lifeline Tea Sachet contains pure *C. militaris* fruit body while each capsule contains 500 mg of *C. militaris* fruit body powder. To prepare tea, one sachet is poured in a cup of hot water and left for 2–4 min; the tea would be ready for consumption. For Lifeline Capsules, the recommended dose is 2–3 capsules per day. These products serve as an immunity booster, help in balancing blood sugar metabolism, provide support to mental health, respiratory system, heart and kidney health, etc. due to the presence of high amounts of Cordycepin in this mushroom species (Fig. 10.1j and k).

Prices: VN Organics Lifeline Capsules: ₹2499 per pack of 60 capsules.

***Cordyceps* Lifeline Tea:** ₹2499 per pack of 20 sachet.

Certifications and warnings: These products have FSSAI certifications. These are not for use by children below 13 years of age. In case of medications, lactating mothers, pregnant women, doctors should be consulted before using these products.

10.2.3.3 UMBRELLA AGRO FARMING DRY CORDYCEPS MILITARIS, CORDYCEPS MILITARIS CAPSULES, POWDER, ORAL LIQUID SOLUTION

An India-based company Umbrella Agro Farming is manufacturing few products made with *Cordyceps militaris* in different forms such as dry fruit body, fruit body powder, capsules, and oral liquid solution. These products work as immunity boosters, maintain cholesterol levels, blood glucose levels, and a lot more (Fig. 10.1l–n).

Prices: Umbrella agro farming dry *Cordyceps militaris*: ₹50,000 per pack of 1 kg.

Cordyceps militaris capsules: ₹2600 per bottle of 60 capsules.

Cordyceps militaris powder: ₹1000.00 per pack of 10 g

Cordyceps militaris oral liquid solution: ₹2999 per bottle of 30 ml

Certifications and warnings: This product has FSSAI certifications. In case of pregnancy, lactating mothers, or in any other medical condition, physicians should be consulted. The product should be kept out of reach of children.

10.2.3.4 OTHER PRODUCTS OF C. MILITARIS

Some other products from *C. militaris* are Nutriyaan advanced *Cordyceps*; healthy Ceps elixir, Avocare SuperFood *Cordyceps-Militaris*; Biotrex Nutraceuticals *Cordyceps*; the mushrooms hub dried *Cordyceps militaris*; CordyGold *Cordyceps* capsules.

10.2.4 INONOTUS OBLIQUUS (ACH. EX PERS.) PILAT AS A SOURCE OF ANTIDIABETIC PRODUCTS

I. obliquus, commonly known as Chaga mushroom, is traditionally used as a medicine particularly in Siberia and Russia.[14] A number of previous studies have shown this species to contain various bioactive compounds including triterpenoids, polysaccharides, and polyphenols which are responsible for the pharamacological activities such as antiviral, anti-diabetic, and hepatoprotective.[48–50] Various market products containing *I. obliquus* are mentioned below.

10.2.4.1 ROOTED ACTIVE NATURALS CHAGA MUSHROOM EXTRACT POWDER PURE FRUIT BODY

This product is a hot water extract of *Inonotus obliquus* prepared using pure powder. It is manufactured and marketed by Manger Health Dynamics Pvt Ltd., Faridabad, India. It is a dietary supplement that may support healthy blood sugar level, cholesterol and fight cancerous tumors due to the presence of essential bioactive compounds such as β-(1,3)(1,6)-glucans; triterpenoids. The manufacturer suggests taking 2 g of this powder daily with or without food. This powder can be added to tea, coffee, soups, juices, or food (Fig. 10.1o).

Price: ₹1332 per pack of 60 g.

Certifications and warnings: This product has ISO and FSSAI certifications. Besides this, the manufacturer warns that this product should be consumed after consulting a physician if pregnant, nursing mother, or with any other medical condition.

10.2.4.2 SIBERIAN CHAGA MUSHROOM

This product is manufactured by Paithan Eco Foods Pvt. Ltd., India. It contains powder of dried fruit bodies of *I. obliquus*. It is rich in antioxidants, prevents cancer cell growth, maintains blood sugar levels, helps in lowering cholesterol, and boosts up immunity. It can be taken by adding 1 tablespoon of powder in one cup of hot water and then by straining the water after 8–10 min. The manufacturer recommends taking 1 cup of this water per day as a dietary supplement (Fig. 10.1p).

Price: ₹720.00 per pack.

Certification and warnings: This product is not evaluated by FDA and FSSAI. This product is not suitable for lactating and pregnant women and those below 18 years of age. In case of people with on diuretics, diabetic medications, and using antihypertensives or blood thinners, they should consult doctors before consuming this product.

10.2.4.3 OTHER PRODUCTS OF INONOTUS OBLIQUUS

These include Swayamacare FIN-CHAGA, Urban Platter Chaga Mushroom Tea.

10.2.5 PLEUROTUS OSTREATUS (JACQ.) P. KUMM. AS A SOURCE OF ANTIDIABETIC PRODUCTS

P. ostreatus belongs to the group of one of the most appreciated edible mushrooms. Besides its flavor and taste, it also possesses various medicinal properties. One of those is its antidiabetic potential. There are various reports presenting the hypoglycemic potential of this species.[51] Zhang et al.[52] demonstrated that *P. ostreatus* polysaccharides lower hyperglycemia and hyperlipidemia levels, enhance glycogen storage, and improve insulin resistance by activating GSK3 phosphorylation and GLUT4 translocation. It also lowers the risk of oxidative damage. Other studies have reported the antidiabetic effects of ergosterol present in *P. ostreatus* which increases glucose uptake and reduces fasting blood glucose and insulin resistance in mice.[53] Some of the products containing *P. ostreatus* are discussed here.

10.2.5.1 OYSTER MUSHROOM EXTRACT POWDER PURE FRUIT BODY

Manger Health Dynamics Pvt. Ltd., Faridabad, India manufactures this product. It is in the form of powder made from hot water extract of fruit bodies of *Pleurotus ostreatus*. It supports healthy blood glucose level, cholesterol level and acts as an immunity booster also. This powder can be taken in various forms such as in hot water, green tea, coffee, juices, shakes, smoothies, food, etc. The manufacturer recommends that 2–3 g of this powder should be taken daily (Fig. 10.1q).

Price: ₹324 per pack of 60 g.

Certifications and warnings: This product has GMP, ISO, and FSSAI certifications. In case of pregnancy, nursing mother, or with any other medical condition, physicians should be consulted before using this product.

10.2.5.2 THE MUSHROOMS HUB OYSTER MUSHROOM POWDER AND DRIED OYSTER MUSHROOM

These products are manufactured by the company "The Mushrooms Hub." These contain dried fruit bodies and powder of dried fruit bodies of *P. ostreatus*. The dried mushroom fruit bodies are required to rehydrate in hot water before use or can be added to dishes while cooking without rehydration. The powder can be added to various dishes, vegetables, pasta, or soups (Fig. 10.1r and s).

Price: The Mushrooms Hub Oyster Mushroom Powder: ₹250 per pack of 100 g.

The Mushrooms Hub Oyster Mushroom Dried Oyster Mushroom: ₹275 per pack of 100 g

Certifications and warnings: These products are approved by FSSAI.

10.2.5.3 OTHER PRODUCTS OF P. OSTREATUS

Mushroom Wala Oyster mushroom protein powder; SOMAZ dry oyster mushroom powder; Sattvic foods dried oyster mushrooms are other such products from oyster mushroom.

10.2.6 HERICIUM ERINACEUS (BULL.) PERS. AS A SOURCE OF ANTIDIABETIC PRODUCTS

H. erinaceus is commonly known as Lion's Mane. The local people of China are traditionally using this mushroom as a source of medicine.[14] Like other medicinal species, this one is also reported to possess antidiabetic properties. *Hericium erinaceus* polysaccharides have been shown to reduce blood glucose level, fasting glucose and increase insulin concentration.[20,21] Some of the products manufactured using *H. erinaceus* are discussed below.

10.2.6.1 LION'S MANE MUSHROOM EXTRACT POWDER

The hot water extract prepared using pure powder of *H. erinaceus* is reported to contain essential bio active compounds such as β-glucans, Hericenones, Anderinacines, Cyathanes, etc. This product is reported to serve as a tonic for brain, nerve health, immunity, cardio & digestion and helps in maintaining blood sugar level. It is manufactured by Manger Health Dynamics Pvt. Ltd., Faridabad, India. According to the manufacturing company, it is recommended to take 2–3 g of this powder daily by adding in coffee, tea, juices, shakes, smoothies, food, or in any other form as a dietary supplement (Fig. 10.1t).

Price: ₹865 per pack of 60 g.

Certifications and warnings: This product has GMP, ISO, and FSSAI certifications. In case of pregnancy, nursing mother, or with any other medical condition, physicians should be consulted before using this product.

10.2.6.2 OTHER PRODUCTS OF H. ERINACEUS

Real Mushrooms Lion's Mane Organic mushroom extract powder; Mind Force Lion's Mane Mushroom Blend; Brainforza Lion's mane mushroom; Organic Naturals Cordy Life; Swanson Lion's Mane Mushroom are some other products from this mushroom.

10.2.7 ANTIDIABETIC PRODUCTS USING MIXTURE OF DIFFERENT MUSHROOMS

Some of the brands have manufactured products containing a blend of various mushroom species. These products provide benefits from the properties of all the species it contains. A few of such products are being discussed below.

10.2.7.1 MYCOBOTANICALS® BLOOD SUGAR CAPSULES

These capsules are made up with the mycelial extracts of three different mushroom species, namely *Grifola frondosa*, *Ganoderma lucidum*, and *Inonotus obliquus* along with some herbs. According to the information provided by the manufacturer, these three mushroom species support insulin sensitivity. Thus, this product helps in maintaining a healthy blood glucose level, which is already in a normal range. It is recommended to take 2 capsules of this product once a day as a dietary supplement (Fig. 10.1u).

Price: $29.95 per pack of 60 capsules.

Certifications and warnings: The product is manufactured with certified organic mushrooms. The company warns if a person is already on medications, pregnant, or nursing then healthcare professionals should be consulted before using this product and it should be kept out of reach of children.

10.2.7.2 ROOTED ACTIVE NATURALS MUSHROOM + SUPER HERBS EXTRACT POWDER (IMMUNITY BOOSTER, BRAIN BOOSTER, AND HEART DEFENSE)

Manger Health Dynamics Pvt Ltd., Faridabad, India has manufactured these three products with name "Rooted Active Naturals Mushroom + Super herbs extract powder," which are in the form of powder made from hot water extracts of *Ganoderma lucidum* along with the combinations of different mushrooms species. One of these three products is "Immunity Booster" which is made from *Ganoderma lucidum* and *Trametes versicolor* as well as some herbs like Ashwagandha, Amla, Tulsi, Noni, Green Coffee, Turmeric, and Giloy. This product provides support to the immune system, cardio health, healthy liver and gut, healthy brain, and blood sugar and helps to fight stress and cancer. Another product "Brain booster" contains powder made from hot water extracts of *Ganoderma lucidum* and *Hericium erinaceus* along with some herbs like Bacopa, Gotu Kola, Lemon Balm, Shankapushpi, Green Tea, Jatamasi, and Rosemary. It supports brain and nerve health, alleviates neurogenerative diseases, improves mood, anxiety, and focus, and also supports healthy blood sugar and cardiac health. Another product "Heart Defense" is a combination of mushrooms *Ganoderma lucidum* and *Lentinula edodes* as well as some herbs namely, *Rhodiona*, *Gracinia*, and Arjuna. It is a formulation made for overall heart health, reduces cholesterol, inflammation, maintains blood sugar, blood pressure, etc. Any of these products can be taken 2 g/day with or without food (Fig. 10.1v–x).

Prices: Rooted active naturals mushroom + super herbs extract powder Immunity booster: ₹383 per pack of 60 g.

Rooted Active Naturals Mushroom+Super herbs extract powder Brain booster: ₹450 per pack of 60 g.

Rooted Active Naturals Mushroom+Super herbs extract powder Heart Defense: ₹383 per pack of 60 g.

Certifications and warnings: These products have GMP, ISO, and FSSAI certifications. In case of pregnancy, nursing mother, or with any other medical condition, physicians should be consulted before using this product. These products should be kept out of reach of children.

10.2.7.3 OTHER PRODUCTS MADE OF MIXED MUSHROOM SPECIES

Dr. Mercola Fermented Mushroom Complex Dietary supplement; Solgar Reishi Shiitake Maitake mushroom extract; Avocare Biotech—4 Mushroom Complex are some such products prepared from mixed mushrooms.

10.2.8 ANTIDIABETIC PRODUCTS MADE OF GANODERMA LUCIDUM (CURTIS) P. KARST.

These include Nature suve *Ganoderma*, DXN Mycovita, DXN Reishilium Powder, DXN Ganocelium® (GL), DXN Reishi Gano (RG), DXN RG Powder & GL Powder, 1 Tree *Ganoderma* capsules, Mahogany Reishi Mushroom Mycelium (GL), Trexgenics *Ganoderma* Reishi Mushroom Extract, Back to Beginnings Reishi Mushroom capsules; Solaray Reishi Mushroom capsules; Amalth Reishi Mushroom capsules, etc. There are many mushroom products available in the market, which can be consumed and used to fight diabetes. Some of the manufacturers have clearly mentioned the use of the product in maintaining a healthy blood glucose level as mentioned above while there are also various products, which are made from the antidiabetic mushroom species but are not labeled as antidiabetic by the manufacturer. Products are mentioned in the content discussed above under the title "Other products."

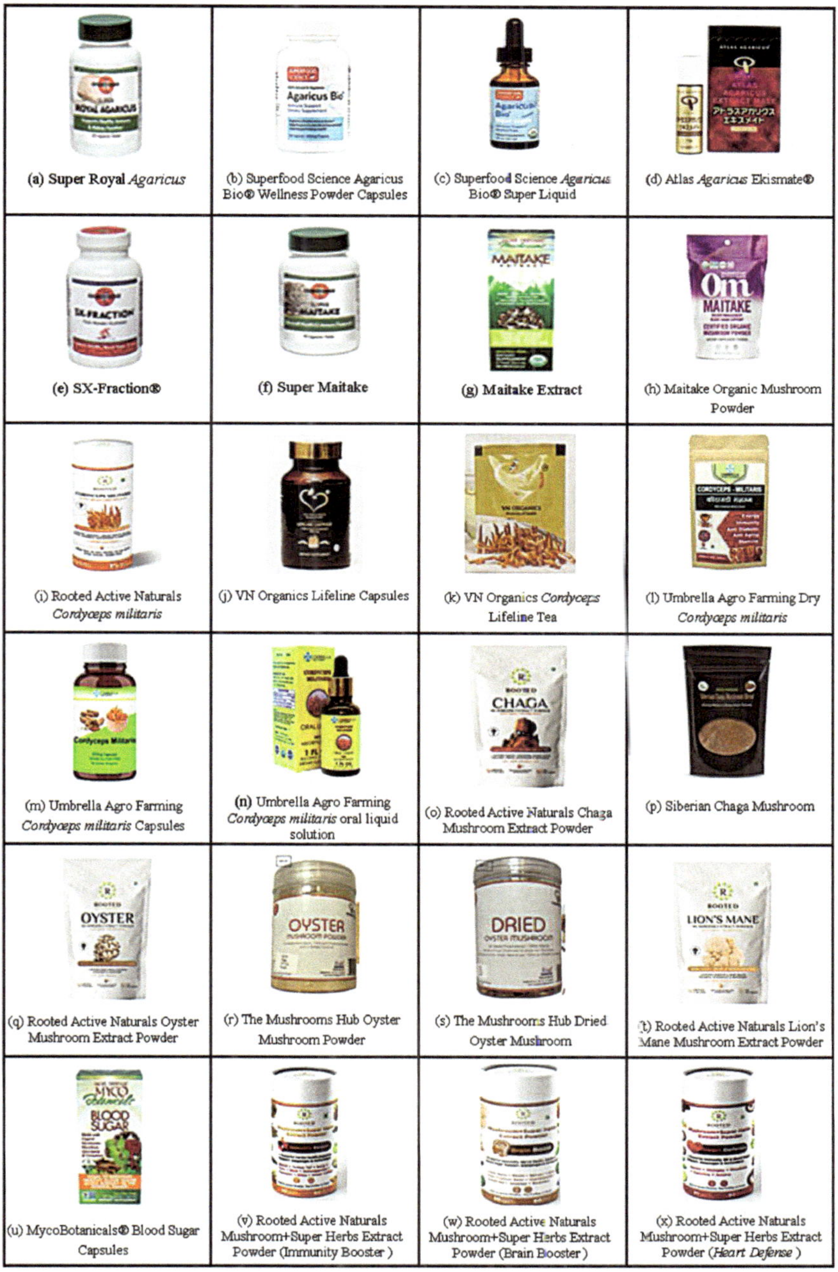
(a) Super Royal *Agaricus*
(b) Superfood Science Agaricus Bio® Wellness Powder Capsules
(c) Superfood Science *Agaricus* Bio® Super Liquid
(d) Atlas *Agaricus* Ekismate®
(e) SX-Fraction®
(f) Super Maitake
(g) Maitake Extract
(h) Maitake Organic Mushroom Powder
(i) Rooted Active Naturals *Cordyceps militaris*
(j) VN Organics Lifeline Capsules
(k) VN Organics *Cordyceps* Lifeline Tea
(l) Umbrella Agro Farming Dry *Cordyceps militaris*
(m) Umbrella Agro Farming *Cordyceps militaris* Capsules
(n) Umbrella Agro Farming *Cordyceps militaris* oral liquid solution
(o) Rooted Active Naturals Chaga Mushroom Extract Powder
(p) Siberian Chaga Mushroom
(q) Rooted Active Naturals Oyster Mushroom Extract Powder
(r) The Mushrooms Hub Oyster Mushroom Powder
(s) The Mushrooms Hub Dried Oyster Mushroom
(t) Rooted Active Naturals Lion's Mane Mushroom Extract Powder
(u) MycoBotanicals® Blood Sugar Capsules
(v) Rooted Active Naturals Mushroom+Super Herbs Extract Powder (Immunity Booster)
(w) Rooted Active Naturals Mushroom+Super Herbs Extract Powder (Brain Booster)
(x) Rooted Active Naturals Mushroom+Super Herbs Extract Powder (*Heart Defense*)

FIGURE 10.1 Images of various antidiabetic market products (images taken from the websites of the manufacturers).

10.3 SAFETY ISSUES AND CHALLENGES OF ANTIDIABETIC MUSHROOM MARKET PRODUCTS

From the commercial perspective, it is always a good idea to change any useful natural herb/plant into its products such as extracts, tablets, capsules, powder, or pellets. It is the case with the mushrooms. As mentioned above there are a number of products available in the market, which help in maintaining a healthy blood glucose level. However, these products are not intended to treat, mitigate, prevent, or cure the diseases, rather they are good dietary supplements, which can help in the prevention of diabetes or can delay its onset. Such a natural nutraceutical is boon for a healthy life in today's changing lifestyle scenario. The products made from mushrooms, especially the antidiabetic ones, are increasing in demand nowadays as they do not affect the body's other systems like the common antidiabetic drugs do. Still, there are so many safety issues as well as certain challenges concerned with the manufacturing, availability, marketing, and demands of such products. All such issues are discussed below.

10.3.1 QUALITY STANDARD REGULATIONS

The usage of these dietary supplements varies in different countries. In some countries, dietary supplements are just a part of a healthy lifestyle while in some regions these are recommended by healthcare professionals as medicines. Due to the increase in the use of dietary supplements, the matter of their quality check is an important issue for the safety of consumers.[54] Different countries have their own agencies that regulate the products marked as dietary supplements such as Food and Drug Administration (FDA) in USA, Therapeutic Goods Administration (TGA) in Australia, Health Canada (HC) in Canada, China Food and Drug Administration (CFDA) in China, Food Safety and Standards Authority of India (FSSAI) in India, European Medicines Agency (EMA) in Europe and European Food Safety Authority (EFSA) in European member countries. All the countries have their own terminologies and classifications for dietary supplements, health foods, herbal medicinal products or nutraceuicals, or functional foods. These regulatory bodies monitor the health-related claims on the labels of the products, manufacturing practices, purity, strength, and composition of the products. But it has been seen that there are many products that are not approved by any of the regulatory agencies. Therefore, the absence of any such seal on a product can be a question mark on its quality.

10.3.2 LACK OF SCIENTIFIC INFORMATION ON DOSAGE

There are a number of evidence demonstrating mushroom products supporting a healthy blood glucose level. Every manufacturing brand recommends a different dose of its product. However, enough scientific information is not available determining an appropriate range of doses to be taken. Taking higher doses of a supplement or taking many different supplements instead of prescribed medicines can lead to other health issues.[55] The dose of a supplement can depend on several factors such as the user's age, health, and several other conditions. Therefore, there should be an authentic parameter to determine the appropriate dose requiring combination of doses, dosage according to various age groups, as well as in various health conditions like pregnancy, lactation, etc. Data regarding the recommended dosages are highly variable due to different formulations.

10.3.3 POTENTIAL SIDE EFFECTS OF MUSHROOM DIETARY SUPPLEMENTS

Mushrooms contain various bioactive components, which are hypoglycemic, but there are several other compounds present in some species, which can cause some side effects. For example, there is a report that states *Agaricus blazei* contains a carcinogen agaritine and a daily intake of this compound can lead to its accumulation in the body. Therefore, this component should be removed from the fruit body extract for safe consumption.[56] Therefore, there is a need for these mushroom products to be examined by a certified mushroom expert or a mycologist for a safe procedure.[57] Besides this, not enough scientific data is available regarding the use of mushrooms or mushroom products during pregnancy and lactating women, that is why most of the mushroom products manufacturers suggest doctor consultation before their use by children and pregnant or breast-feeding women.

10.3.4 MUSHROOM ALLERGIES

There are various articles showing food allergies due to intake of mushrooms. For example, there is a report demonstrating a case of allergy with *Lentinula edodes*, *Grifola frondosa*, and *Lyophyllum decastes* (Fr.) Singer in an 18-year-old female.[57] White and coworkers[58] have proposed a new clinical classification for mushroom poisoning in which some medicinally important mushroom species are also included such as *Morchella* spp., *Lentinula edodes*, and *Ganoderma neojaponicum* Imazeki. Although mushroom species-specific allergy is rare, still antidiabetic mushroom products should be consumed carefully.

10.3.5 LACK OF STANDARDIZED PREPARATIONS

There are many limitations when efforts are made to extrapolate or demonstrate biological effects of mushrooms in human health or disease. Therefore, to check out the efficacy of *Agaricus blazei* as a therapeutic agent trials that are more clinical are required using legitimate statistical methods and standardized protocols.[59] However, specific standards for their use in hyperglycemia are lacking, probably due to insufficient data regarding the potency of mushroom species on diabetes and lack of an evident molecular mechanism to ensure their antidiabetic potential. Hence, there is a need to focus toward investigation of exact molecular mechanisms that can illustrate their antidiabetic potential. Maximum evidence concerning the curative activities of medicinal mushrooms has been procured from animal studies. Additionally, controlled human testing, particularly for long run use, is necessary. Safety matters on the intake of mushrooms on a long-term basis, and their interaction with other medicines, require more explanation. Hence, future investigations focused toward aforementioned issues are essential to justify the utilization of mushrooms and their products as possible drugs or nutraceuticals for the treatment of diabetes.

10.3.6 CORRECT IDENTIFICATION AND NOMENCLATURE OF SPECIES USED

There are many records available, which document the cases of mushroom poisoning due to intake of inedible or poisonous wild mushrooms mistakenly. This happens due to the confusion between the similar morphology of edible and inedible ones. Therefore, a correct identification by an expert is a necessary step to be taken before consuming the mushrooms. Similar accidents can also take place when an inedible mushroom is wrongly identified as edible.[60] For instance, it has been reported that most of the species identified and published as *Ganoderma lucidum* are actually some other species.[60] Another important information published by Wasser[60] is regarding the mistaken use of the name of *Agaricus blazei* as a medicinal mushroom. According to his report, *A. blazei* is considered medicinal and commonly named as Royal Sun *Agaricus* or the Himematsutake mushroom. Actually it is not a medicinal mushroom, the correct name of a medicinal mushroom Royal Sun *Agaricus* is *A. brasiliensis* Fr. These kinds of mistakes are a risk to the health of consumers. Therefore, it is very important that the fruit body or the mycelium used for the manufacturing of antidiabetic mushroom products should be correctly identified by an expert with the help of the latest techniques as well as latest rules of classification and nomenclature.

10.3.7 PURITY OF CULTURES OF MEDICINAL MUSHROOMS USED

More investigation must be endowed to the study of culinary medicinal mushrooms in pure cultures. It is necessary to analyze the cultures to provide proper maintenance in scientific work. The teleomorph stage is the most important feature for the identification of cultures; sometimes, these mushrooms do not produce carpophores in pure culture. Vegetative mycelia of these mushrooms in pure culture have received little emphasis in mycological literature. Mushrooms cannot be identified correctly without the proper study of their vegetative mycelia. In the pure cultures of these mushrooms, the vegetative mycelia are masses of branched hyphae, which are isolated only based on narrow limits of hyphal width, number of nuclei, thickness of cell wall, branching, etc. Procuring information on a number of taxonomic studies of vegetative mycelia of these mushroom species provides new matter for the comparative studies of morphological features of mycelia and for the assessment of their potential use for taxonomic purposes and purity control in biotechnological processes.[17,60] For the reason that there are no type strains of medicinal mushrooms, which is correctly identified type strain, this issue must be discussed with the World Federation of Culture Collections (WFCC).[17,60]

10.3.8 UNEXPLORED ANTIDIABETIC MUSHROOM SPECIES

As discussed above, a large number of mushroom species have been reported in the literature, which has the antidiabetic potential. However, among them, only a few have been used to manufacture products at commercial level such as *Agaricus blazei, Grifola frondosa, Cordyceps militaris*, and *Ganoderma lucidum*. But there are hardly any or a very few products available which are made by using antidiabetic mushrooms like *Phellinus linteus*, *Agaricus subrufescens*, *Lentinula edodes*, *Auricularia auricula-judae*, *Pleurotus florida*, and *Catathelasma ventricosum*. Therefore, there is a need to utilize these underused sources.

10.3.9 SOME COMMON CONSTRAINTS IN USE

Even though consumption of wild mushrooms for food and medicinal purposes is a common and traditional practice all around the world, still, in many countries especially the developing ones or some underdeveloped regions, people are unaware about the availability of antidiabetic mushroom products in the market. That is why such products are less in demand in these regions. Advertisements through various sources of media are important channels through which a commodity reaches to the consumers. However, ads regarding mushroom products are very rare. This is another reason for lesser demand for such products. In many countries, doctors or physicians hardly prescribe the dietary supplements made with mushrooms to the patients. Because of being unaware people do not prefer to take such products of mushroom origin. In many civilizations, cultures, and traditions of different regions in the world, mushrooms are considered edible, inedible, poisonous, hallucinogenic, magical, and even mysterious or sanctified.[61–65] There are various perceptions and myths associated with mushrooms due to which some people do not prefer consuming the mushrooms or their products.[66] The dietary supplements containing mushrooms are available at very high prices which are difficult to afford by lower- or middle-income people.

10.4 CONCLUSION

Antidiabetic mushrooms provide a great opportunity for the development of therapeutic substances and probiotics. There are many mushroom-based bioactive components such as β-(1 → 3)-D-glucans and polyphenols, which exhibit antidiabetic activity. Many brands are already manufacturing various forms of products using such mushroom species and many others are coming forward to develop such dietary supplements at commercial scale. However, specific standards and precise recommendations for the utilization of such products in lowering the blood glucose level are lacking probably due to inadequate data regarding the efficacy of mushroom species on diabetes and lack of clear molecular mechanism to ensure their antidiabetic potential. Hence, there is a need to focus on the investigation at an advanced level to demonstrate their antidiabetic potential. There is a need for more clinical trials on humans to make certain the safe use of such products. The production of dietary supplements can be very beneficial for human health if some of the challenges and issues associated with it could be solved. Various medicinal mushrooms are not available in all the regions of the world, so people can be benefited by recommending the use of products made from them. Second, the commercial forms of these products like powder, capsules, or tablets are easy to take orally with or without food. The field of commercial production of antidiabetic market products bears a great potential and scientists as well as industrialists need to work in tandem with one another. These products should also be recommended by the physicians and doctors. Besides this, making the common people aware of antidiabetic mushrooms, their products, and the benefits associated with them is the need of the time.

KEYWORDS

- **bioactive constituents**
- **commercialization**
- **diabetes mellitus**
- **medicinal mushrooms**

REFERENCES

1. Lima-Martínez, M. M.; Carrera Boada, C.; Madera-Silva, M. D.; Marín, W.; Contreras, M. COVID-19 and Diabetes: A Bidirectional Relationship. *Clin. Investig. Arterioscler.* **2021,** *33* (3), 151–157.

2. John, T. M.; Jacob, C. N.; Kontoyiannis, D. P. When Uncontrolled Diabetes Mellitus and Severe COVID-19 Converge: The Perfect Storm for Mucormycosis. *J. Fungus* **2021,** *7* (4), 298.
3. Soković, M.; Ćirić, A.; Glamočlija, J.; Stojković, D. The Bioactive Properties of Mushrooms. In *Wild Plants, Mushrooms and Nuts: Functional Food Properties and Applications*; Ferreira, I. C. F. R., Morales, P., Barros, L., Eds.; John Wiley & Sons, Ltd.: Chichester, UK, 2016; pp 83–122.
4. Kalac, P. *Edible Mushrooms: Chemical Composition and Nutritional Value*; Academic Press: London, 2016.
5. Barros, L.; Cruz, T.; Baptista, P.; Estevinho, L. E.; Ferreira; I. C. F. R. Wild and Commercial Mushrooms as Source of Nutrients and Nutraceuticals. *Food Chem. Toxicol.* **2008,** *46*, 2742–2747.
6. Chatterjee, S.; Sarma, M. K.; Deb, U.; Steinhauser, G.; Walther, C.; Gupta, D. K. Mushrooms: from Nutrition to Mycoremediation. *Environ. Sci. Pollut. Res.* **2017,** *24* (24), 19480–19493.
7. Mattila, P. H.; Marnila, P.; Pihlanto, A. Wild and Cultivated Mushrooms. *Fruit and Vegetable Phytochemicals: Chemistry and Human Health*, 2nd ed.; John Wiley & Sons, Ltd.: Hoboken, NJ, 2017; pp 1279–1304.
8. Brown, A. C.; Waslien, C. I. Stress and Nutrition. *Encyclopedia of Food Sciences and Nutrition*, 2nd ed.; Academic Press: London, 2003; pp 5628–5636.
9. Sarikurkcu, C.; Tepe, B.; Yamac, M. Evaluation of the Antioxidant Activity of Four Edible Mushrooms from the Central Anatolia, Eskisehir—Turkey: *Lactarius deterrimus*, *Suillus collitinus*, *Boletus edulis*, *Xerocomus chrysenteron*. *Bioresour. Technol.* **2008,** *99*, 6651–6655.
10. Chang, S. T.; Wasser, S. P. The Role of Culinary-Medicinal Mushrooms on Human Welfare with a Pyramid Model for Human Health. *Int. J. Med. Mushrooms* **2012,** *14*, 95–134.
11. Carneiro, A. A. J.; Ferreira, I. C. F. R.; Duenas, M.; Barros, L.; da Silva, R.; Gomes, E.; Santos-Buelga, C. Chemical Composition and Antioxidant Activity of Dried Powder Formulations of *Agaricus blazei* and *Lentinus edodes*. *Food Chem.* **2013,** *138*, 2168–2173.
12. Venturella, G.; Ferraro, V.; Cirlincione, F.; Gargano, M. L. Medicinal Mushrooms: Bioactive Compounds, Use, and Clinical Trials. *Int. J. Mol. Sci.* **2021,** *22* (2), 634.
13. Gulati, V.; Singh, M. D.; Gulati, P. Role of Mushrooms in Gestational Diabetes Mellitus. *AIMS Med. Sci.* **2019,** *6* (1), 49–66.
14. Khursheed, R.; Singh, S. K.; Wadhwa, S.; Gulati, M.; Awasthi, A. Therapeutic Potential of Mushrooms in Diabetes Mellitus: Role of Polysaccharides. *Int. J. Biol. Macromol.* **2020,** *164*, 1194–1205.
15. De Silva, D. D.; Rapior, S.; Hyde, K. D.; Bahkali, A. H. Medicinal Mushrooms in Prevention and Control of Diabetes Mellitus. *Fung. Divers.* **2012,** *56* (1), 1–29.
16. Kaur, H.; Kaur, M.; Malik, N. A. New Additions to the Genus *Agaricus* (*Agaricaceae*, *Agaricales*) from Northwest India. *Kavaka* **2017,** *48* (2), 84–94.
17. Al-Faqeeh, L. A. S.; Naser, R.; Kagne, S. R.; Khan, S. W. Activity of Mushrooms against Diabetic and Inflammation: A Review. *GSC Biol. Pharm. Sci.* **2021,** *14* (2), 037–044.

18. Srivastva, A.; Attri, B. L.; Sharma, V. P. Status Report on Mushroom Products *Technical Bulletin*; ICAR-Directorate of Mushroom: Chambaghat, Solan, India, 2019.
19. Liang, B.; Guo, Z.; Xie, F.; Zhao A. Antihyperglycemic and Antihyperlipidemic Activities of Aqueous Extract of *Hericium erinaceus* in Experimental Diabetic Rats. *BMC Complement. Altern. Med.* **2013,** *13* (1), 253.
20. Chaiyasut, C.; Sivamaruthi, B. S. Anti-hyperglycemic Property of *Hericium erinaceus*—A Mini Review. *Asian Pac. J. Trop. Biomed.* **2017,** *7* (11), 1036–1040.
21. Cai, W. D.; Ding, Z. C.; Wang, Y. Y.; Yang, Y.; Zhang, H. N.; Yan, J. K. Hypoglycemic Benefit and Potential Mechanism of a Polysaccharide from *Hericium erinaceus* in Streptozotoxin-induced Diabetic Rats. *Process. Biochem.* **2020,** *88*, 180–188.
22. Kim, H. M.; Kang, J. S.; Kim, J. Y.; Park, S. K.; Kim, H. S.; Lee, Y. J.; Yun, J.; Hong, J. T.; Kim, Y.; Han, S. B. Evaluation of Antidiabetic Activity of Polysaccharide Isolated from *Phellinus linteus* in Non-obese Diabetic Mouse. *Int. Immunopharmacol.* **2010,** *10* (1), 72–78.
23. Feng, H.; Zhang, S.; Wan, J. M. F.; Gui, L.; Ruan, M.; Li, N.; Zhang, H.; Liu, Z.; Wang, H. Polysaccharides Extracted from *Phellinus linteus* Ameliorate High-fat High-fructose Diet Induced Insulin Resistance in Mice. *Carbohydr. Polym.* **2018,** *200*, 144–153.
24. Shen, M.; Fang, Z.; Chen, Y.; Chen, Y.; Xiao, B.; Guo, L.; Xu, Y.; Wang, G.; Wang, W.; Zhang, Y. Hypoglycemic Effect of the Degraded Polysaccharides from the Wood Ear Medicinal Mushroom *Auricularia auricula-judae* (*Agaricomycetes*). *Int. J. Med. Mushrooms* **2019,** *21* (10), 1033–1042.
25. Liu, Y.; Sun, J.; Rao, S.; Su, Y.; Yang, Y. Antihyperglycemic, Antihyperlipidemic and Antioxidant Activities of Polysaccharides from *Catathelasma ventricosum* in Streptozotocin-induced Diabetic Mice. *Food Chem. Toxicol.* **2013,** *57*, 39–45.
26. Friedman, M. Mushroom Polysaccharides: Chemistry and Antiobesity, Antidiabetes, Anticancer, and Antibiotic Properties in Cells, Rodents, and Humans. *Foods* **2016,** *5* (4), 80.
27. Ganeshpurkar, A.; Kohli, S.; Rai, G. Antidiabetic Potential of Polysaccharides from the White Oyster Culinary—Medicinal Mushroom *Pleurotus florida* (Higher Basidiomycetes). *Int. J. Med. Mushrooms* **2014,** *16* (3), 207–217.
28. Jeong, S. C.; Jeong, Y. T.; Yang, B. K.; Islam, R.; Koyyalamudi, S. R.; Pang, G.; Cho, K. Y.; Song, C. H. White Button Mushroom (*Agaricus bisporus*) Lowers Blood Glucose and Cholesterol Levels in Diabetic and Hypercholesterolemic Rats. *Nutr. Res.* **2010,** *30* (1), 49–56.
29. Wang, P. C.; Zhao, S.; Yang, B. Y.; Wang, Q. H.; Kuang, H. X. Anti-diabetic Polysaccharides from Natural Sources: A Review. *Carbohydr. Polym.* **2016,** *148*, 86–97.
30. Jia, J.; Zhang, X.; Hu, Y. S.; Wu, Y.; Wang, Q. Z.; Li, N. N.; Guo, Q. C.; Dong, X. C. Evaluation of In Vivo Antioxidant Activities of *Ganoderma lucidum* Polysaccharides in STZ-Diabetic Rats. *Food Chem.* **2009,** *115*, 32–36.
31. Wasser, S. P.; Weis, A. L. Therapeutic Effects of Substances Occurring in Higher Basidiomycetes Mushrooms: A Modern Perspective. *Crit. Rev. Immunol.* **1999,** *19*, 65–96.

32. Hetland, G.; Johnson, E.; Lyberg, T.; Bernardshaw, S.; Tryggestad, A. M. A.; Grinde, B. Effects of the Medicinal Mushroom *Agaricus blazei* Murill on Immunity, Infection and Cancer. *Scand. J. Immunol.* **2008,** *68* (4), 363–370.
33. Wei, Q.; Zhan, Y.; Chen, B.; Xie, B.; Fang, T.; Ravishankar, S.; Jiang, Y. Assessment of Antioxidant and Antidiabetic Properties of *Agaricus blazei* Murill Extracts. *Food Sci. Nutr.* **2020,** *8* (1), 332–339.
34. Chinese Herbalism Editorial Board. *Zhonghua Bencao*; Shanghai Science and Technology Press: Shanghai, 1999; pp 548–549.
35. He, X.; Wang, X.; Fang, J.; Chang, Y.; Ning, N.; Guo, H.; Huang, L.; Huang, X.; Zhao, Z. Polysaccharides in *Grifola frondosa* Mushroom and Their Health Promoting Properties: A Review. *Int. J. Biol. Macromol.* **2017,** *101*, 910–921.
36. Pang, F. Chemical Constituents and Antiproliferative of *Grifola frondosa* on Cancer Cell Line, Thesis for the Degree of Master of Science, East China Normal University, Shanghai, 2010; pp 9–10.
37. Su, C. H.; Lai, M. N.; Lin, C. C.; Ng, L. T. Comparative Characterization of Physicochemical Properties and Bioactivities of Polysaccharides from Selected Medicinal Mushrooms. *Appl. Microbiol. Biotechnol.* **2016,** *100*, 4385–4393.
38. Kodama, N.; Komuta, K.; Nanba, H. Can Maitake MD-Fraction Aid Cancer Patients? *Sci. Rev. Altern. Med.* **2002,** *7* (3), 236–239.
39. Masuda, Y.; Kodama, N; Nanba, H. Macrophage J774. 1 Cell Is Activated by MZ-Fraction (Klasma-MZ) Polysaccharide in *Grifola frondosa*. *Mycoscience* **2006,** *47* (6), 360–366.
40. Konno, S.; Alexander, B.; Zade, J.; Choudhury, M. Possible Hypoglycemic Action of SX-Fraction Targeting Insulin Signal Transduction Pathway. *Int. J. Gen. Med.* **2013,** *6*, 181–187.
41. Manohar, V.; Talpur, N. A.; Echard, B. W.; Lieberman, S. Preuss, H. G. Effects of a Water-Soluble Extract of Maitake Mushroom on Circulating Glucose/Insulin Concentrations in KK Mice. *Diabetes Obes. Metab.* **2002,** *4*, 43–48.
42. Mehra, A.; Zaidi, K. U.; Mani, A.; Thawani, V. The Health Benefits of *Cordyceps militaris*—A Review. *Kavaka* **2017,** *48* (1), 27–32.
43. Liu, R. M.; Dai, R.; Luo, Y.; Xiao, J. H. Glucose-lowering and Hypolipidemic Activities of Polysaccharides from *Cordyceps taii* in Streptozotocin-induced Diabetic Mice. *BMC Complement. Altern. Med.* **2019,** *19* (1), 1–10.
44. Wu, J. Y.; Siu, K. C.; Geng, P. Bioactive Ingredients and Medicinal Values of *Grifola frondosa* (Maitake). *Foods* **2021,** *10* (1), 95.
45. Zhao, H.; Lai, Q.; Zhang, J.; Huang, C.; Jia, L. Antioxidant and Hypoglycemic Effects of Acidic-extractable Polysaccharides from *Cordyceps militaris* on Type 2 Diabetes Mice. *Oxid. Med. Cell Longev.* **2018,** *2018*, 1–15.
46. Shang, X. L.; Pan, L. C.; Tang, Y.; Luo, Y.; Zhu, Z. Y.; Sun, H. Q.; Meng, M.; Zhang, Y. M. 1H NMR-based Metabonomics of the Hypoglycemic Effect of Polysaccharides from *Cordyceps militaris* on Streptozotocin-induced Diabetes in Mice. *Nat. Prod. Res.* **2020,** *34* (10), 1366–1372.
47. Sun, H.; Zhu, Z.; Tang, Y.; Ren, Y.; Song, Q.; Tang, Y.; Zhang, Y. Structural Characterization and Antitumor Activity of a Novel Se-Polysaccharide from Selenium-Enriched *Cordyceps gunnii*. *Food Funct.* **2018,** *9* (5), 2744–2754.

48. Ying, Y. M.; Zhang, L. Y.; Zhang, X.; Bai, H. B.; Liang, D. E.; Ma, L. F.; Shan, W. G.; Zhan, Z. J. Terpenoids with Alpha-glucosidase Inhibitory Activity from the Submerged Culture of *Inonotus obliquus*. *Phytochemistry* **2014,** *108*, 171–176.
49. Wang, J.; Wang, C.; Li, S.; Li, W.; Yuan, G.; Pan, Y.; Chen, H. Anti-diabetic Effects of *Inonotus obliquus* Polysaccharides in Streptozotocin-induced Type 2 Diabetic Mice and Potential Mechanism Via PI3K-Akt Signal Pathway. *Biomed. Pharmacother.* **2017,** *95*, 1669–1677.
50. Stojkovic, D.; Smiljkovic, M.; Ciric, A.; Glamoclija, J.; Van Griensven, L.; Ferreira, I. C.; Sokovic, M. An Insight into Antidiabetic Properties of Six Medicinal and Edible Mushrooms: Inhibition of α-Amylase and α-Glucosidase Linked to Type-2 Diabetes. *S. Afr. J. Bot.* **2019,** *120*, 100–103.
51. Deepalakshmi, K.; Sankaran, M. *Pleurotus ostreatus*: An Oyster Mushroom with Nutritional and Medicinal Properties. *J. Biochem. Technol.* **2014,** *5* (2), 718–726.
52. Zhang, Y.; Hu, T.; Zhou, H.; Zhang, Y.; Jin, G.; Yang, Y. Antidiabetic Effect of Polysaccharides from *Pleurotus ostreatus* in Streptozotocin-induced Diabetic Rats. *Int. J. Biol. Macromol.* **2016,** *83*, 126–132.
53. Xiong, M.; Huang, Y.; Liu, Y.; Huang, M.; Song, G.; Ming, Q.; Ma, X.; Yang, J.; Deng, S.; Wen, Y.; Shen, J. Antidiabetic Activity of Ergosterol from *Pleurotus ostreatus* in KK-Ay Mice with Spontaneous Type 2 Diabetes Mellitus. *Mol. Nutr. Food Res.* **2018,** *62* (3), 1700444.
54. Thakkar, S.; Anklam, E.; Xu, A.; Ulberth, F.; Li, J.; Li, B.; Hugas, M.; Sarma, N.; Crerar, S.; Swift, S.; Hakamatsuka, T. Regulatory Landscape of Dietary Supplements and Herbal Medicines from a Global Perspective. *Regul. Toxicol. Pharmacol.* **2020,** *114*, 104647.
55. Sorimachi, K.; Nakamoto, T. Alternative Medicine Safety: *Agaricus blazei* and Propolis. *Comb. Chem. High Throughput Screen.* **2011,** *14* (7), 616–621.
56. Feeney, M. J.; Dwyer, J.; Hasler-Lewis, C. M.; Milner, J. A ; Noakes, M.; Rowe, S.; Wach, M.; Beelman, R. B.; Caldwell, J.; Cantorna, M. T.; Castlebury, L. A.; Chang, S. T.; Cheskin, L. J.; Clemens, R.; Drescher, G.; Fulgoni, V. L.; Haytowitz, D. B.; Hubbard, V. S.; Law, D.; Myrdal Miller, A.; Minor, B.; Percival, S. S.; Riscuta, G.; Schneeman, B.; Thornsbury, S.; Toner, C. D.; Woteki, C. E.; Wu, D. Mushrooms and Health Summit Proceedings. *J. Nutr.* **2014,** *144* (7), 1128S–36S. doi: 10.3945/jn.114.190728.
57. Ito, T.; Kobayashi, T.; Egusa, C.; Maeda, T.; Abe, N.; Okubo, Y.; Tsuboi, R.; Niitsuma, T. A Case of Food Allergy Due to Three Different Mushroom Species. *Allergol. Int.* **2020,** *69* (1), 152–153.
58. White, J.; Weinstein, S. A.; De Haro, L.; Bédry, R.; Schaper, A.; Rumack, B. H.; Zilker, T. Mushroom Poisoning: A Proposed New Clinical Classification. *Toxicon* **2019,** *157*, 53–65.
59. da Silva, C.; de Souza, A.; Gesser Correa, V.; de Almeida Goncalves, G.; Assuncao Soares, A.; Bracht, A.; Marina Peralta, R. *Agaricus blazei* Bioactive Compounds and Their Effects on Human Health: Benefits and Controversies. *Curr. Pharm. Des.* **2017,** *23* (19), 2807–2834.
60. Wasser, S. Medicinal Mushroom Science: Current Perspectives, Advances, Evidences, and Challenges. *Biomed. J.* **2014,** *7* (6), 345–356.

61. Pegler, D. N. *A Preliminary Agaric flora of East Africa. Kew Bulletin Additional Series. 6*; Her Majesty Stationary Office, 1977; p 615.
62. Purkayastha, R. P.; Chandra, A. *Manual of Indian Edible Mushrooms*; Jagmander Book Agency: New Delhi, 1985.
63. Singer, R. *The Agaricales in Modern Taxonomy*, 4th ed.; Sven Koeiltz Scientific Books: Germany, 1986; p 981.
64. Rai, R. D.; Arumuganathan, T. Nutritive Value of Mushrooms. In *Frontiers in Mushroom Biotechnology*; National Research Centre for Mushroom: Solan, 2005; pp 27–36.
65. Arora, D.; Shepard, G. H. Mushrooms and Economic Botany. *Econ. Bot.* **2008,** *62*, 207–212.
66. Atri, N. S.; Mridu. Mushrooms—Some Ethnomycological and Sociobiological Aspects. *Kavaka* **2018,** *51*, 11–19.

WEBSITES FOLLOWED

http://www.who.int/diabetes/global-report
https://www.who.int/news-room/fact-sheets/detail/diabetes (accessed on June 15th, 2021).
https://www.mushroomshub.com/product/oyster-mushroom-powder-100-gm/
https://rootedactives.com/product/lions-mane-mushroom-extract-powder-pure-fruit-body/
https://hostdefense.com/collections/capsules/products/blood-sugar
https://rootedactives.com/product/immunity-booster-mushrooms-super-herbs-extract-powder-blend/
https://rootedactives.com/product/brain-boost-mushroom-super-herbs-extract-powder-blend/
https://rootedactives.com/product/heart-defense-mushroom-super-herbs-extract-powder-blend/
https://rootedactives.com/product/buy-chaga-mushroom-powder-pack/
https://www.paithanecofoods.com/product/siberian-chaga-mushroom/
https://rootedactives.com/product/cordyceps-militaris-mushroom-pure-fruit-body-15gm
https://vnorganicshealth.com/product-detail.php?pid=2)
http://www.umbrellaagrofarming.com/10gm-cordyceps-militaris-6473639.html
https://hostdefense.com/collections/in-stock/products/maitake-extract
https://ommushrooms.com/products/maitake?variant=18554016563296
https://ods.od.nih.gov/factsheets/WYNTK-Consumer/
http://www.mushroomwisdom.com
https://www.superfoodscience.com

Index

B

C

D

E

F

G